# Artificial Intelligence in PET/CT Oncologic Imaging

John A. Andreou
Paris A. Kosmidis
Athanasios D. Gouliamos
Editors

# Artificial Intelligence in PET/CT Oncologic Imaging

Springer

*Editors*
John A. Andreou
Radiologic Imaging
Hygeia Hospital
Athens, Greece

Paris A. Kosmidis
Medical Oncology
Hygeia Hospital
Athens, Greece

Athanasios D. Gouliamos
Medical School
National and Kapodistrian University of Athens
Athens, Greece

ISBN 978-3-031-10089-5 ISBN 978-3-031-10090-1 (eBook)
https://doi.org/10.1007/978-3-031-10090-1



This Springer imprint is published by the registered company Springer Nature Switzerland AG
The registered company address is: Gewerbestrasse 11, 6330 Cham, Switzerland

*This book is dedicated to all cancer patients and their families.*
*We are grateful to our teachers and thankful to our staff.*

# Foreword

Artificial Intelligence, aka AI, is a term that became very familiar to us in recent years. Indeed AI is part of our daily life, with a number of applications almost impossible to count, and now incorporated in most technological innovations. The relevance and impact of AI is hard to estimate, due to its incredibly rapid growth and diffusion, and this is true also for AI in medicine.

Proposal of using AI in medicine started in the 1950s, mainly as futuristic prediction, while a real boom occurred with the new millennium, and now counting thousands of papers and proposals every year, making difficult to stay updated, especially in areas where AI has been intensively studied, such as medical imaging.

For those reasons, it is very important to have reference reviews that make possible to understand the state of the art, and this is the scope of this book from J.Andreou, P. Kosmidis and A.Gouliamos, covering the applications of Artificial Intelligence in Oncological PET/CT.

The book is focused on the use of AI in the most advanced functional imaging method, and it covers all oncological clinical indications for PET/CT, being at the same time exhaustive and synthetic, while updated. Different perspectives are presented, as AI in PET/CT is clearly a very multidisciplinary field, bringing together the expertise of medical doctors, informatics, physics and many other professionals. The book is useful and recommended for all those specialists who will surely benefit from such a comprehensive text.

Diagnostic Imaging
University of Bologna,
Bologna, Italy
5 May 2022

Stefano Fanti

# Preface

The content of this book is mainly updated chapters from the second edition of *Imaging in Clinical Oncology* (2017) with addition of an introductory chapter about AI systems for Oncology.

Originally positioned as a means for noninvasive molecular phenotyping and quantification in the 1970s, PET's technological improvements in the 2000s and PET/CT fusion imaging generated renewed interest in quantification, which has grown over the last 5 years for cancer treatment planning. With fusion imaging radiologists and oncologists can combine anatomical and metabolic information and estimate the response to therapy. This progress is parallel with the development of artificial intelligence (AI) systems for Oncology which is an AI system with the aim of providing the best possible treatment to patients suffering from lung, breast, brain, prostate, liver and other types of cancer.

Applications of AI systems in imaging modalities have the following trends:

1. Artificial intelligence applications may help in detection of disease, tissue characterisation (benign vs malignant), staging and correlation with molecular biomarkers.
2. Radiomic signatures may help in prediction of response to therapy, risk scores for recurrence and classification of patients based on prognosis.
3. Correlation of data sets with imaging findings and pathology findings.
4. AI is under intensive research for massive screening for early diagnosis of cancer. More specifically, radiological screening for lung and breast cancer is more advanced. Additionally, colorectal polyps screening is another attractive examination through colonoscopy for early diagnosis of cancer.

Considering how different things were 10 or 20 years ago can we imagine or foresee the advancements in medical technology in the next 10 years? We should be thankful to the many pioneers who have made PET/CT during the past 20 years what is today: a useful tool for depiction of anatomy and pathology for the benefit of millions of patients around the world.

Although technical difficulties were encountered at the beginning, limited applications of AI in PET/CT are already here and appear promising in the near future as have been in other imaging modalities. There is no doubt that

AI can help radiologists lessen their workload and oncologists develop novel tools.

Athens, Greece John A. Andreou
Athens, Greece Paris A. Kosmidis
Athens, Greece Athanasios D. Gouliamos
March 2022

# Acknowledgements

We would like to express our gratitude to the staff of Springer Milan and especially to Ms. Antonella Cerri for their enormous support to get this book published. Project coordinator Ms. Niveka Somasundaram and project manager N. Priyadarsiny provided outstanding book production services.

We would also like to thank Ms. Argyro Loula for her secretarial assistance.

October, 2022.

The Editors.

# Contents

# Introduction: Artificial Intelligence (AI) Systems for Oncology

**1**

João Santinha, Ana Castro Verde, and Nikolaos Papanikolaou

## 1.1 Introduction

Artificial intelligence (AI) is a topic of growing interest in various fields, including finance, entertainment, transports, agriculture, and healthcare. The application of **machine learning (ML)** and **deep learning (DL)** algorithms in medicine was enabled by three essential aspects: the increase in data availability, the development of innovative software technologies, and the capacity improvement of the computing systems [1]. The former was most evident in radiology and nuclear medicine due to the accessibility of digitised images, but it also impacted dermatology, ophthalmology, histopathology, and clinical and genetic data. Although plenty of research was conducted several decades before, in the 2012 ImageNet Challenge—a natural image classification competition with more than 14 million images of more than 20,000 categories—a convolutional neural network (CNN) model named AlexNet was able to substantially reduce the classification error showing the potential of DL-based models in comparison with traditional computer vision approaches [2]. By this time, the limitation in transposing this work to medicine was the insufficient labelled data. Two facilitators for this were, in 2015/2016, the emergence of transfer learning algorithms [3]—where DL networks pre-trained on non-medical images are used and/or finetuned for medical imaging applications—and, in 2017/2018, the development of synthetic data augmentation—mainly, using Generative Adversarial Networks (GANs) to generate synthetic images that are visually mistaken with real medical images and, when fed into CNN, can increase the performance of these models in

João Santinha and Ana Castro Verde contributed equally with all other contributors.

J. Santinha
Computational Clinical Imaging Group, Champalimaud Experimental Clinical Research Programme, Champalimaud Foundation, Av. Brasília, Lisbon, Portugal

Instituto Superior Técnico, Universidade de Lisboa, Av. Rovisco Pais 1, Lisbon, Portugal
e-mail: joao.santinha@research.fchampalimaud.org

A. C. Verde
Computational Clinical Imaging Group, Champalimaud Experimental Clinical Research Programme, Champalimaud Foundation, Av. Brasília, Lisbon, Portugal
e-mail: ana.castroverde@research.fchampalimaud.org

N. Papanikolaou (✉)
Computational Clinical Imaging Group, Champalimaud Experimental Clinical Research Programme, Champalimaud Foundation, Av. Brasília, Lisbon, Portugal

Department of Radiology, Royal Marsden Hospital Downs Road, Sutton, UK
e-mail: nickolas.papanikolaou@research.fchampalimaud.org


J. A. Andreou et al. (eds.), *Artificial Intelligence in PET/CT Oncologic Imaging*, https://doi.org/10.1007/978-3-031-10090-1_1

medical tasks. Besides those, additional contributions to the field were the UNet architecture for image segmentation in 2015 [4] and, in 2015/2016, the advent of multiple medical imaging DL challenges.

In parallel to the emergence of DL solutions for medical problems and as an extension of computer-aided diagnosis and detection (CAD) systems, **radiomics** (Fig. 1.1) was first coined in 2012 [5]. It is based on the principle that images contain unexplored information on the tumour phenotype and microenvironment that can only be identified through quantitative analysis [6]. Radiomics refers to the extraction of high-dimensional features reflecting intensity, shape, size or volume, and texture—from computer tomography (CT), magnetic resonance (MR), and positron emission tomography (PET) images. These features are to be combined with additional information from multiple data sources and used for hypothesis generation and testing. The number of radiomics publications (Fig. 1.2) has seen a drastic increase over the past 10 years, with more developments in oncology due to support from the National Cancer Institute (NCI) Quantitative Imaging Network (QIN). Although we verify this trend, further work is still necessary for tackling multiple challenges in the field (see Sect. 1.3 for a more detailed description) to achieve reproducible results with the end goal of clinical translation [7].

Overall, the establishment of validated imaging biomarkers is an opening opportunity to drive **precision medicine** forward by characterising a patient's tumoral heterogeneity across space and time [8].

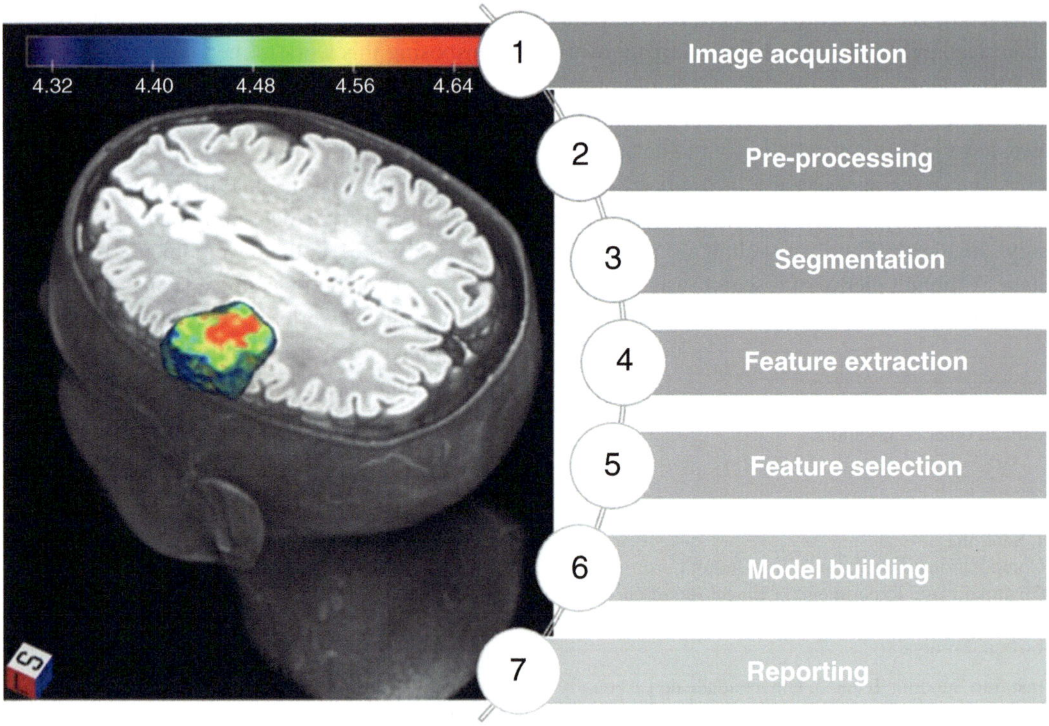


**Fig. 1.1** The main steps of a Radiomics study, illustrated on the left by a 3D Radiomics map of the "'Entropy"' feature from a patient with a brain tumour

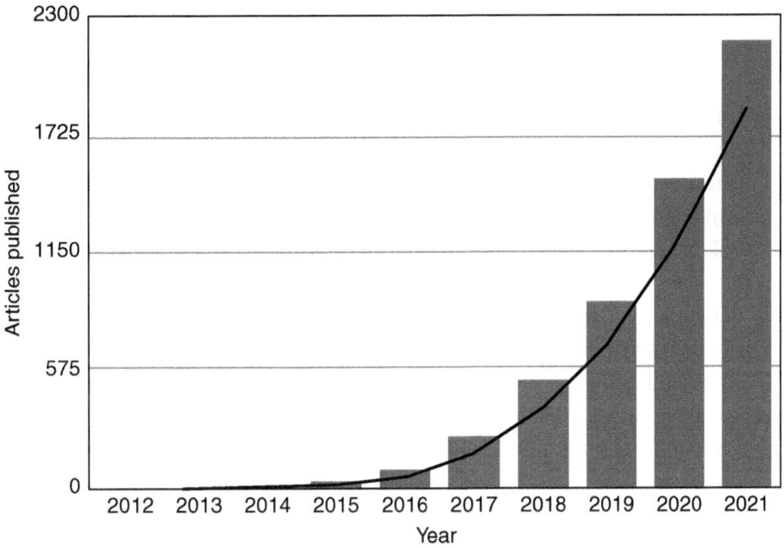


**Fig. 1.2** Number of radiomics articles over time (in years) until 2021. (Data source: Pubmed)

## 1.2 Applications

Artificial intelligence (AI) has been applied to different fields with considerable success, and oncology is no exception. The utilisation of AI applications in oncology allows the optimisation of multiple tasks contributing to cancer detection, diagnosis, staging, treatment planning, and prognosis. Cancer imaging, encompassing digital pathology, radiographic imaging, and clinical photographs, is the area within AI in oncology where the most promising work has been done [1]. While in digital pathology and clinical pictures, the main focus has been to automate and improve image analysis and diagnostic performance, in radiology, the application of AI is also being widely applied to image reconstruction and enhancement, segmentation, and registration, and computer-aided detection (CADe) and computer-aided diagnosis (CADx) tasks with promising results. Improvements in image reconstruction and enhancement, segmentation, and registration may also improve results obtained in CADe and CADx tasks. Furthermore, these applications are expected to facilitate the radiologists' work by decreasing the variability inherent to interpretation and reducing human errors due to the short time to evaluate medical images and increased workload [9].

Regarding the use of AI in PET-CT images, several studies have already demonstrated that the use of AI in image reconstruction and enhancement allows faster acquisitions (low-count acquisitions) while providing better diagnostic images [10–14]. In the study performed by Arabiand Zaidi, a deep learning-based metal artefact reduction algorithm reduced the adverse effects of metal artefacts on PET images by improving the generation of accurate attenuation maps in the presence of CT images corrupted due to the presence of metallic implants [14]. Chaudhari and colleagues demonstrated that deep learning could reconstruct images from low-count whole-body PET acquisition (fourfold count reduction), restoring diagnostic image quality and maintaining SUV accuracy [11]. Furthermore, the authors showed that the method generalised on an external dataset comprised patients from multiple institutions and scanner types [11]. Gong et al. proposed an iterative reconstruction neural network that can improve PET image quality, outperforming denoising neural networks used as postprocessing tools and conventional penalised maximum likelihood methods [10]. More recently, Sanaat et al. and Feng et al. also investigated the use of deep learning methods to reconstruct PET images with 1/ eighth of standard injected activity or acquisition time and within the limits of the current hardware, respectively [12, 13]. Some AI commercial applications like SubtlePET™ [15] and OncoFreeze AI [16] are already available for image reconstruction and enhancement.

In terms of AI-based segmentation, Edenbrandt and colleagues demonstrated the benefits of using convolutional neural networks to segment lesions in PSMAPET/CT images which reduced variability between readers [17]. In the studies by Zhao et al. and Moe et al., a multi-modality convolutional neural network with both PET and CT images as input showed significant improvements over methods that use only PET or CT [18, 19].

Several studies also investigated the use of AI for CADe and CADx in PET/CT images. Kawauchi and colleagues investigated the use of CNNs to classify patients into benign, malignant, or equivocal using FDG PET/CT examinations [20]. Peng et al. evaluated the prognostic value of DL PET/CT-based radiomics for individual induction chemotherapy in advanced nasopharyngeal carcinoma [21]. In another study by Polymeri et al., the authors assessed the association between DL-based quantification of PET/CT prostate gland uptake and overall survival [22], which was followed by a study by Borrelli and colleagues in which an AI method was developed to automatically detect lymph node metastasis that was shown to be associated with prostate cancer-specific survival [23]. Sibille and colleagues used DL to localise and classify uptake patterns into foci suspicious and non-suspicious in lymphoma and lung cancer [24]. An automatic method to detect abnormal lung lesions and calculate the total lesion glycolysis (TLG) on FDG PET-CT was developed by Borrelli and colleagues [25]. As for the use of texture-based analysis, the studies by Fan, Satoh, and Zheng assessed its performance for the differential diagnosis in spinal metastases, for comparing diagnosis of primary breast cancer using whole-body PET/CT and high-resolution dedicated breast PET, and to predict mediastinal node metastasis in non-small cell lung cancer patients, respectively [26–28].

## 1.3 Challenges

In combination with the growing number of applications of AI in oncology, some challenges need to be addressed for achieving the end goal of implementation into clinical practice. One can broadly divide these challenges into three topics: Data, AI Model, and AI Framework, as shown in Fig. 1.3. Firstly, challenges with Data come from the fact that the training data used to feed the algorithms can be **biased**, under-representing specific age, gender, and racial populations or perpetuating social biases, possibly leading to undertreatment of specific races and/or socioeconomic groups, known as under-served populations, by perpetuating systematic mistakes in inpatient care [29]. Potential solutions to this problem are, on the one hand, the utilisation of large *real-world* datasets that are representative across patient groups, time (historically vs. recently treated patients), and data sources (data obtained at different institutes, using different scanner models and manufacturers), and on the other hand, the development of methods to estimate and eliminate preexisting biases in the training data. However, the advent of larger datasets coming from multiple institutions is still hindered by the need to protect patient information, which may be overcome with federated learning. Furthermore, multiple institution datasets, acquired using different equipment, parameters, and/or reconstruction algorithms and settings, pose the challenge of data **heterogeneity**, leading to variability in algorithms' performance. Individual variations in the images can be observed in multi-centre studies, as shown in Fig. 1.4, resulting in a shift in data distribution across various settings. For the case of radiomics—mentioned previously in Sect. 1.1, different harmonisation methods can be applied to ensure repeatability and/or reproducibility of the radiomics features across diverse settings [30]. One possible scenario is to harmonise the image/intensities domain, whether by using guidelines for the acquisition and reconstruction parameters' standardisation or by utilising meth-

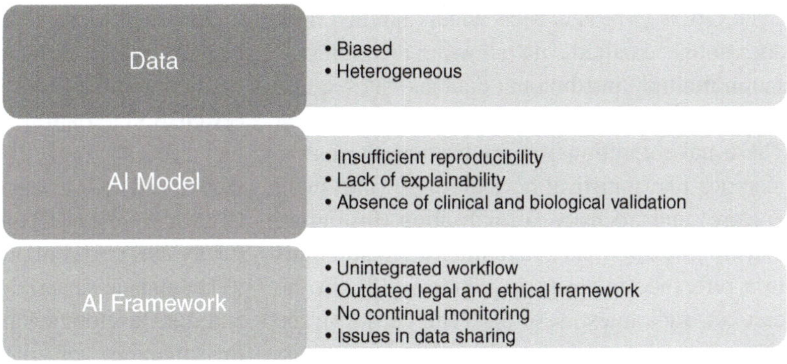


**Fig. 1.3** Schematic on the current challenges of AI in oncology

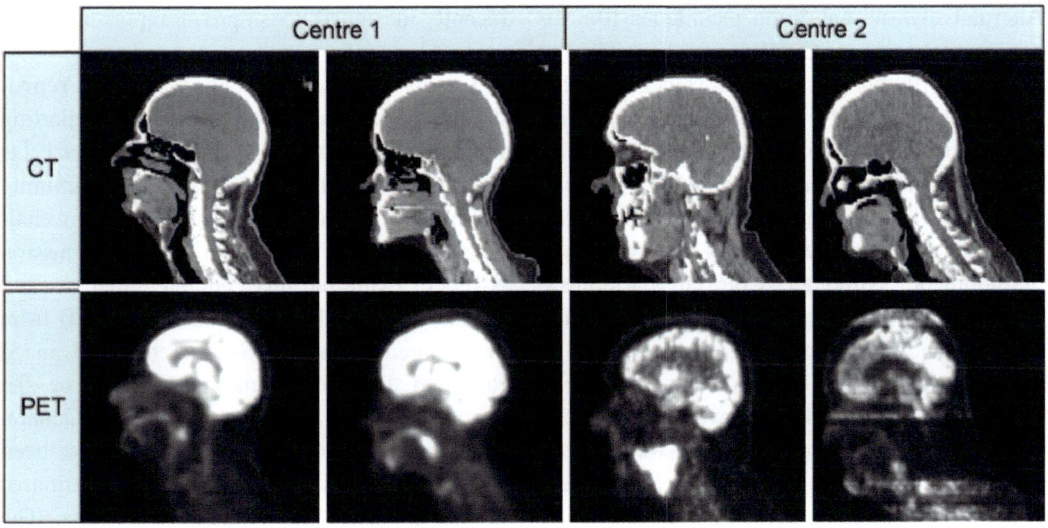


**Fig. 1.4** Multi-center centre variability of PET and CT slices of four different patients, taken from [30]

ods on the raw or reconstructed image data. For PET imaging standardisation, the European Association of Nuclear Medicine (EANM) launched the EARL (EANM Research Ltd.) [31]. For more than one modality, the RSNA's Quantitative Imaging Biomarkers Alliance (QIBA) [32] and the Image Biomarker Standardisation Initiative (IBSI) [33] provide common nomenclature and definitions for image biomarkers, benchmarks for image processing and feature extraction, and reporting guidelines. Since guidelines may be insufficient to accommodate the number of scanner and protocol combinations, postprocessing of raw sensor-level data, data augmentation techniques using generative adversarial networks (GANs), or the style transfer methods can be employed to overcome such variability. In the first case, studies have shown similar performance when using raw data and the reconstructed images [34], so one possible methodology is to use the raw data's latent information to reduce the variability introduced by image reconstruction. As for GANs, which are formed by two adversarial networks, a generator that learns to synthesise "realistic" data capable of "fooling" the discriminator, which in turn learns how to discriminate real and synthesised data better, has been used to generate new data [35]. In the case of style transfer, images are translated from one domain to another (e.g., from Philips to Siemens data, from low to high resolution, to normalise slice thickness and dosage in CT, from one CT reconstruction kernel to another [36]), a particular type of GANs, called

CycleGANs [37], has been widely studied as it does not need paired data, allowing the harmonisation multiple institutional data and subsequent improvement of AI models generalizability. These have traditional normalisation alternative methods like statistical normalisation (min-max, *Z*-score) and intensity normalisation (histogram matching to align the image intensity histograms to a reference intensity histogram) [38]. In the case of radiomics, several techniques can be applied in the feature domain, where non-robust features across institutions may be disregarded. Alternatively, normalisation techniques like the min-max, *Z*-score, or ComBat may be applied to minimise differences in features values from different institutions. Several studies using phantoms and patients have proposed workflows for identifying reproducible features in MRI [39] and PET-CT [40], allowing the selection of repeatable and reproducible features for AI model development. Although ComBat harmonisation—a methodology developed for genomic analysis that eliminates batch effects by scaling and shifting the values of each feature—has been extensively used and frameworks to obtain "ComBatable" radiomics features were established [41], it fails to generalise to new unseen cases. On the other hand, using a simple neural network to learn a non-linear normalisation transformation allows generalisation to unseen textures and scanners, representing a future direction in harmonisation when validated on real patients.

When developing AI models, large-scale annotated datasets comprising data acquired from multiple institutions with different scanner models and manufacturers and different patient demographics will likely result in more generalisable models. Nonetheless, models shall be **evaluated** using internal (via temporal partitioning of the dataset to provide insights into temporal variability of the model performance) and external datasets. Furthermore, reporting best practices shall be followed to ensure that research and development of these AI models are appropriately conducted.

Several reporting guidelines are being developed to define these best practices for AI algorithms. The Transparent Reporting of a multivariable prediction model of Individual Prognosis Or Diagnosis (TRIPODAI), the Prediction model Risk Of Bias ASsessment Tool (PROBAST-AI) [42], the Reporting Guidelines for Clinical Trial Protocols for Interventions (SPIRITAI) [43], the Reporting Guidelines for Clinical Trial Reports for Interventions (CONSORT-AI) [44], the Standards for Reporting of Diagnostic Accuracy Study (STARD-AI) [45], and the Developmental and Exploratory Clinical Investigation of DEcision-support systems (DECIDE-AI) [46] are some of these guidelines recently designed to improve reporting when using AI models.

Concerning the latter, to ensure model **reproducibility**, it is crucial to establish AI reporting standards on the model's source code, datasheets describing the utilised datasets [47], and training conditions [1]. Furthermore, a significant challenge that has been a thriving topic of discussion is model **explainability**. Global initiatives and regulations, like the Explainable AI (XAI) from the United States (US) Defense Advanced Research Projects Agency (DARPA) or the European Union (EU) regulation on General Data Protection Regulation (GDPR), have been established to restrain the clinical utilisation of noninterpretable highly complex models. The solutions for delivering explainable models can range from developing transparent models with low complexity to black-box models that can be explained a posteriori using textual or visual maps of explanations. The latter includes saliency maps that highlight relevant image components explaining the model's predictions but need further validation due to its questionable trustworthiness [48]. However, some argue that current explainability techniques are seen as insufficient for decision support at the individual patient level [49] and that if the model is useful and shows accurate predictions, a detailed explanation of its functioning may not be necessary [50]. The latter is especially true in medicine, where the principle behind effective drugs routinely prescribed by clinicians is not entirely understood.

Moreover, humans are biased to trust a wrong model's decision because it is interpretable. So, the need for interpretability depends on the con-

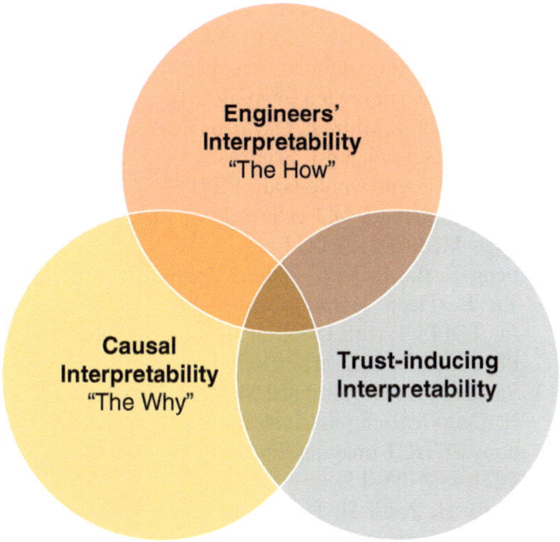


**Fig. 1.5** Types of AI interpretability

text, and different individuals may look at different types of interpretability (Fig. 1.5). Whereas engineers are interested in revealing factors to boost models' predictive power, clinicians are keener on causality and trust. Presenting an explanation outside of the area of interest can result in a loss of trust in a potential accurate and useful model. From the point of view of the model's **clinical validation** and cost-effectiveness, randomised controlled trials (RCTs) are the gold standard of care to evaluate whether a new prediction tool using traditional statistics (TS), ML, or DL provides an improvement compared to the clinical standard of care. By evaluating 65 RCTs, a review [9] has shown that good performance in model development is not a sign of a clinical benefit to patients since two-fifths of trials did not present a clinical benefit compared to standard care. Although DL and ML solutions have demonstrated a higher percentage of positive results, this difference decreased or disappeared after stratifying by the risk of bias when considering only trials with low risk-of-bias. To our knowledge, only six RCTs of DL in medicine have been conducted so far. There is a paramount need to increase the number of high-quality RCTs to estimate the benefits of new AI medical technologies in realistic settings [51]. Besides, **biological validation** of the findings is vital to promote a clinical translation of the models. Indeed, current models may have high predictive power but lack a clear causal relationship between the extracted features and the clinical outcome. To trust model decisions, there are different strategies to select features that are biologically meaningful, including selecting only semantic features that are accepted by radiologists and describe morphologic and location characteristics, combining the extracted features with mutation information coming from genetic analysis and with histopathologic findings and immunohistochemistry (IHC), and identifying functional sub-regions within the tumour, known as habitat imaging [52].

Thirdly, most current AI applications are **not integrated** into the clinical workflow from the AI framework's perspective. Although some of these applications are not created to be directly used by clinicians, for instance, clinical decision support systems (CDSS) for oncologists require interactive and explanatory environments [1]. As mentioned before, regarding explainability, the level of understanding that needs to be provided will depend on the use case and AI methodology. Moreover, existing **legal and ethical frameworks are outdated** and fail to accompany AI solutions' progress and self-learning characteristics. The system should minimise automation complacency so that the end user does not blindly accept the clinical recommendations or overlook alternatives when the algorithm confirms its initial assumptions. Most consider it insufficient to regulate AI in oncology with existing legislative frameworks, so a new regulatory framework needs to be developed. Source data has a **dynamic distribution**, with constant updates on the data standards and ontologies and on the scanner's technology and protocol, which is likely to cause drifts in the algorithm's performance. Continual learning solves this problem, with deployed models in the production environment being automatically retrained when new data input is entered to maintain high-performing models [53]. Finally, there is the challenge of **data sharing** across multiple sites that can be overcome by creating large centralised repositories—with limited permissions or personal information removed from data—or by implementing federated approaches, with each institution maintaining individual data and only sending out the models, or with a single honest broker assessing data for all the involved institutions [6].

For all the mentioned challenges for AI in oncology, efforts should be made by multidisciplinary professionals (clinicians, epidemiologists, computer scientists,biomedic alengineers,informaticians,ethicists,andleg islators)toaddress them to deliver robust, explainable, and reproducible AI models that can be implemented into clinical practice.

## References


1. Chua I, Yablowitz M, Korach Z, Kehl K, Levitan N, Arriaga Y, Jackson G, Bates D, Hassett M. Artificial intelligence in oncology: path to implementation. Cancer Med. 2021;10:4138–49.
2. Krizhevsky A, Sutskever I, Hinton G. Imagenet classification with deep convolutional neural networks. Adv Neural Inf Proces Syst. 2012;25:1097–105.
3. Bar Y, Diamant I, Wolf L, Lieberman S, Konen E, Greenspan H. Chest pathology detection using deep learning with non-medical training. In: 2015 IEEE 12th International Symposium on Biomedical Imaging (ISBI); 2015. p. 294–7.
4. Ronneberger O, Fischer P, Brox T. U-net: convolutional networks for biomedical image segmentation. In: International Conference on Medical Image Computing and Computer-assisted Intervention; 2015. p. 234–41.
5. Lambin P, Rios-Velazquez E, Leijenaar R, Carvalho S, Van Stiphout R, Granton P, Zegers C, Gillies R, Boellard R, Dekker A, et al. Radiomics: extracting more information from medical images using advanced feature analysis. Eur J Cancer. 2012;48:441–6.
6. Gillies R, Kinahan P, Hricak H. Radiomics: images are more than pictures, they are data. Radiology. 2016;278:563–77.
7. Dos Santos D, Dietzel M, Baessler B. A decade of radiomics research: are images really data or just patterns in the noise? Eur Radiol. 2020;31:1–4.
8. Papanikolaou N, Santinha J. An introduction to radiomics: capturing tumour biology in space and time. Hellenic J Radiol. 2018;3.
9. Zhou Q, Chen Z, Cao Y, Peng S. Clinical impact and quality of randomized controlled trials involving interventions evaluating artificial intelligence prediction tools: a systematic review. NPJ Digit Med. 2021;4:154.
10. Gong K, Guan J, Kim K, Zhang X, Yang J, Seo Y, El Fakhri G, Qi J, Li Q. Iterative PET image reconstruction using convolutional neural network representation. IEEE Trans Med Imaging. 2018;38:675–85.
11. Chaudhari A, Mittra E, Davidzon G, Gulaka P, Gandhi H, Brown A, Zhang T, Srinivas S, Gong E, Zaharchuk G. Low-count whole-body PET with deep learning in a multicenter and externally validated study. NPJ Digit Med. 2021;4:1–11.
12. Feng T, Yao S, Xi C, Zhao Y, Wang R, Wu S, Li C, Xu B. Deep learning-based image reconstruction for TOFPET with DIRECT data partitioning format. Phys Med Biol. 2021;66:165007.
13. Sanaat A, Shiri I, Arabi H, Mainta I, Nkoulou R, Zaidi H. Deep learning-assisted ultra-fast/low-dose whole-body PET/CT imaging. Eur J Nucl Med Mol Imaging. 2021;48:2405–15.
14. Arabi H, Zaidi H. Deep learning–based metal artefact reduction in PET/CT imaging. Eur Radiol. 2021;31(8):6384–96.
15. Medical S. Subtle PET. https://subtlemedical.com/subtlepet/. Accessed 21 Dec 2021.
16. Healthineers S. Oncofreeze AI. https://www.siemens-healthineers.com/molecularimaging/options-and-upgrades/software-applications/oncofreeze. Accessed 21 Dec 2021.
17. Edenbrandt L, Borrelli P, Ulen J, Enqvist O, Tragardh E. Automated analysis of PSMA-PET/CT studies using convolutional neural networks. MedRxiv. 2021.
18. Zhao X, Li L, Lu W, Tan S. Tumor co-segmentation in PET/CT using multi-modality fully convolutional neural network. Phys Med Biol. 2018;64:015011.
19. Moe Y, Groendahl A, Mulstad M, Tomic O, Indahl U, Dale E, Malinen E, Futsaether C. Deep learning for automatic tumour segmentation in PET/CT images of patients with head and neck cancers. ArXiv Preprint ArXiv:1908.00841. 2019.
20. Kawauchi K, Furuya S, Hirata K, Katoh C, Manabe O, Kobayashi K, Watanabe S, Shiga T. A convolutional neural network-based system to classify patients using FDG PET/CT examinations. BMC Cancer. 2020;20:1–10.
21. Peng H, Dong D, Fang M, Li L, Tang L, Chen L, Li W, Mao Y, Fan W, Liu L, et al. Prognostic value of deep learning PET/CT-based radiomics: potential role for future individual induction chemotherapy in advanced nasopharyngeal carcinoma. Clin Cancer Res. 2019;25:4271–9.
22. Polymeri E, Sadik M, Kaboteh R, Borrelli P, Enqvist O, Ulén J, Ohlsson M, Trägardh E, Poulsen M, Simonsen J, et al. Deep learning-based quantification of PET/CT prostate gland uptake: association with overall survival. Clin Physiol Funct Imaging. 2020;40:106–13.
23. Borrelli P, Larsson M, Ulén J, Enqvist O, Träg E, Poulsen M, Mortensen M, Kjölhede H, Høilund-Carlsen P, Edenbrandt L. Artificial intelligence-based detection of lymph node metastases by PET/CT predicts prostate cancer-specific survival. Clin Physiol Funct Imaging. 2021;41:62–7.

24. Sibille L, Seifert R, Avramovic N, Vehren T, Spottiswoode B, Zuehlsdorff S, Schafers M. 18F-FDG PET/CT uptake classification in lymphoma and lung cancer by using deep convolutional neural networks. Radiology. 2020;294:445–52.
25. Borrelli P, Ly J, Kaboteh R, Ulén J, Enqvist O, Träg E, Edenbrandt L. AI-based detection of lung lesions in [18 F] FDG PET-CT from lung cancer patients. EJNMMI Phys. 2021;8:1–11.
26. Fan X, Zhang H, Yin Y, Zhang J, Yang M, Qin S, Zhang X, Yu F. Texture analysis of 18F-FDG PET/CT for differential diagnosis spinal metastases. Front Med. 2021;7:605746.
27. Satoh Y, Hirata K, Tamada D, Funayama S, Onishi H. Texture analysis in the diagnosis of primary breast cancer: comparison of high-resolution dedicated breast positron emission tomography (dbPET) and whole-body PET/CT. Front Med. 2020;7:603303.
28. Zheng K, Wang X, Jiang C, Tang Y, Fang Z, Hou J, Zhu Z, Hu S. Pre-operative prediction of mediastinal node metastasis using Radiomics model based on 18F-FDG PET/CTof the primary tumorin non-small cell lung cancer patients. Front Med. 2021;8:673876.
29. Pierson E, Cutler D, Leskovec J, Mullainathan S, Obermeyer Z. An algorithmic approach to reducing unexplained pain disparities in underserved populations. Nat Med. 2021;27:136–40.
30. Mali S, Ibrahim A, Woodruff H, Andrearczyk V, Müller H, Primakov S, Salahuddin Z, Chatterjee A, Lambin P. Making radiomics more reproducible across scanner and imaging protocol variations: a review of harmonization methods. J Pers Med. 2021;11:842.
31. Boellaard R, Delgado-Bolton R, Oyen W, Giammarile F, Tatsch K, Eschner W, Verzijlbergen F, Barrington S, Pike L, Weber W, et al. FDG PET/CT: EANM procedure guidelines for tumour imaging: version 2.0. Eur J Nucl Med Mol Imaging. 2015;42:328–54.
32. Sullivan D, Obuchowski N, Kessler L, Raunig D, Gatsonis C, Huang E, Kondratovich M, McShane L, Reeves A, Barboriak D, et al. Metrology standards for quantitative imaging biomarkers. Radiology. 2015;277:813–25.
33. Zwanenburg A, Leger S, Vallières M, Löck S. Image biomarker standardisation initiative. ArXiv Preprint. 2016.
34. Lee H, Huang C, Yune S, Tajmir S, Kim M, Do S. Machine friendly machine learning: interpretation of computed tomography without image reconstruction. Sci Rep. 2019;9:1–9.
35. Islam J, Zhang Y. GAN-based synthetic brain PET image generation. Brain Inform. 2020;7:1–12.
36. Yang S, Kim E, Ye J. Continuous conversion of CT Kernel using switchable CycleGAN with AdaIN. In: IEEE transactions on medical imaging. Piscataway, NJ: IEEE; 2021.
37. Zhu J, Park T, Isola P, Efros A. Unpaired image-to-image translation using cycle-consistent adversarial networks. In: Proceedings of the IEEE International Conference on Computer Vision; 2017. p. 2223.
38. Nyúl L, Udupa J. On standardizing the MR image intensity scale. Magn Reson Med. 1999;42:1072–81.
39. Bianchini L, Santinha J, Loução N, Figueiredo M, Botta F, Origgi D, Cremonesi M, Cassano E, Papanikolaou N. A multicenter study on radiomic features from T2-weighted images of a customized MR pelvic phantom setting the basis for robust radiomic models in clinics. Magn Reson Med. 2020;85:1713–26.
40. Shiri I, Rahmim A, Ghaffarian P, Geramifar P, Abdollahi H, Bitarafan-Rajabi A. The impact of image reconstruction settings on 18F-FDG PET radiomic features: multi-scanner phantom and patient studies. Eur Radiol. 2017;27:4498–509.
41. Ibrahim A, Primakov S, Beuque M, Woodruff H, Halilaj I, Wu G, Refaee T, Granzier R, Widaatalla Y, Hustinx R. Radiomicsforprecisio nmedicine: currentchallenges, future prospects, and the proposal of a new framework. Methods. 2021;188:20–9.
42. Collins G, Dhiman P, Navarro C, Ma J, Hooft L, Reitsma J, Logullo P, Beam A, Peng L, Van Calster B, et al. Protocol for development of a reporting guideline (TRIPOD-AI) and risk of bias tool (PROBAST-AI) for diagnostic and prognostic prediction model studies based on artificial intelligence. BMJ Open. 2021;11:e048008.
43. Rivera S, Liu X, Chan A, Denniston A, Calvert M. Guidelines for clinical trial protocols for interventions involving artificial intelligence: the SPIRIT-AI extension. Lancet Digit Health. 2020;2(10):e549–60.
44. Liu X, Rivera S, Moher D, Calvert M, Denniston A. Reporting guidelines for clinical trial reports for interventions involving artificial intelligence: the CONSORT-AI extension. BMJ. 2020;370:m3164.
45. Sounderajah V, Ashrafian H, Golub R, Shetty S, De Fauw J, Hooft L, Moons K, Collins G, Moher D, Bossuyt P, et al. Developing a reporting guideline for artificial intelligence-centred diagnostic test accuracy studies: the STARD-AI protocol. BMJ Open. 2021;11:e047709.
46. Watkinson P, Clifton D, Collins G, Mcculloch P, Morgan L, Group, D. DECIDE-AI: new reporting guidelines to bridge the development-to-implementation gap in clinical artificial intelligence. Nat Med. 2021;27(2):186–7.
47. Gebru T, Morgenstern J, Vecchione B, Vaughan J, Wallach H, Au H, Crawford K. Datasheets for dlatasets. ArXiv.2021.
48. Arun N, Gaw N, Singh P, Chang K, Aggarwal M, Chen B, Hoebel K, Gupta S, Patel J, Gidwani M, Adebayo J, Li M, Kalpathy-Cramer J. Assessing the (un)trustworthiness of saliency maps for localizing abnormalities in Medical imaging. Radiol Artif Intell. 2021;3(6):e200267.
49. Ghassemi M, Oakden-Rayner L, Beam A. The false hope of current approaches to explainable artificial intelligence in health care. Lancet Digit Health. 2021;3:e745–50.

50. Miller K. Should AI models be explainable? That depends. 2021. https://hai.stanford.edu/news/should-ai-models-be-explainable-depends. Accessed 16 Mar 2021.
51. Genin K. Grote T. Randomized controlled trialsin medical AIA methodological critique. Philosophy Med. 2021;2.
52. Tomaszewski M, Gillies R. The biological meaning of radiomic features. Radiology. 2021;298:505–16.
53. Lee C, Lee A. Clinical applications of continual learning machine learning. Lancet Digit Health. 2020;2:e279–81.

# Positron Emission Tomography in Bone and Soft Tissue Tumors

2

Nikoletta K. Pianou

## 2.1 Introduction

Positron emission tomography/computed tomography (PET/CT) with the use of $^{18}$F-fluorodeoxyglucose ($^{18}$F-FDG) is an imaging modality that combines both functional and anatomical information. The combination of PET with CT has been established as an imaging modality and is currently widely used in oncology. Bone and soft tissue tumors, as of course the majority of tumors, are characterized by multiple metabolic and molecular alterations, which allow us imaging with positron emitters. These alterations include increased glycolysis, increased amino acid and increased nucleic acid metabolic activity.

There are several radiotracers available for PET imaging, but the most widely used tracer in oncology is $^{18}$F-fluorodeoxyglucose ($^{18}$F-FDG) which is a glucose analogue. Contemporary PET scanners are equipped also with CT (PET/CT scanners) and very recently with MRI (PET/MRI scanners), thus allowing a comprehensive functional and an anatomical assessment of tumors.

$^{18}$F-FDG follows the pathways of glucose into the cells, meaning that it enters into the cells through membrane glucose transporters (GLOUT 1–GLOUT 7). After its entrance into the cell, it is phosphorylated by an enzyme called hexokinase and converted to FDG-6-phosphate. The difference from glucose is that $^{18}$F-FDG is not further metabolized, and it is metabolically trapped into the cell. Taking advantage of the fact that tumors are characterized by increased glycolysis, we can depict images of the tumor. During tumor proliferation, the glucose transporters, especially GLUT 1, are over-expressed, bur other changes as well, like increased hexokinase activity and reduced glucose-6-phosphatase activity, make tumors "visible" to PET.

$^{18}$F-FDG is injected intravenously to the patient and then the patient remains at rest for about 1 h. Hydration and fasting for at least 6 h prior to the examination are mandatory. Blood glucose levels should also be measured as it is preferred that the glucose level remains <160 mg/dL. Then the patient initially undergoes CT imaging and then PET imaging, usually from the base of the skull to the thighs. In selected patients, the extremities may be in the field of interest. PET images are attenuation corrected with the CT and both images are fused.

## 2.2 Positron Emission Tomography in Sarcomas

Sarcomas are relatively rare and account for about 1% of all malignancies. They arise from tissue of mesenchymal origin and are very heterogeneous group of malignancies comprising

N. K. Pianou (✉)
Division of Nuclear Medicine, Department of PET/CT, "EVANGELISMOS" General Hospital of Athens, Athens, Greece


J. A. Andreou et al. (eds.), *Artificial Intelligence in PET/CT Oncologic Imaging*,
https://doi.org/10.1007/978-3-031-10090-1_2

bone sarcomas (BS) and soft tissue sarcomas (STS). However, sarcomas can develop from many types of tissue such as bone, cartilage, muscle, connective tissue, fat, peripheral nerves or vessels, occurring almost anywhere in the body. They usually grow locally, infiltrating surrounding tissues. They occur in both children and elderly. Ewing's sarcoma, which is a malignant primary bone tumor, and rhabdomyosarcoma usually occur in children and adolescents, but osteosarcoma may occur in the elderly also. Lungs are the most frequent site for metastases, as sarcomas tend to spread hematogenously, although lymphatic spread is also possible. Extremities, especially lower limbs, are usual sites where sarcomas grow up, but some of them may occur intra-abdominally, like gastrointestinal stromal tumors (GIST), which are the most common sarcomas (mesenchymal tumors) of the gastrointestinal tract.

When the disease is initially diagnosed, there are some parameters which are very important for the management of these tumors, such as the exact location of the tumor, the size and grade of the tumor and the accurate staging. The conventional imaging modalities (CIM) which are used to determine the location and the size of the primary tumor are the magnetic resonance imaging (MRI) and the CT. However, benign soft tissue masses and STS may be difficult to separate with the use of CIM, while sarcomas show very heterogeneous character. Biopsy remains the method of choice for the diagnosis and grading of sarcomas. The biopsy site determines the result which is dependent and directed by anatomical imaging. A problem which often arises when biopsy is performed is that the site of the biopsy taken may not represent the "behavior" of the whole mass; therefore, clinically significant high-grade areas of the tumor may be missed. $^{18}$F-FDG PET/CT can help improve the localization of the biopsy site, helping for a more accurate staging (Fig. 2.1). However, there are substantial differences in $^{18}$F-FDG uptake values between low-

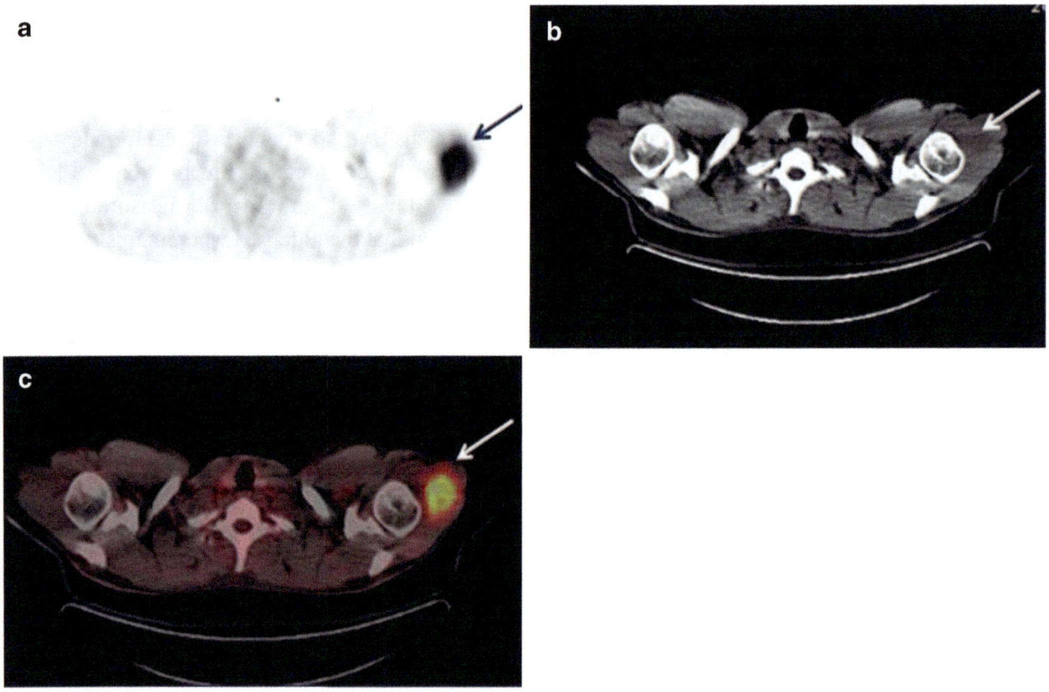


**Fig. 2.1** (**a**–**c**) Young patient with fever of unknown origin. There is focally increased $^{18}$F-FDG uptake at left humeral soft tissues. Biopsy revealed sarcoma. ((**a**) $^{18}$F-FDG PET, black arrow; (**b**) CT, white arrow;(**c**) Fusion PET/CT, white arrow)

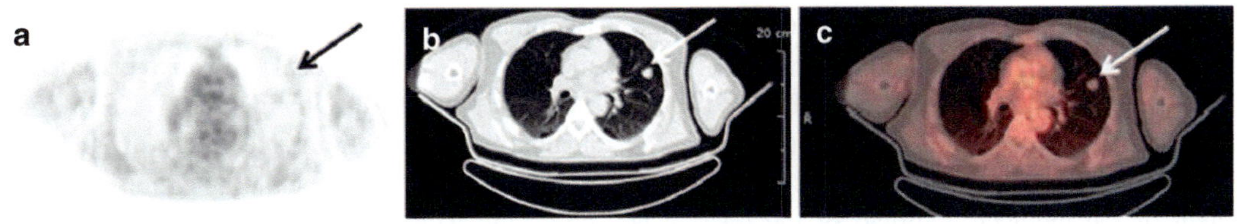


**Fig. 2.2** (**a**–**c**) Male patient with history of resected low-grade synovial sarcoma of the right lower extremity. Lung metastases on CT images showing mildly increased. $^{18}$F-FDG uptake on PET images ((**a**) $^{18}$F-FDG PET, black arrow; (**b**) CT, white arrow; (**c**) fusion PET/CT, white arrow)

and high-grade BS and STS, while $^{18}$F-FDG uptake correlates with histological grade in heterogeneous sarcomas.

High-grade sarcomas show more intense $^{18}$F-FDG uptake, while low-grade sarcomas the opposite, leading sometimes to false negative result (Fig. 2.2). Nevertheless, in clinical practice, the noninvasive assessment of the sites with the highest grade of malignancy is very important for the guidance of biopsy.

$^{18}$F-FDG uptake is not pathognomonic for malignancy. Some benign lesions, such as giant cell tumors of the bones, inflammatory changes, as well as bone fractures may present a high level of tracer accumulation. Among these, inflammatory disease is the most common cause of a false positive $^{18}$F-FDG PET/CT scan and malignant lesions should always be confirmed either with histopathology examination or with a follow-up. False negative $^{18}$F-FDG PET/CT results may also occur. Malignant diseases may show nonspecific or asymmetric $^{18}$F-FDG uptake, while the limited spatial resolution of $^{18}$F-FDG PET/CT scan may be a reason for some occult or sub-centimeter lesions to be missed [1].

A semiquantitative method which is used to determine the $^{18}$F-FDG uptake by the primary tumor is the maximum standardized uptake value (SUVmax). SUVmax of the primary tumor seems to be a prognostic factor of survival and high SUVmax values indicate a poor prognosis. In a recent study of 74 patients with STS, Schwarzbach et al. divided the patients into three groups based on SUVmax, those with values <1.59, values >1.59 but <3.6 and > 3.6, with 5-year survival rate 84, 45, and 38%, respectively [2].

Recently, Chen et al. evaluated the usefulness of $^{18}$F-FDG PET/CT-derived parameters to differentiate STS and BS from benign lesions, in a total of 70 patients. SUVmax index is a marker of glucose metabolism of a single integrin in the tumor. On the other hand, Metabolic Tumor Volume (MTV) and Total Lesion Glycolysis (TLG) reflect the global metabolic activity of the tumor. Another parameter is the intratumoral heterogeneity of glucose metabolism, which is expressed by the heterogeneous factor (HF). As it was expected, the tumor size, SUVmax, MTV, TLG, and HF in the STS and BS group were all significantly higher than in the benign lesions group. Additionally, only SUVmax and HF were identified as independent risk factors for malignant tumors. Despite the usual false positive causes, six false negative malignant lesions were also determined. For example, myxofibrosarcomas, as well as other malignancies which were rich in mucous matrix, usually exhibited insufficient glucose transporter expression and showed low FDG uptake [3].

RHR Marles et al. conducted a retrospective study on patients diagnosed with STS, which included 83 patients. The most common tumor types were adipocytic tumors (31%), smooth muscle tumors (16%), fibroblastic/myofibroblastic tumors (13%), and undifferentiated or unclassified sarcomas (13%). Several metabolic parameters were also calculated, like SUV, MTV, and TLG. The SUVmax remains the most accurate parameter to distinguish between high-grade and low-grade STS, which is also correlated with the histological grade measured in the baseline PET/CT. However, when considering the relationship between MTV and TLG parameters with the tumor grade, the authors concluded that these parameters do not allow defining a significant cut off point to discriminate high- from low-grade STS.

In the same study, the authors concluded that patients with high SUVmax, SUVpeak, MTV, and TLG values of baseline $^{18}$F-FDG PET/CT have significantly lower Overall Survival (OS) [4].

During staging procedure a total body assessment of the metastatic spread of the disease is also important, concerning either the lymph nodes metastases or the distant metastases (Figs. 2.3, and 2.4). $^{18}$F-FDG PET/CT has high accuracy for staging lymph node metastases and shows high sensitivity and specificity, although lymph node metastases are not very frequent. In a recent study by Fuglo et al. [5] which included 89 sarcoma patients, the $^{18}$F-FDG PET/CT revealed a sensitivity of 100%, a specificity of 90%, and an accuracy of 91% for the detection of lymph node metastases. Nevertheless, false negative results may occur if the cancer has low glucose metabolism, if the metastatic lymph nodes are small in size, or a focus may be missed if it is located adjacent to an area of high physiological or pathological.

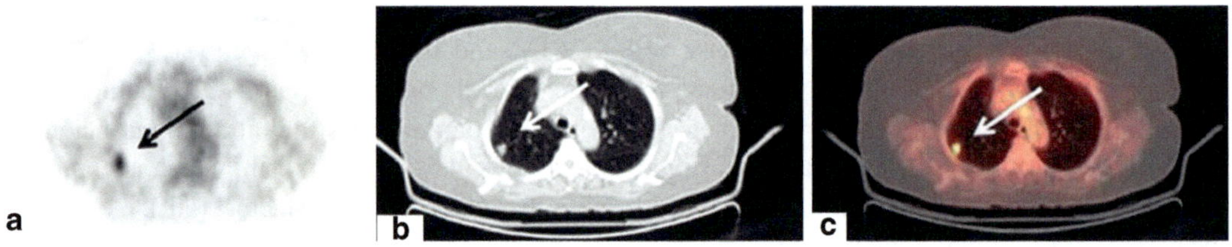


**Fig. 2.3** (**a**–**c**) Female patient with history of resected uterine leiomyosarcoma. Right pulmonary nodule shows increased $^{18}$F-FDG uptake on PET/CT consistent with metastasis. ((**a**) $^{18}$F-FDG PET, black arrow; (**b**) CT, white arrow; (**c**) fusion PET/CT, white arrow)

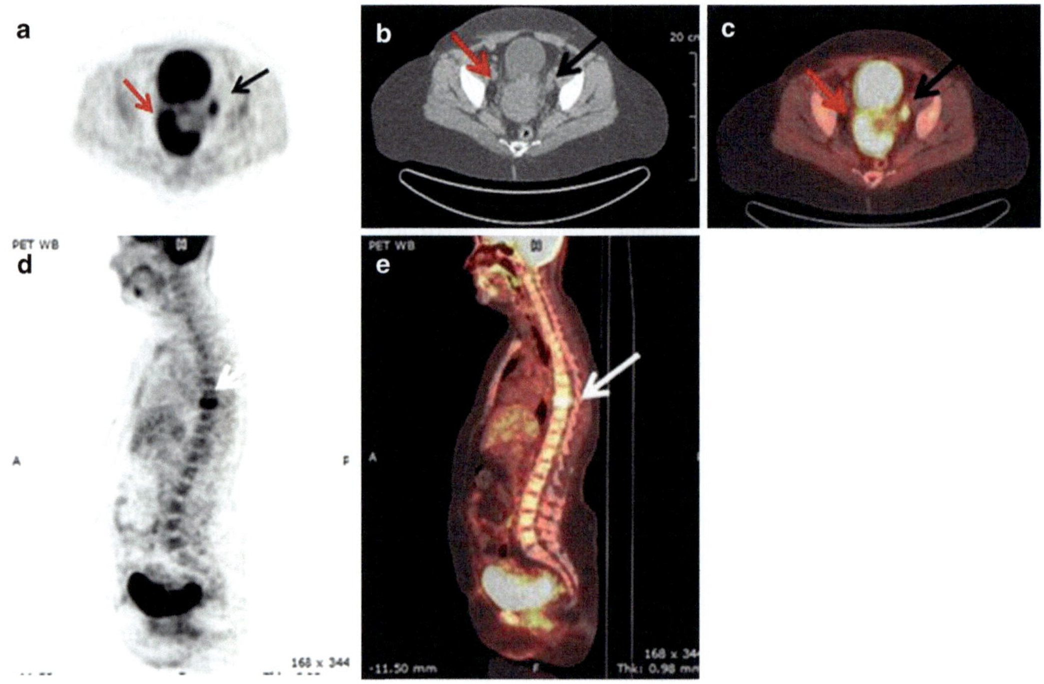


**Fig. 2.4** **a**–**e** Female patient with uterine leiomyosarcoma. $^{18}$F-FDG PET/CT performed at initial staging shows increased $^{18}$F-FDG uptake at the primary mass (red arrows), at left iliac lymph node compatible with metastasis (black arrows) and at T8 vertebra compatible with metastasis (white arrows). (Transverse views: (**a**) $^{18}$F-FDG PET, (**b**) CT, (**c**) fusion PET/CT; Sagittal views: (**d**) $^{18}$F-FDG PET, (**e**) fusion PET/CT)

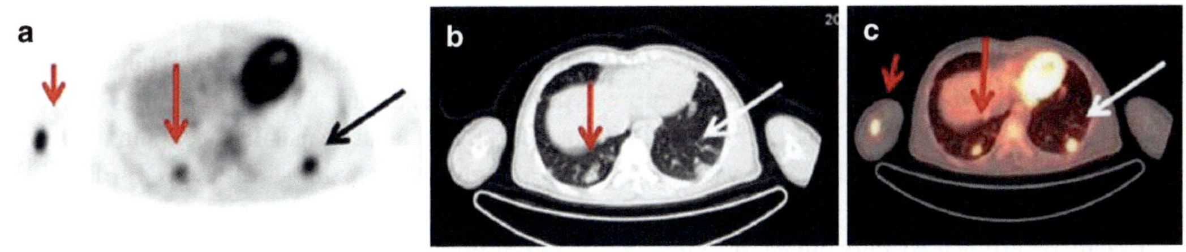


**Fig. 2.5** (**a–c**) Male patient at initial staging of angiosarcoma of the left lung (black and white arrows). There is increased $^{18}$F-FDG uptake at a right pulmonary nodule consistent with metastasis (long red arrow) and at the shaft of the right humerus consistent with bone metastasis (short red arrow) ((**a**) $^{18}$F-FDG PET; (**b**) CT; (**c**) fusion PET/CT)

$^{18}$F-FDG uptake. On the other hand, false positive results may occur due to reactive/inflammatory lymph nodes, as increased glucose metabolism is not specific only to cancer cells but in activated leukocytes and macrophages as well. In situations such as following biopsy, tumor resection, or during infection we may have a false positive $^{18}$F-FDG uptake in lymph nodes. The tumor itself may also lead to reactive $^{18}$F-FDG uptake in the regional lymph nodes due to inflammation. $^{18}$F-FDG PET/CT may be used to guide sampling of sites of unexpected nodal metastases.

As for the distant metastases, $^{18}$F-FDG PET/CT seems to be a very accurate method of staging (Fig. 2.5). In the study by Fuglo et al. [5], the $^{18}$F-FDG PET/CT detected distant metastases with a sensitivity of 95%, a specificity of 96%, and an accuracy of 95%. In this study, the positive predictive value was 87%, which shows moderate to high ability of $^{18}$F-FDG PET/CT to diagnose distant metastases, with not too many false positive results. However, the negative predictive value was high (98%), which means that $^{18}$F-FDG PET/CT may exclude with confidence the presence of distant metastatic disease. In another study by Tateishi et al. [6], which included 117 patients with BS and STS combined PET/CT and CIM helped to avoid surgical resection in 13% of patients and to alter management in additional 14% of patients. In the same study the sensitivity, specificity, and accuracy of $^{18}$F-FDG PET/CT were found to be 92, 91, and 91%, respectively. Another advantage of $^{18}$F-FDG PET/CT is that the whole-body imaging may also reveal incidental findings, such as other malignancies.

In a study of Franzius et al. [7] $^{18}$F-FDG PET was compared to bone scintigraphy in the detection of osseous metastases in 38 patients with Ewing Sarcoma (ES). The sensitivity, specificity, and accuracy of $^{18}$F-FDG PET was 100, 96, and 97%, respectively, on a patient-based analysis. The comparable values for bone scintigraphy were 68, 87, and 82%. On a lesion-based analysis, the sensitivity of $^{18}$F-FDG PET was 88% and for bone scintigraphy was 69%. The superiority of $^{18}$F-FDG PET over bone scintigraphy for the detection of osseous metastases from ES may be explained by the fact that $^{18}$F-FDG PET depicts the increased glucose metabolism of the metastases before bone scintigraphy shows increased osteoblastic activity. Also, $^{18}$F-FDG PET has a better spatial resolution than bone scintigraphy. Small metastases adjacent to the growth plates in children, which are areas of normal radiotracer accumulation in a bone scintigraphy, might be missed giving a false negative result. The only exception where bone scintigraphy is superior to $^{18}$F-FDG PET is the depiction of metastases to the skull because $^{18}$F-F-FDG normally accumulates in the adjacent cerebral cortex which uses glucose. Bone scintigraphy is more sensitive in that case than $^{18}$F-FDG PET. In addition, $^{18}$F-FDG PET may detect soft tissue metastases, while bone scintigraphy may not. As for pediatric sarcoma patients, Volker et al. [8] evaluated the impact of $^{18}$F-FDG PET in 46 pediatric patients with ES, osteosarcoma, and rhabdomyosarcoma at initial staging, compared to other CIM. Authors concluded that $^{18}$F-FDG PET and CIM were equally effective in the detection of primary tumors, while $^{18}$F-FDG PET was superior to CIM concerning the correct detection of lymph node involvement (sensitivity 95% vs. 25%, respectively) and bone manifestations (sensitivity 90% vs. 57%, respectively). However, CT was more reliable than $^{18}$F-FDG PET in depicting lung metastases (sensitivity 100% vs. 25%, respectively).

Local recurrence occurs in approximately 10–15% of patients with STS, while distant recurrence develops in 35–45% of patients, even when treated suitably. Surgical resection usually disturbs the normal anatomy of the area and as a result, local recurrence is difficult to be detected (Figs. 2.6, and 2.7). In addition, radiotherapy may disturb the anatomy of the area, leading to difficulties in detecting local recurrence and $^{18}$F-FDG PET/CT may be false positive due to post radiation inflammatory changes. On the other hand, CIM are most prone to errors and CT and MRI, although they are more suitable techniques for visualization of anatomy, usually cannot differentiate a scar from local recurrence. $^{18}$F-FDG PET/CT depicts the increased metabolism associated with abnormal tissues enabling visualization of recurrences. Nevertheless, the study should be performed at least 4–6 months after radiation therapy and the results should be interpreted with caution.

Distant recurrence usually occurs in the lungs. In a study by Franzius et al. [9], $^{18}$F-FDG PET was compared to spiral thoracic CT for the detection of pulmonary metastases in 39 patients with ES. There was no patient with a true positive $^{18}$F-FDG PET and a false negative CT, and no pulmonary metastasis was detected earlier with $^{18}$F-FDG PET than with spiral CT, giving a clear superiority to CT for detecting pulmonary metastases in ES patients. On an examination-based analysis, $^{18}$F-FDG PET had a sensitivity of 56%, a specificity of 91%, and an accuracy of 82%, while the same values for CT were 88, 100, and 97%, respectively. In conclusion, an $^{18}$F-FDG PET should not be recommended to exclude lung metastases when the lung CT is negative. However, a positive $^{18}$F-FDG PET result can be used to confirm lesions seen on CT as metastatic disease because of its high specificity.

$^{18}$F-FDG PET may also be used in evaluation of treatment response after neoadjuvant chemo-

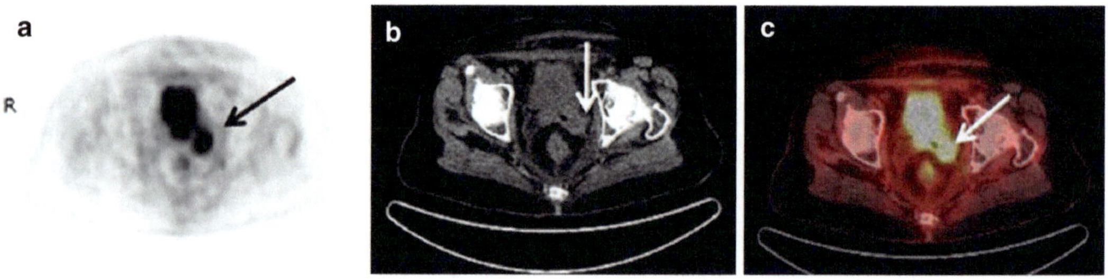


**Fig. 2.6** (**a**–**c**) Female patient with history of resected uterine leiomyosarcoma. $^{18}$F-FDG PET/CT during restaging shows increased $^{18}$F-FDG uptake in anatomical position of the uterus, consistent with local recurrence ((**a**) $^{18}$F-FDG PET, black arrow; (**b**) CT, white arrow; (**c**) fusion PET/CT, white arrow)

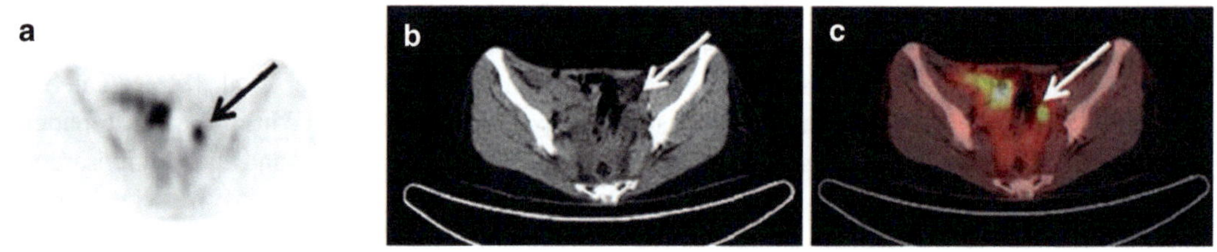


**Fig. 2.7** (**a**–**c**) Female patient with history of resected uterine leiomyosarcoma. $^{18}$F-FDG PET/CT during restaging shows increased $^{18}$F-FDG uptake in a left iliac lymph nodes compatible with recurrence ((**a**) $^{18}$F-FDG PET, black arrow; (**b**) CT, white arrow; (**c**) fusion PET/CT, white arrow)

therapy in patients with STS. Herrmann et al. evaluated prospectively whether $^{18}$F-FDG PET imaging after one cycle of neoadjuvant therapy could predict overall survivor in patients with primary high-grade STS. They pointed out that $^{18}$F-FDG PET can potentially serve as an intermediate end point biomarker in clinical research and patient care [10]. Fendler et al. also evaluated 73 patients with STS after chemotherapy with regional hyperthermia (RHT). All patients underwent a baseline $^{18}$F-FDG PET and after two to four cycles of neoadjuvant chemotherapy with RHT. PET Response Criteria in Solid Tumors (PERCIST 1.0) and Response Evaluation Criteria in Solid Tumors (RECIST 1.1) were applied. Metabolic response by PERCIST ($n = 44/73$) was an independent predictor of Progression-Free Survival (PFS) ($P = 0.002$) and time to local or distant progression [11]. More recently Koshkin et al. analyzed assessments made during a clinical trial of a novel IGF1R antibody in patients with Ewing sarcoma. $^{18}$F-FDG PET studies were conducted at baseline and on day 9 of treatment. Functional imaging assessment of progressive disease could be identified as early as day 9 versus at 6 weeks by using any of the anatomic imaging criteria, giving PET a superiority to anatomic imaging in identification of responders [12].

## 2.3 Positron Emission Tomography in Gastrointestinal Stromal Tumors

As for the monitoring of treatment, $^{18}$F-FDG PET/CT seems to have the most important role in GIST therapy [13]. GIST have a common molecular pathogenesis with activating mutations in the gene encoding Kit (a tyrosine kinase and stem cell factor receptor). For that reason, treatment of GIST is currently regarded as the paradigm of molecular-targeted therapy in solid tumors, and targeted therapies by means of the tyrosine kinase inhibitor imatinib mesylate and other similar drugs have been introduced in clinical practice. Conventional cytotoxic chemotherapy and radiotherapy are not effective in this kind of tumors [13].

Most GIST show increased metabolic activity in $^{18}$F-FDG PET/CT at initial diagnosis and decreased $^{18}$F-FDG uptake during treatment, which is related to a positive treatment result. Treatment with c-Kit inhibitors causes some changes in the tumor structure, such as decreased vascularity, hemorrhage, necrosis, cystic or myxoid degeneration, which may not alter the tumor volume. For that reason the morphologic criteria only, meaning the tumor size, as it is depicted by CT imaging, is not the optimal way to assess treatment response of GIST to drugs, usually underestimating the treatment result. The metabolism of the tumor cell is reflected by the decrease of $^{18}$F-FDG uptake, which usually precedes changes in tumor size. There are many studies showing that $^{18}$F-FDG PET/CT may identify GIST patient responders to imatinib or other drugs, earlier than CT, while in others $^{18}$F-FDG PET/CT is considered as the gold standard technique for the assessment of treatment response in patients with GIST.

Holdsworth et al. [14], studied 63 patients with advanced GIST disease and compared CT bidimensional measurements and $^{18}$F-FDG PET/CT SUVmax values to determine response to imatinib treatment. The authors concluded that after 1 month of treatment, the SUVmax cut off value of 3.4, the reduction of the SUVmax value of 40% compared to the baseline PET, and the absence of growth of the tumor are optimal criteria for treatment response.

Unfortunately, 14% of GIST patients may show primary imatinib resistance, while 50% of those who responded initially might develop secondary resistance. In these patients, the alteration of therapy with newer tyrosine kinase inhibitors is mandatory [13]. $^{18}$F-FDG PET seems to be the most significant independent predictor of PFS predicting patient outcome. Demetri et al. [15] studied 97 patients with imatinib-resistant GIST and bulky metastatic disease who were treated with sunitinib. A baseline $^{18}$F-FDG PET was performed initially and follow-up $^{18}$F-FDG PET scans were performed at several points during treatment. In the majority of patients, a partial metabolic response was evident on $^{18}$F-FDG PET within 1 week of starting sunitinib. On the contrary, objective responses on CT took much longer to detect. In another study by Fuster et al. [16], 21 patients with locally advanced and/or metastatic GIST refractory to imatinib, treated with doxorubicin (four cycles), followed by imatinib maintenance, were evaluated with CT and $^{18}$F-FDG PET at baseline and after completion of therapy. A correlation was found between PET response and PFS. A residual SUVmax <5 after treatment correlated with improved PFS while survival curves showed a significant association between PET response and PFS.

Recently, Fendler et al. investigated the SUV-based parameters with the tumor grade of STS. SUVpeak and SUVpeak/SUVliver showed diagnostic accuracy separating between low- and high-grade GIST tumors [17]. Miyake et al. retrospectively evaluated 46 patients with primary GIST who received preoperatively $^{18}$F-FDG PET followed by complete resection without any neoadjuvant therapy. They concluded that ring-shaped $^{18}$F-FDG uptake preoperatively may be a potential predictor of postoperative tumor recurrence of localized primary GISTs [18].

## 2.4 Artificial Intelligence

Artificial intelligence (AI) is a growing field of research that is emerging as a promising adjunct to assist physicians in detection and management of patients with cancer. AI applications are mathematical techniques and programs that use a variety of approaches (e.g., convolutional analysis, various types of neural networks and deep learning) in order to analyze datasets of base or raw data after scientists or radiologists set up parameters about the data. This process allows the AI application to learn on its own by recognizing patterns in the data sets by using many layers of processing to yield the same results as an expert radiologist or nuclear medicine specialist. AI is a complex field, mostly applicable in patients with lung cancer and lymphoma [19].

A recent study by Peng et al. included $^{18}$F-FDG PET/CT images of 48 patients with pathology-proven STS from a publicly available dataset (24 with distant metastases and 24 without metastatic disease). The aim of the study was to develop a deep multi-modality collaborative learning (DMCL) model to predict distant metastases. The model provided higher accuracy, sensitivity, and area under the ROC curve (AUC) in comparison with other state-of-the-art models including single-modality PET convolutional neural network (CNN) and multi-modality CNN [20]. Further studies are needed to establish the utility of AI in patients with STS and BS.

## 2.5 Conclusion

Conclusively, $^{18}$F-FDG PET/CT is a useful imaging modality in the management of bone and soft tissue tumors. At the initial staging, its role is primarily to indicate the site of biopsy, to characterize a lesion, and to detect metastatic disease. During restaging, the differentiation between viable tumor and necrosis is the most important advantage of $^{18}$F-FDG PET/CT for the detection of local recurrence, but distant recurrence may be depicted as well. As for the monitoring of therapy, $^{18}$F-FDG PET/CT seems to be an important tool to evaluate treatment efficacy primarily in GIST. The role of artificial intelligence is also under evaluation.

## References

1. Liu F, Zhang Q, Zhou D, Dong J. Effectiveness of 18F-FDG PET/CT in the diagnosis and staging of osteosarcoma: a meta-analysis of 26 studies. BMC Cancer. 2019;19:323.
2. Schwarzbach MHM, Hinz U, Dimitrakopoulou-Strauss A, et al. Prognostic significance of preoperative (18-F)fluorodeoxyglucose (FDG) positron emission tomography (PET) imaging in patients with resectable soft tissue sarcomas. Ann Surg. 2005;241:286–94.
3. Chen B, Feng H, Xie J, et al. Differentiation of soft tissue and bone sarcomas from benign lesions utilizing 18F-FDG PET/CT-derived parameters. BMC Med Imaging. 2020;20:85.
4. Marlés RHR, Fernández JLN, García-Sandoval JPP, et al. Clinical value of baseline 18F-FDG PET/CT in soft tissue sarcomas. Eur J Hybrid Imaging. 2021;5:16.
5. Fuglø HM, Jørgensen SM, Loft A, et al. The diagnostic and prognostic value of 18F-FDG PET/CT in the

initial assessment of high-grade bone and soft tissue sarcoma. A retrospective study of 89 patients. Eur J Nucl Med Mol Imag. 2012;39:1416–24.
6. Tateishi U, Yamaguchi U, Seki K, et al. Bone and soft-tissue sarcoma: preoperative staging with fluorine 18 fluorodeoxyglucose PET/CT and conventional imaging. Radiology. 2007;245(3):839–47.
7. Franzius C, Sciuk J, Daldrup-Link HE, et al. FDG-PET for detection of osseous metastases from malignant primary bone tumours: comparison with bone scintigraphy. Eur J Nucl Med. 2000;27:1305–11.
8. Völker T, Denecke T, Steffen I, et al. Positron emission tomography for staging of pediatric sarcoma patients: results of a prospective multicenter trial. J Clin Oncol. 2007;25:5435–41.
9. Franzius C, Daldrup-Link HE, Sciuk J, et al. FDG-PET for detection of pulmonary metastases from malignant primary bone tumors: comparison with spiral CT. Ann Oncol. 2001;12:479–86.
10. Herrmann K, Benz M, Czernin J, et al. 18F-FDG-PET/CT imaging as an early survival predictor in patients with primary high-grade soft tissue sarcomas undergoing neoadjuvant therapy. Clin Cancer Res. 2012;18:2024–31.
11. Fendler WP, Lehmann M, Todica A, et al. PET response criteria in solid tumors predicts progression-free survival and time to local or distant progression after chemotherapy with regional hyperthermia for soft-tissue-sarcoma. J Nucl Med. 2015;56:530–7.
12. Koshkin V, Bolejack V, Schwartz L, et al. Assessment of imaging modalities and response metrics in Ewing sarcoma: correlation with survival. J Clin Oncol. 2016;34:3680–5.
13. Treglia G, Mirk P, Stefanelli A, et al. 18F-Fluorodeoxyglucose positron emission tomography in evaluating treatment response to imatinib or other drugs in gastrointestinal stromal tumors: a systematic review. Clin Imag. 2012;36:167–75.
14. Holdsworth CH, Badawi RD, Manola JB, et al. CT and PET: early prognostic indicators of response to imatinib mesylate in patients with gastrointestinal stromal tumor. AJR Am J Roentgenol. 2007;189:W324–30.
15. Demetri GD, Heinrich MC, Fletcher JA, et al. Molecular target modulation, imaging, and clinical evaluation of gastrointestinal stromal tumor patients treated with sunitinib malate after imatinib failure. Clin Cancer Res. 2009;15:5902–9.
16. Fuster D, Ayuso JR, Poveda A, et al. Value of FDG-PET for monitoring treatment response in patients with advanced GIST refractory to high- dose imatinib. A multicenter GEIS study. Q J Nucl Med Mol Imag. 2011;55:680–7.
17. Fendler WP, Chalkidis RP, Ilhan H, et al. Evaluation of several FDG parameters for prediction of soft tissue tumor grade at primary diagnosis and recurrence. Eur Radiol. 2015;25:2214–21.
18. Miyake KK, Nakamoto Y, Mikami Y, et al. The predictive value of preoperative $^{18}$F-fluorodeoxyglucose PET for postoperative recurrence in patients with localized primary gastrointestinal stromal tumor. Eur Radiol. 2016;26:4664–74.
19. Sadaghiani MS, Rowe SP, Sheikhbahaei S. Applications of artificial intelligence in oncologic 18F-FDG PET/CT imaging: a systematic review. Ann Transl Med. 2021;9(9):823.
20. Peng Y, Bi L, Guo Y, et al. Deep multi-modality collaborative learning for distant metastases predication in PET-CT soft-tissue sarcoma studies. Annu Int Conf IEEE Eng Med Biol Soc. 2019;2019:3658–88.

# 3 PET/CT in Brain Tumors: Current Artificial Intelligence Applications

Julia V. Malamitsi

## 3.1 Introduction

The best anatomic study of brain tumors is acquired by conventional magnetic resonance imaging (MRI). **However**, by offering metabolic information, Positron Emission Tomography (PET) has been extensively used in the study of brain tumors. Co-registration of PET with MRI data is nowadays possible, either by software fusion of PET/CT images with MR images or on integrated PET/MR tomographs. The role of radiomics in acquiring valuable quantitative information on almost any aspect of glioma and brain metastases management is presented. The focus is set on gliomas, because they represent the majority of primary brain tumors, and on brain metastases because they are more common than primary brain tumors.

## 3.2 Radiopharmaceuticals

Radiopharmaceuticals used for brain tumor imaging are mainly markers of glucose metabolism, amino acid transport, proliferation rate, membrane synthesis, hypoxia, and angiogenesis. Molecular imaging tracers are being developed to select patients for targeted therapies.

J. V. Malamitsi (✉)
Medical Physics, Medical School, National and Kapodistrian University of Athens, Athens, Greece

**Glucose Metabolism** 2-[18F] fluoro-2-deoxy-D-glucose (FDG), the most frequently used radiopharmaceutical for PET, is taken up by 3–6% of low-grade and 21–47% of high-grade gliomas [1]. FDG is taken up by normal brain tissue, a fact that compromises the detection and delineation of an adjacent brain tumor, and by inflammatory cells. FDG uptake correlates with tumor cell density, grading, and malignancy of the tumor.

**Amino Acid Transport** Radiolabeled amino acids, being a marker of amino acid transport which is increased in malignant transformation, are taken up by both high- and low-grade gliomas and to a minor degree by normal brain tissue. [11C]methionine ([11C]MET), [18F]fluoroethyl-tyrosine ([18F] FET) [2], and [18F]fluorodopa ([18F]DOPA) [3] are the most widely used amino acids. Radiolabeled tryptophan [11C]AMT which can be metabolized not only via the serotonin but also via the kynurenine pathway shows increased uptake in gliomas [4]. [18F]fluciclovine, a cyclic amino acid, is taken up by brain tumors and not by normal brain [5], by targeting the overexpression of L-type amino acid transporter (LAT) system subtypes LAT1 and LAT2.

**Proliferation Rate** Proliferation markers are taken up by both high- and low-grade gliomas. [18F]fluorothymidine (FLT), a marker of DNA replication, is an index of malignant transformation and therefore of tumor progression and ther-


J. A. Andreou et al. (eds.), *Artificial Intelligence in PET/CT Oncologic Imaging*,
https://doi.org/10.1007/978-3-031-10090-1_3

apy response [6]. FLT is practically not taken up by normal brain tissue, due to low neuronal cell division and intact blood-brain barrier (BBB).

**Membrane Synthesis** [18F]fluorocholine, an index of cell membrane biosynthesis and hence of cell proliferation, has been used in distinguishing malignant from benign brain lesions [7].

**Hypoxia** [18F]fluoromisonidazole ([18F] FMISO) is a marker of hypoxia and therefore of aggressiveness of the brain tumor. Its metabolites are trapped exclusively in hypoxic cells [8]. Various radioisotopes of copper have been used to label ATSM, another hypoxia marker. [64Cu] seems to be the most appropriate copper radionuclide. Radiolabeled ATSM diffuses freely in tumor cells, and under hypoxic conditions, its metabolite is trapped by intracellular proteins [9].

**Angiogenesis** Peptides are eligible ligands for imaging gliomas. Arginine-glycine-aspartic acid (RGD) peptides, markers for alphavbeta3 ($\alpha\nu\beta3$) integrin expression, monitor response to antiangiogenic treatment and detect early recurrence. They are labeled with 18F ([18F]Galacto-RGD) and more recently with 68Ga ([68Ga]-PRGD2), a generator-produced radionuclide [10, 11].

**Other Tracers** Radiolabeled with PET tracers antisense oligonucleotides, small chains of nucleic acids, have been used to trace specific mRNA in vivo and hence any endogenous gene for imaging and treatment purposes [12]. A novel small molecule tracer for apoptosis [18F]-ML-10 has been used to monitor response to radiation therapy of brain metastases [13]. A [68Ga] bombesin analog [68Ga]-BZH3, associated with gastrin-releasing peptide receptor expression, is used in gliomas in the framework of quantitative dynamic PET [14].

## 3.3 Radiomics in the Study of Brain Malignancies

Radiomics in Neurooncology, an application of Artificial Intelligence, is the way of extracting a significant amount of quantitative information concerning brain tumors (primary or metastatic), which is also associated with biological features, and is taken either from MRI images, conventional or advanced, or from PET images or both. In addition radiomics' purpose is to set up models for predicting clinical results with the aid of selected features and this is accomplished through machine learning [15].

The information acquired through radiomics, concerning inner heterogeneity and microenvironment of the tumor lesion, can lead to a more efficient and personalized handling of brain malignancies [16]. Radiomics is implicated in predicting molecular subtypes of primary tumors, in differential diagnosis, grading, tumor proliferation and mutation status, treatment response, as well as in issues of recurrence vs. pseudoprogression or necrosis concerning both gliomas and brain metastases.

Furthermore, radiogenomics combines gene expression with features extracted from radiomics. This may explain how genetic changes by inducing changes to the phenotype can lead to radiomics' features alterations [17].

## 3.4 Identification of Brain Tumors, Molecular Markers, Grading and Prognosis

The 2021 WHO Classification of Tumors of the Central Nervous System, an update of the 2016 WHO version, has put great emphasis on the role of molecular diagnosis in classifying brain tumors, while remaining committed to histology and immunohistochemistry [18]. The most significant molecular biomarkers in classifying gliomas are Isocitrate Dehydrogenase (IDH) genotype and the loss of heterozygosity of the 1p/19q chromosome arms. O6-methylguanine-DNA-methyltransferase (MGMT) promoter methylation status is an independent prognostic factor in treated by temozolamide and radiation high risk-low grade gliomas [19].

### 3.4.1 FDG PET

FDG is taken up mainly by high-grade tumors and anaplastic areas of low-grade tumors [20, 21]. In low-grade tumors on repeat FDG scans, newly appearing areas of increased FDG uptake must be interpreted as areas of anaplastic transformation and therefore of higher grading and worse prognosis.

FDG PET radiomics has been used for predicting glioma proliferation. In a retrospective study 123 patients with primary glioma were assigned randomly into the primary cohort ($n = 82$) and validation cohort ($n = 41$). Tumor proliferative activity was known from the Ki-67 index on immunohistochemical examination. The derived radiomics signature based on 9 features stratified the patients into two prognostic groups, the results being similar to those obtained with Ki-67 on immunochemistry; however a less satisfactory accuracy was found in the validation cohort [22].

In addition FDG PET radiomics has been used in detecting Isocitrate Dehydrogenase (IDH) genotype and overall survival (OS) in gliomas preoperatively. In a retrospective study with 127 patients, by using a combined model applied for IDH genotyping, where age and type of metabolism (cystic vs. solid) were included, the obtained radiomic signature was associated with IDH genotype (wild type vs. mutant) to a statistically significant degree ($p < 0.05$), the derived areas under the ROC curve being 0.911 and 0.900 on the training and validation cohorts, respectively. Moreover, the results predicted from this combined model could reliably differentiate high- from low-risk groups. OS differed to a statistically significant degree between these two groups ($p < 0.001$) and was similar to the actual survival of the patients with the respective genotypes. This combined model acted as an independent risk factor for prognosis and could become a promising biomarker [23].

High-grade glioma patients with methylated MGMT promoter show a higher uptake of FDG than those with unmethylated MGMT promoter. Although high uptake is a sign of worse prognosis, the former patients have a better response to temozolomide compared to the latter who develop resistance [24].

FDG PET radiomics has been applied in studying MGMT promoter methylation status. In a retrospective study 107 glioma patients were assigned randomly to the primary ($n = 71$) and the validation cohort ($n = 36$). The MGMT promoter methylation status was assessed by pyrosequencing. A radiomics signature constructed by five radiomics features stratified the patients in two significantly different prognostic groups, which however did not differ significantly from the MGMT methylation status predicted groups in terms of prognosis. Area under the curve for the primary cohort was 0.94 and for the validation cohort 0.86, which were higher than in the case of the fused (clinical and radiomics) signature and definitely higher than the clinical signature [25].

### 3.4.2 MET PET

The uptake of FDG by inflammatory cells makes differentiation between neoplastic and non-neoplastic lesions difficult. In contrast to FDG, all amino acid tracers are taken up by both low- and high-grade gliomas. A comparison between FDG and MET has shown that, by reflecting the biology of gliomas, MET PET is more accurate than FDG PET in identifying active tumors [26].

The potential for MET-PET/MRI in classifying gliomas according to the revised WHO classification using a machine learning model was studied on a patient cohort preoperatively. Postoperatively patients were divided into the following subtypes: IDH wild-type glioblastoma (GBM), IDH wild-type grade II/III glioma (GII/III-IDHwt), IDH mutant grade II/III glioma with co-deletion of 1p/19q (GII/III-IDHmut1p/19qcod) or without 1p/19q-co-deletion (GII/III-IDHmut1p/19qnc). Maximum tumor-to-brain ratio (TBR max) proved highest in GBM patients (TBRmax =3.83 + 1.30) and significantly higher from GII/III-IDHmut 1p/19q non-co-deleted group which had a TBRmax of 2.05 ± 0.94 ($P = 0.004$). In the GII/III-IDHmut 1p/19q co-deleted group, TBR values were mildly elevated compared with the IDHmut1p/19q non-co-deleted group. Area under the ROC curve for predicting IDH status proved higher (0.79), than for predicting glioma subtyping, which was 0.62 respectively [27].

### 3.4.3 FDOPA PET

Tumor uptake of FDOPA is similar to that of MET [28]. In order to predict MGMT promoter methylation status in high-grade gliomas, a radiomics model was constructed based on FDOPA PET images. With extraction of three features an accuracy for the prediction of MGMT status of 80% ± 10% (for 95% confidence level) was achieved. Median overall survival was found to be 18 months for the patients with predicted unmethylated MGMT status and 39 months for the patients with predicted methylated status respectively. This model proved to be of high predictive accuracy [29].

### 3.4.4 FET PET

FET uptake does not depend on the blood-brain barrier integrity; therefore FET PET is also eligible for non-contrast enhancing lesions. FET PET detects anaplastic foci and can differentiate histologically grade II from grade III within the same lesion, when dynamic analysis is applied [30]. On a meta-analysis on 462 patients with a newly diagnosed brain lesion, FET PET, used for initial assessment prior to treatment, demonstrated a pooled sensitivity of 82% and specificity of 76% respectively [31]. Besides, increased amino acid uptake in remnant glioma tissue goes along with worse survival [32].

IDH genotype plays a significant role in the response to therapy and the assessment of prognosis, IDH wild-type gliomas being of worse prognosis than the IDH mutated variant [33]. FET PET radiomics has been applied to noninvasively predict IDH genotype in gliomas (i.e., IDH wild-type vs. IDH mutant), complementing in this way radiomics-derived information from MRI.

FET PET textural features have been used in combination with static and dynamic FET PET parameters preoperatively for differentiating IDH mutant from IDH wild-type gliomas. Standard PET parameters combined with textural features increased the diagnostic accuracy significantly. The highest diagnostic accuracy (93%) for prediction of IDH genotype was achieved with the Hybrid PET/MR scanner, compared to standalone PET, acquired after combination of TBRmean with a specific textural feature (SZHGE) [34].

Multiparametric FET PET-MRI and MR fingerprinting have been used on patients with suspected brain tumor preoperatively, to produce radiomics signatures for predicting mutational status of IDH1, 1p/19q, ATRX (alpha-thalassemia mental retardation syndrome X-linked), and MGMT and for differentiation of low-grade vs. high-grade gliomas. Areas under the curve in predicting mutations of ATRX, MGMT, IDH1, and 1p/19q were 85.1%, 75.7%, 88.7%, and 97.8% respectively. The area under the curve for the differentiation between low-grade and high-grade glioma was 85.2% [35].

### 3.4.5 FLT PET and Other Tracers

Although FDG uptake in brain tumors has prognostic significance (Fig. 3.1), the most reliable prognostic information is given by FLT PET, in cases however with disrupted BBB [6] (Fig. 3.2). Kaplan-Meier curves show that a negative FLT PET scan shows an excellent survival, whereas a positive scan goes along with a fast-declining curve. Tumor/cortex SUV values and kinetic analysis of radiolabeled tryptophan (AMT) can differentiate glioblastoma from brain metastases with an accuracy of over 90% for ring-enhancing lesions [4]. On a Phase IIa clinical study in preoperative patients, 18F-fluciclovine demarcated areas of malignant extent greater than those seen on CE-T1WMRI and even disclosed areas not seen on CE-T1WMRI, as proven by histopathological specimen taken during surgery [5].

RGD peptides markers for tumor angiogenetic integrin imaging are taken up by brain tumors but not by normal brain, except choroid plexus. SUVmax of [68Ga]RGD correlates well with tumor grade [36]. [68Ga]-BNOTA-PRGD2, a marker for alphavbeta3 ($\alpha\nu\beta 3$) integrin, showed on a prospective study better differentiation between high-grade and low-grade gliomas than FDG [11].

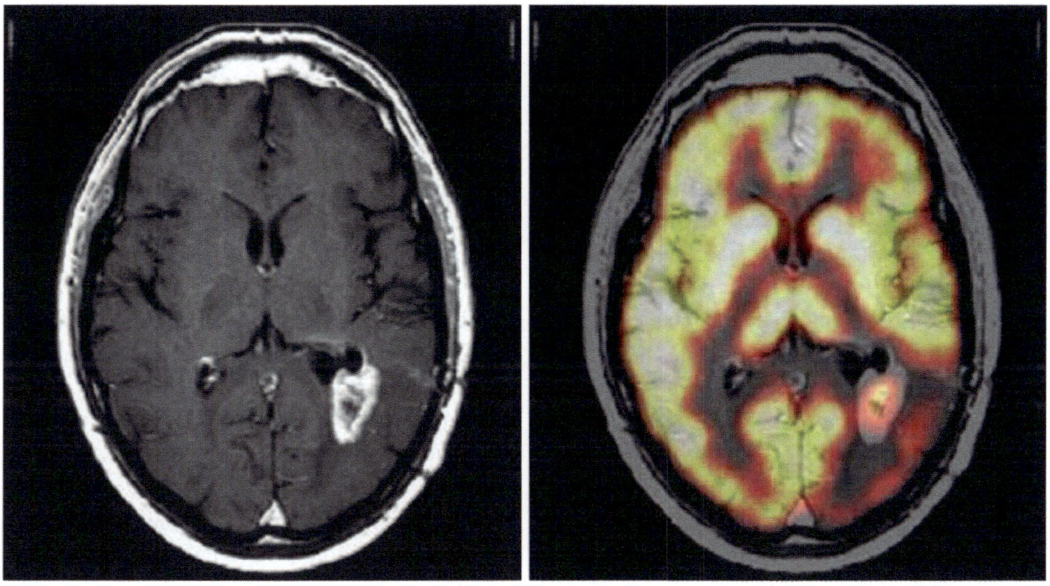

**Fig. 3.1** Glioblastoma multiforme in the left parietal lobe postsurgery and chemoradiotherapy. The treated area appears on MRI as contrast enhanced (left) and on FDG PET co-registered with MRI as hypermetabolic (right), suggestive of recurrence. The patient died 4 months after the PET/CT study. (Courtesy of Dr. V. Prassopoulos)

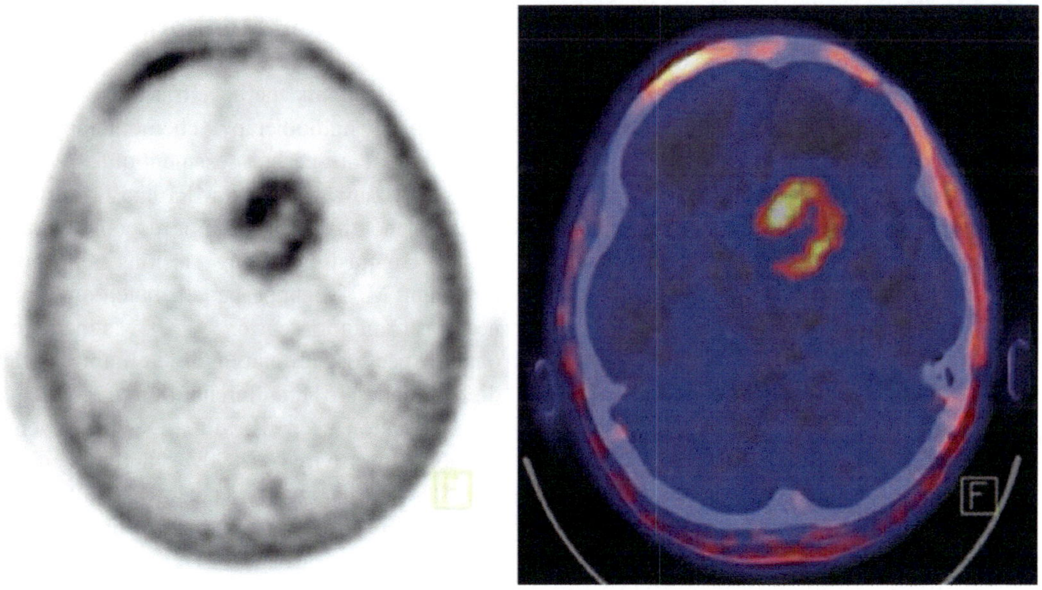


**Fig. 3.2** FLT uptake in the left frontal lobe, suggestive of recurrent tumor in the treated area of a glioblastoma. FLT PET (left) and FLT PET/CT (right). (Courtesy of Dr. V. Prassopoulos)

([18F]FMISO) shows a high uptake in high-grade and not low-grade gliomas, since hypoxia characterizes the more malignant tissues, is capable of predicting pathological necrosis, and correlates with HIF-1alpha and VEGF expression in newly diagnosed and recurrent malignant gliomas [8, 37]. [62Cu] ATSM uptake in gliomas can help differentiate tumor grade, since it correlates with the presence of necrosis, uptake within contrast-enhanced regions on MRI, and HIF-1alpha expression on immunohistochemistry [38].

## 3.5 Biopsy Guiding

MRI/CT biopsy guidance may be misleading in cases of high-grade gliomas and anaplastic astrocytomas when contrast enhancement on gadolinium T1, necessary for stereotactic biopsy, is absent [39], as well as in cases of low-grade gliomas with peritumoral edema and contrast enhancement [40]. As brain tumors can be heterogeneous, PET is able to define the most malignant area for a biopsy specimen and help select anaplastic specimens on previously characterized as low-grade gliomas. For stereotactic biopsy, microsurgery, and radiotherapy purposes, neuronavigation relies on fusion of MRI/CT with PET, diffusion tensor imaging (DTI), and functional MRI (fMRI) data. FDG is better in selecting site for stereotactic biopsy compared with CT or MRI alone, but worse than amino acids especially in low-grade gliomas [41]. Although amino acids are useful in biopsy planning and patient selection, they are not adequate to replace histology in order to assess recurrence or progression.

However, tissue sampling taken on biopsy represents only a minor part of the tumor in contrast to diagnostic imaging which assesses the tumor in its entirety. Quantitative mapping accomplished by radiomics techniques possesses a higher predictive potential, considering its ability to detect mutations of significant biomarkers present, which determine prognosis [42].

## 3.6 Radiation Therapy Planning

PET data are valuable in all forms of radiotherapy planning, i.e., stereotactic radiotherapy, radiosurgery, intensity-modulated radiotherapy, and brachytherapy, because they reveal tumor biology. Biological tumor volume (BTV) based on PET imaging has been proposed for radiotherapy planning, since morphological gross tumor volume (GTV) does not cover adequately the area of the tumor [43]. BTV is promising in sparing normal tissue, reducing toxicity, and better defining the target volume; therefore, it has been suggested to identify areas for conformal boost [44]. Treatment planning based on amino acid PET combined with CT/MRI was associated with improved survival than when CT/MRI were used alone [45]. Hypoxia may drive the peripheral growth of glioblastoma. Combined with MRI, images of hypoxia may reveal areas of tumor neoangiogenesis [46], which are radioresistant and thus help individualize treatment.

Applications of radiomics in the field of glioma radiotherapy planning are preliminary and concern tumor segmentation [47], differentiation of recurrence from chemoradiation effects (pseudoprogression or radiation necrosis) [48], as well as predicting the site of glioma first recurrence, so to contribute to a more personalized approach in dose escalation [49]. The above-mentioned applications are accomplished by applying radiomics on the combined use of FET PET and contrast-enhanced MRI scans.

## 3.7 Treatment Monitoring

With multimodality therapy strategies available, i.e., surgery, radiotherapy, chemotherapy, and novel treatments, early assessment of response is necessary. **However**, with MRI and CT it takes weeks or months to show tumor response to treatment. Contrast-enhancing lesions on post-treatment MRI cannot be attributed to tumor necrosis or tumor recurrence [50]. Magnetic resonance spectroscopy and PET are eligible for this discrimination [51]. Differentiation of recurrence from radiation necrosis with FDG has given a variable sensitivity (40–90%) and specificity (40–80%), respectively [1]. However FDG can help in clinical decision-making of brain tumors post-radiosurgery because FDG uptake depends on lesion metabolism and not on histological findings suggestive of recurrence [52].

Since radiolabeled amino acid tracers are not taken up by inflammatory cells, they are more eligible to discriminate recurrence or progression from post-treatment changes. FET PET with dynamic data analysis has a sensitivity of 100%

and a specificity of 93% in discriminating the two entities [53]. In patients scheduled for radiotherapy and temozolomide treatment, FET PET-based biological tumor volume (BTV) was a strong independent prognostic factor for overall survival [54, 55]. Increasing BTV, poor performance status, MGMT promoter methylation status, and high age in glioblastoma patients are independent prognostic factors for overall survival [54]. FET PET with dynamic analysis has been used to monitor antiangiogenic treatment (bevacizumab/irinotecan) in cases with recurrent high-grade glioma and has given more reliable results concerning antiangiogenic treatment failure than MRI [56]. Rising time activity curves (TAC) of FET in glioblastomas before radiochemotherapy are consistent with a longer overall survival [55].

Changes in FLT kinetic parameters early during treatment are a criterion of the efficacy of the applied therapy [57]. Since FLT uptake is BBB breakdown dependent, FLT should only be used to evaluate high-proliferating tumors and not for treated low-grade gliomas with disrupted BBB.

Effectiveness of therapeutic agents in gliomas such as antivascular endothelial-like growth factor receptor-1 antibody bevacizumab and topoisomerase I inhibitor irinotecan has been evaluated by FLT PET; the metabolic response as assessed by FLT PET was a better predictor of survival than gadolinium contrast MRI response [58]. Radiolabeled RGD peptides are useful in assessing tumor response to antiangiogenic treatment. In addition after radiolabeling with therapeutic radionuclides like [177Lu] and [90Y], RGD peptides can become therapeutic agents, another application of theragnosis [36].

Concerning radiomics and treatment monitoring, MET PET differentiated recurrent tumor from radiation necrosis in treated gliomas and brain metastases, on the basis of 42 PET extracted features, with a sensitivity of 90.1%, and a specificity of 93.9%, the area under the ROC curve being 0.98. T/N (tumor-to-normal cortex) ratio with a cut-off value 2.83 gave definitely lower scores [59].

An FET PET radiomics model could reliably differentiate progression from pseudoprogression in a cohort of 34 IDH wild-type glioblastomas with a sensitivity 100% and a negative predictive value also 100%, while static parameter TBRmax had lower scores (sensitivity 81% and a negative predictive value also 80%) [48].

## 3.8 Role of PET/CT in Brain Metastases

PET has been used post chemo−/radiotherapy of the whole brain or stereotactic radiosurgery, to discriminate between tumor recurrence and radiation injury (radiation necrosis, pseudoprogression), since this is not possible on the basis of CT and MRI. FDG PET has been used extensively to differentiate tumor recurrence from radiation necrosis of brain metastases (Fig. 3.3). Dual phase FDG PET differentiates the two entities in a more reliable manner [60]. Cerebral metastases are mostly associated with high amino acid uptake; therefore, differentiation between recurrence and necrosis is preferable with them. [11C] AMT kinetic analysis can differentiate brain metastases from glioblastomas [4]. Due to its low uptake by normal brain, FLT has been used to assess the presence of brain metastases [61] (Fig. 3.4). Lastly [18]F-ML-10 is used to monitor response to radiation therapy of brain metastases [13].

As far as radiomics in brain metastases is concerned, MET PET has been used in a mixed population of gliomas and brain metastases to discriminate between recurrence and radiation necrosis. Radiomics and T/N ratio evaluation had a sensitivity of 90.1% and a specificity of 93.9%, and an area under the curve of 0.98; T/N ratio gave much lower values [59]. In another study with brain metastases treated mainly with radiosurgery FET PET radiomics and MRI radiomics were applied separately and combined, in order to discriminate between recurrence and radiation injury; the combination of the two gave the highest diagnostic accuracy (89%) [62].

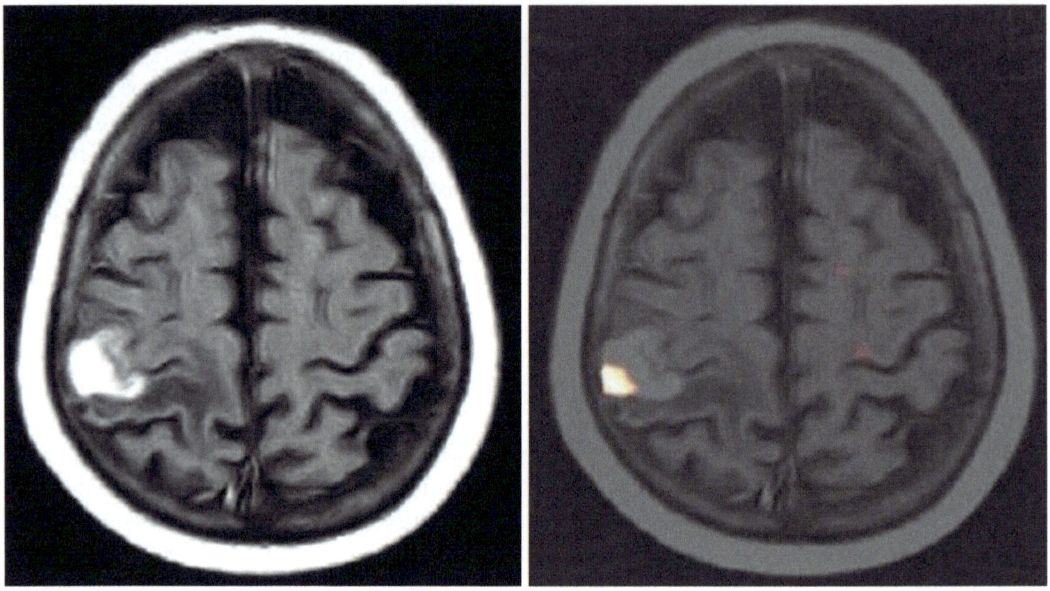

**Fig. 3.3** Contrast enhancement on MRI scan (left) after gamma knife radiosurgery of a Ca breast cerebral metastasis in the R parietal area. FDG PET/CT scan co-registered with MRI (right) shows hypermetabolism in the treated area, suggestive of recurrence. Physiological uptake by normal brain tissue has been suppressed for better distinction of the hypermetabolic lesion. (Courtesy of Dr. V. Prassopoulos)

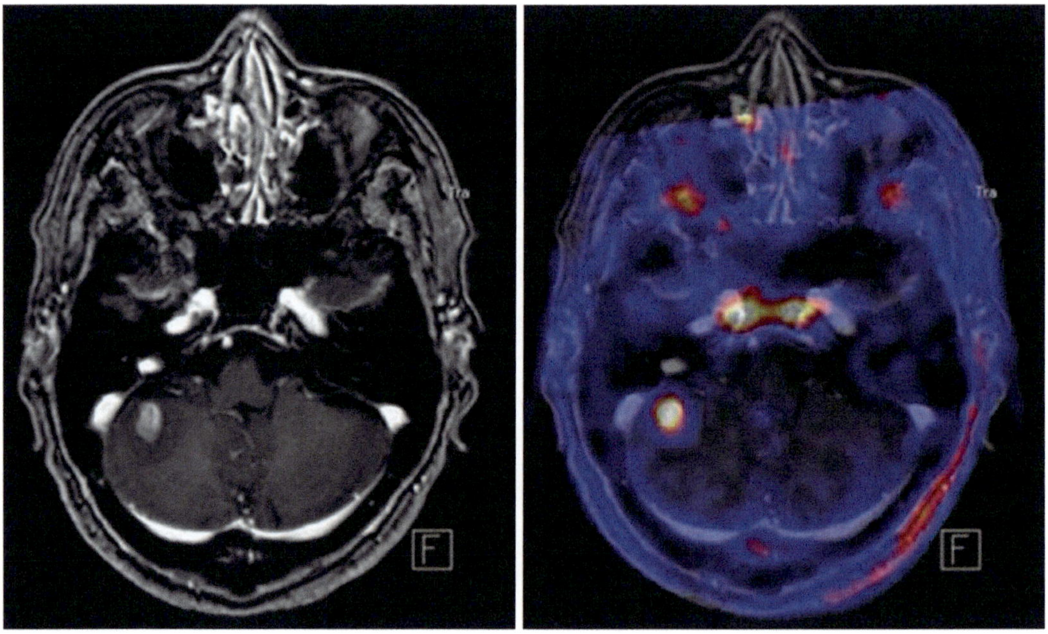


**Fig. 3.4** MRI (left) shows contrast enhancement of a brain metastasis in the right cerebellum, treated with gamma knife radiosurgery. FLT PET/CT co-registered with MRI shows hypermetabolism in the contrast-enhanced area, suggestive of tumor recurrence. (Courtesy of Dr. V. Prassopoulos)

## References


1. La Fougère C, Suchorska B, Bartenstein P, et al. Molecular imaging of gliomas with PET: opportunities and limitations. Neuro Oncol. 2011;13:806–19.
2. Heiss P, Mayer S, Herz M, et al. Investigation of transport mechanism and uptake kinetics of O-(2-[18F] fluoroethyl)-L-tyrosine in vitro and in vivo. J Nucl Med. 1999;40:1367–73.
3. Chen W, Silverman DH, Delaloye S, et al. 18F-FDOPA PET imaging of brain tumors: comparison study with 18F-FDG PET and evaluation of diagnostic accuracy. J Nucl Med. 2006;47:904–11.
4. Kamson DO, Mittal S, Buth A, et al. Differentiation of glioblastomas from metastatic brain tumors by tryptophan uptake and kinetic analysis: a PET study with MRI comparison. Mol Imaging. 2013;12:327–37.
5. Kondo A, Ishii H, Aoki S, et al. Phase IIa clinical study of [18F] fluciclovine: efficacy and safety of a new PET tracer for brain tumors. Ann Nucl Med. 2016;30:608–18.
6. Chen W, Cloughesy T, Kamdar N, et al. Imaging proliferation in brain tumors with 18F-FLT PET: comparison with 18F-FDG. J Nucl Med. 2005;46:945–52.
7. Kwee SA, Ko JP, Jiang CS, et al. Solitary brain lesions enhancing at MR imaging: evaluation with fluorine 18 fluorocholine PET. Radiology. 2007;244(2):557–65.
8. Toyonaga T, Hirata K, Yamaguchi S, et al. (18) F-fluoromisonidazole positron emission tomography can predict pathological necrosis of brain tumors. Eur J Nucl Med Mol Imaging. 2016;43:1469–76.
9. Dealing JLJ, Lewis JS, Mc Carthy DW. Redox-active metal complexes for imaging hypoxic tissues: structure activity relationships in copper (II)bis (thiosemicarbazone) complexes. Chem Commun (Camb). 1998;22:2531–2.
10. Schnell O, Krebs B, Carlsen J, et al. Imaging of integrin $\alpha_v\beta_3$ expression in patients with malignant glioma by [$^{18}$F] Galacto-RGD positron emission tomography. Neuro Oncol. 2009;11:861–70.
11. Li D, Zhao X, Zhang L, et al. 68Ga-PRGD2 PET/CT in the evaluation of glioma: a prospective study. Mol Pharm. 2014;11:3923–9.
12. Lendvai G, Estrada S, Bergström M, et al. Radiolabelled oligonucleotides for imaging of gene expression with PET. Curr Med Chem. 2009;16:4445–61.
13. Allen AM, Ben-Ami M, Reshef A, et al. Assessment of response of brain metastases to radiotherapy by PET imaging of apoptosis with 18F-ML-10. Eur J Nucl Med Mol Imaging. 2012;39:1400–8.
14. Strauss LG, Koczan D, Seiz M, et al. Correlation of the Ga-68-bombesin analog Ga-68-BZH3 with receptors expression in gliomas as measured by quantitative dynamic positron emission tomography (dPET) and gene arrays. Mol Imaging Biol. 2012;14:376–83.
15. Zhou M, Scott J, Chaudhury B, Hall L, Goldgof D, Yeom KW, Iv M, Ou Y, Kalpathy-Cramer J, Napel S, Gillies R, Gevaert O, Gatenby R. Radiomics in brain tumor: image assessment, quantitative feature descriptors, and machine-learning approaches. AJNR Am J Neuroradiol. 2018;39(2):208–16. Epub 2017 Oct 5. PMID: 28982791; PMCID: PMC5812810. https://doi.org/10.3174/ajnr.A5391.
16. Yi Z, Long L, Zeng Y, Liu Z. Current advances and challenges in radiomics of brain tumors. Front Oncol. 2021;11:732196. PMID: 34722274; PMCID: PMC8551958. https://doi.org/10.3389/fonc.2021.732196.
17. Panth KM, Leijenaar RT, Carvalho S, Lieuwes NG, Yaromina A, Dubois L, Lambin P. Is there a causal relationship between genetic changes and radiomics-based image features? An in vivo preclinical experiment with doxycycline inducible GADD34 tumor cells. Radiother Oncol. 2015;116(3):462–6. https://doi.org/10.1016/j.radonc.2015.06.013.
18. Louis DN, Perry A, Wesseling P, Brat DJ, Cree IA, Figarella-Branger D, Hawkins C, Ng HK, Pfister SM, Reifenberger G, Soffietti R, von Deimling A, Ellison DW. The 2021 WHO classification of tumors of the central nervous system: a summary. Neuro Oncol. 2021;23(8):1231–51. PMID: 34185076; PMCID: PMC8328013. https://doi.org/10.1093/neuonc/noab106.
19. Bell EH, Zhang P, Fisher BJ, Macdonald DR, McElroy JP, Lesser GJ, Fleming J, Chakraborty AR, Liu Z, Becker AP, Fabian D, Aldape KD, Ashby LS, Werner-Wasik M, Walker EM, Bahary JP, Kwok Y, Yu HM, Laack NN, Schultz CJ, Gray HJ, Robins HI, Mehta MP, Chakravarti A. Association of mgmt promoter methylation status with survival outcomes in patients with high-risk glioma treated with radiotherapy and temozolomide: an analysis from the nrg oncology/rtog 0424 trial. JAMA Oncol. 2018;4(10):1405–9. PMID: 29955793; PMCID: PMC6117103. https://doi.org/10.1001/jamaoncol.2018.1977.
20. Goldman S, Levivier M, Pirotte B, et al. Regional methionine and glucose uptake in high—grade gliomas: a comparative study on PET-guided stereotactic biopsy. J Nucl Med. 1997;38:1459–62.
21. Yamaguchi S, Kobayashi H, Hirata K, et al. Detection of histological anaplasia in gliomas with oligodendroglial components using positron emission tomography with (18)F-FDG and (11)C-methionine: report of two cases. J Neurooncol. 2011;101:335–41.
22. Kong Z, Li J, Liu Z, Liu Z, Zhao D, Cheng X, Li L, Lin Y, Wang Y, Tian J, Ma W. Radiomics signature based on FDG-PET predicts proliferative activity in primary glioma. Clin Radiol. 2019;74(10):815.e15–23. https://doi.org/10.1016/j.crad.2019.06.019.
23. Li L, Mu W, Wang Y, Liu Z, Liu Z, Wang Y, Ma W, Kong Z, Wang S, Zhou X, Wei W, Cheng X, Lin Y, Tian J. A Non-invasive radiomic method using 18F-FDG PET predicts isocitrate dehydrogenase genotype and prognosis in patients with glioma. Front Oncol. 2019;14(9):1183. PMID: 31803608; PMCID: PMC6869373. https://doi.org/10.3389/fonc.2019.01183.

24. Park CK, Kim JE, Kim JY, Song SW, Kim JW, Choi SH, Kim TM, Lee SH, Kim IH, Park SH. The Changes in MGMT promoter methylation status in initial and recurrent glioblastomas. Transl Oncol. 2012;5(5):393–7. Epub 2012 Oct 1. PMID: 23066447; PMCID: PMC3468928. https://doi.org/10.1593/tlo.12253.
25. Kong Z, Lin Y, Jiang C, Li L, Liu Z, Wang Y, Dai C, Liu D, Qin X, Wang Y, Liu Z, Cheng X, Tian J, Ma W. 18F-FDG-PET-based radiomics signature predicts MGMT promoter methylation status in primary diffuse glioma. Cancer Imaging. 2019;19(1):58. PMID: 31426864; PMCID: PMC6701097. https://doi.org/10.1186/s40644-019-0246-0.
26. Pirotte B, Goldman S, Massager N, et al. Comparison of 18F-FDG and 11C-methionine for PET-guided stereotactic brain biopsy of gliomas. J Nucl Med. 2004;45:1293–8.
27. Kebir S, Weber M, Lazaridis L, Deuschl C, Schmidt T, Mönninghoff C, Keyvani K, Umutlu L, Pierscianek D, Forsting M, Sure U, Stuschke M, Kleinschnitz C, Scheffler B, Colletti PM, Rubello D, Rischpler C, Glas M. Hybrid 11C-MET PET/MRI combined with "machine learning" in glioma diagnosis according to the revised glioma WHO classification 2016. Clin Nucl Med. 2019;44(3):214–20. PMID: 30516675. https://doi.org/10.1097/RLU.0000000000002398.
28. Becherer A, Karanikas G, Szabó M, et al. Brain tumour imaging with PET: a comparison between [18F]fluorodopa and [11C]methionine. Eur J Nucl Med Mol Imaging. 2003;30:1561–7.
29. Qian J, Herman MG, Brinkmann DH, Laack NN, Kemp BJ, Hunt CH, Lowe V, Pafundi DH. Prediction of MGMT Status for glioblastoma patients using radiomics feature extraction from 18F-DOPA-PET Imaging. Int J Radiat Oncol Biol Phys. 2020;108(5):1339–46. Epub 2020 Jul 4. PMID: 32634544; PMCID: PMC7680434. https://doi.org/10.1016/j.ijrobp.2020.06.073.
30. Kunz M, Thon N, Eigenbrod S, et al. Hot spots in dynamic (18)FET-PET delineate malignant tumor parts within suspected WHO grade II gliomas. Neuro Oncol. 2011;13:307–16.
31. Dunet V, Rossier C, Buck A, et al. Performance of 18F-fluoro-ethyL-tyrosine (18F-FET) PET for the differential diagnosis of primary brain tumor: a systematic review and metaanalysis. J Nucl Med. 2012;53:207–14.
32. Nariai T, Tanaka Y, Wakimoto H, et al. Usefulness of L-[methyl-11C] methionine-positron emission tomography as a biological monitoring tool in the treatment of glioma. J Neurosurg. 2005;103:498–507.
33. Hartmann C, Hentschel B, Wick W, Capper D, Felsberg J, Simon M, Westphal M, Schackert G, Meyermann R, Pietsch T, Reifenberger G, Weller M, Loeffler M, von Deimling A. Patients with IDH1 wild type anaplastic astrocytomas exhibit worse prognosis than IDH1-mutated glioblastomas, and IDH1 mutation status accounts for the unfavorable prognostic effect of higher age: implications for classification of gliomas. Acta Neuropathol. 2010;120(6):707–18. https://doi.org/10.1007/s00401-010-0781-z.
34. Lohmann P, Lerche C, Bauer EK, Steger J, Stoffels G, Blau T, Dunkl V, Kocher M, Viswanathan S, Filss CP, Stegmayr C, Ruge MI, Neumaier B, Shah NJ, Fink GR, Langen KJ, Galldiks N. Predicting IDH genotype in gliomas using FET PET radiomics. Sci Rep. 2018;8(1):13328. PMID: 30190592; PMCID: PMC6127131. https://doi.org/10.1038/s41598-018-31806-7.
35. Haubold J, Demircioglu A, Gratz M, Glas M, Wrede K, Sure U, Antoch G, Keyvani K, Nittka M, Kannengiesser S, Gulani V, Griswold M, Herrmann K, Forsting M, Nensa F, Umutlu L. Non-invasive tumor decoding and phenotyping of cerebral gliomas utilizing multiparametric 18F-FET PET-MRI and MR Fingerprinting. Eur J Nucl Med Mol Imaging. 2020;47(6):1435–45. https://doi.org/10.1007/s00259-019-04602-2.
36. Eo JS, Jeong JM. Angiogenesis imaging using 68Ga-RGD PET/CT: therapeutic implications. Semin Nucl Med. 2016;46:419–27.
37. Kawai N, Lin W, Cao WD, et al. Correlation between [18F] fluoromisonidazole PET and expression of HIF-1alpha and VEGF in newly diagnosed and recurrent malignant gliomas. Eur J Nucl Med Mol Imaging. 2014;41:1870–8.
38. Tateishi K, Tateishi U, Sato M, et al. Application of [62Cu]-diacetyl-bis(N4-methylthiosemicarbazone) PET imaging to predict highly malignant tumor grades and hypoxia-inducible factor 1a expression in patients with glioma. AJNR Am J Neuroradiol. 2013;34:92–9.
39. Barker FG 2nd, Chang SM, Huhn SL, et al. Age and the risk of anaplasia in magnetic resonance-nonenhancing supratentorial cerebral tumors. Cancer. 1997;80:936–41.
40. Law M, Yang S, Wang H, et al. Glioma grading: sensitivity, specificity, and predictive values of perfusion MR imaging and proton MR spectroscopic imaging compared with conventional MR imaging. AJNR Am J Neuroradiol. 2003;24:1989–98.
41. Pirotte BJ, Lubansu A, Massager N, et al. Results of positron emission tomography guidance and reassessment of the utility of and indications for stereotactic biopsy in children with infiltrative brainstem tumors. J Neurosurg. 2007;107:392–9.
42. Pinker K, Shitano F, Sala E, Do RK, Young RJ, Wibmer AG, Hricak H, Sutton EJ, Morris EA. Background, current role, and potential applications of radiogenomics. J Magn Reson Imaging. 2018;47(3):604–20. Epub 2017 Nov 2. PMID: 29095543; PMCID: PMC5916793. https://doi.org/10.1002/jmri.25870.
43. Ling CC, Humm J, Larson S, et al. Towards multidimensional radiotherapy (MD-CRT): biological imaging and biological conformality. Int J Radiat Oncol Biol Phys. 2000;47:551–60.
44. Lee IH, Piert M, Gomez-Hassan D, et al. Association of 11C-methionine PET uptake with site of failure after concurrent temozolomide and radiation for pri-

mary glioblastoma multiforme. Int J Radiat Oncol Biol Phys. 2009;73:479–85.

45. Grosu AL, Weber WA, Franz M, et al. Reirradiation of recurrent high-grade gliomas using amino acid PET (SPECT)/CT/MRI image fusion to determine gross tumor volume for stereotactic fractionated radiotherapy. Int J Radiat Oncol Biol Phys. 2005;63:511–9.
46. Swanson KR, Chakraborty G, Wang CH, et al. Complementary but distinct roles for MRI and 18F-fluoromisonidazole PET in the assessment of human glioblastomas. J Nucl Med. 2009;50:36–44.
47. Blanc-Durand P, Van Der Gucht A, Schaefer N, Itti E, Prior JO. Automatic lesion detection and segmentation of 18F-FET PET in gliomas: a full 3D U-Net convolutional neural network study. PLoS One. 2018;13(4):e0195798. . PMID: 29652908; PMCID: PMC5898737. https://doi.org/10.1371/journal.pone.0195798.
48. Lohmann P, Elahmadawy MA, Gutsche R, Werner JM, Bauer EK, Ceccon G, Kocher M, Lerche CW, Rapp M, Fink GR, Shah NJ, Langen KJ, Galldiks N. FET PET Radiomics for differentiating Pseudoprogression from early tumor progression in glioma patients post-chemoradiation. Cancers (Basel). 2020;12(12):3835. PMID: 33353180; PMCID: PMC7766151. https://doi.org/10.3390/cancers12123835.
49. Lipkova J, Angelikopoulos P, Wu S, Alberts E, Wiestler B, Diehl C, Preibisch C, Pyka T, Combs SE, Hadjidoukas P, Van Leemput K, Koumoutsakos P, Lowengrub J, Menze B. Personalized radiotherapy design for glioblastoma: integrating mathematical tumor models, multimodal scans, and Bayesian inference. IEEE Trans Med Imaging. 2019;38(8):1875–84. Epub 2019 Feb 27. PMID: 30835219; PMCID: PMC7170051. https://doi.org/10.1109/TMI.2019.2902044.
50. Brandsma D, Stalpers L, Taal W, et al. Clinical features, mechanisms, and management of pseudoprogression in malignant gliomas. Lancet Oncol. 2008;9:453–61.
51. Shah R, Vattoth S, Jacob R, et al. Radiation necrosis in the brain: imaging features and differentiation from tumor recurrence. Radiographics. 2012;32:1343–59.
52. Torrens M, Malamitsi J, Karaiskos P, et al. Although non diagnostic between necrosis and recurrence, FDG PET/CT assists management of brain tumors after radiosurgery. In Vivo. 2016;30:513–20.
53. Rachinger W, Goetz C, Pöpperl G, et al. Positron emission tomography with O-(2-[18F]fluoroethyl)-L-tyrosine versus magnetic resonance imaging in the diagnosis of recurrent gliomas. Neurosurgery. 2005;57:505–11. (discussion 505–511).
54. Poulsen SH, Urup T, Grunnet K, et al. The prognostic value of FET PET at radiotherapy planning in newly diagnosed glioblastoma. Eur J Nucl Med Mol Imaging. 2017;44:373–81.
55. Suchorska B, Jansen NL, Linn J, et al. Biological tumor volume in 18FET-PET before radiochemotherapy correlates with survival in GBM. Neurology. 2015;84:710–9.
56. Galldiks N, Rapp M, Stoffels G, et al. Response assessment of bevacizumab in patients with recurrent malignant glioma using [18F]Fluoroethyl-L-tyrosine PET in comparison to MRI. Eur J Nucl Med Mol Imaging. 2013;40:22–33.
57. Wardak M, Schiepers C, Dahlbom M, et al. Discriminant analysis of 18F-fluorothymidine kinetic parameters to predict survival in patients with recurrent high-grade glioma. Clin Cancer Res. 2011;17:6553–62.
58. Chen W, Delaloye S, Silverman DH, et al. Predicting treatment response of malignant gliomas to bevacizumab and irinotecan by imaging proliferation with [18F] fluorothymidine positron emission tomography: a pilot study. J Clin Oncol. 2007;25:4714–21.
59. Hotta M, Minamimoto R, Miwa K. 11C-methionine-PET for differentiating recurrent brain tumor from radiation necrosis: radiomics approach with random forest classifier. Sci Rep. 2019;9(1):15666. PMID: 31666650; PMCID: PMC6821731. https://doi.org/10.1038/s41598-019-52279-2.
60. Horky LL, Hsiao EM, Weiss SE, et al. Dual phase FDG-PET imaging of brain metastases provides superior assessment of recurrence versus post-treatment necrosis. J Neurooncol. 2011;103:137–46.
61. Dittmann H, Dohmen BM, Paulsen F, et al. [18F]FLT PET for diagnosis and staging of thoracic tumours. Eur J Nucl Med Mol Imaging. 2003;30:1407–12.
62. Lohmann P, Kocher M, Ceccon G, et al. Combined FET PET/MRI radiomics differentiates radiation injury from recurrent brain metastasis. Neuroimage Clin. 2018;20:537–42. https://doi.org/10.1016/j.nicl.2018.08.024.

# Artificial Intelligence in Head and Neck Cancer Patients

4

T. Pipikos, M. Vogiatzis, and V. Prasopoulos

## 4.1 Introduction

Positron emission tomography (PET) has a major role in patients with head and neck cancer (HNC), and this group of malignancies was identified as one of the first clinical indications for the performance of PET [1]. $^{18}$F-fluoro-deoxy-glucose ($^{18}$F-FDG) PET–computed tomography (CT) can be used in the diagnostic investigation of patients with a malignant neck lymph node, without any other evidence of cancer in the upper aerodigestive tract mucosa. Moreover, $^{18}$F-FDG-PET can contribute to the staging of HNC patients, the detection of residual or recurrent disease, as well as the follow-up of HNC survivors. Apart from $^{18}$F-FDG, there are additional PET tracers that have been investigated using PET-CT techniques, under certain clinical questions [2]. Hypoxia-specific PET radiotracers, such as $^{18}$F-fluoromisonidazole, $^{18}$F-fluoro-azomycin arabinoside, and $^{18}$F-flortanidazole, may add useful information regarding the biological characteristics of these malignancies, like foci of tumour hypoxia. Furthermore, a more accurate differentiation between post-radiotherapy inflammation and residual or recurrent disease may be feasible with the administration of radiolabelled amino acid PET tracers, showing increased uptake by tumour cells but limited accumulation in inflammatory tissues. On the other hand, $^{18}$F-fluoro-thymidine activity evaluation, following therapy, may serve as an early indicator of treatment response. Finally, according to recent research evidence, PET–magnetic resonance (MR) techniques could offer multi-parametric imaging data that may be useful in terms of head and neck malignancies characterization and patient prognostication [3]. Figures 4.1 and 4.2 show fused PET–MRI images in two patients with HNC referred to our department.

T. Pipikos · M. Vogiatzis (✉) · V. Prasopoulos
Department of Nuclear Medicine, Hygeia Hospital, Athens, Greece


J. A. Andreou et al. (eds.), *Artificial Intelligence in PET/CT Oncologic Imaging*, https://doi.org/10.1007/978-3-031-10090-1_4

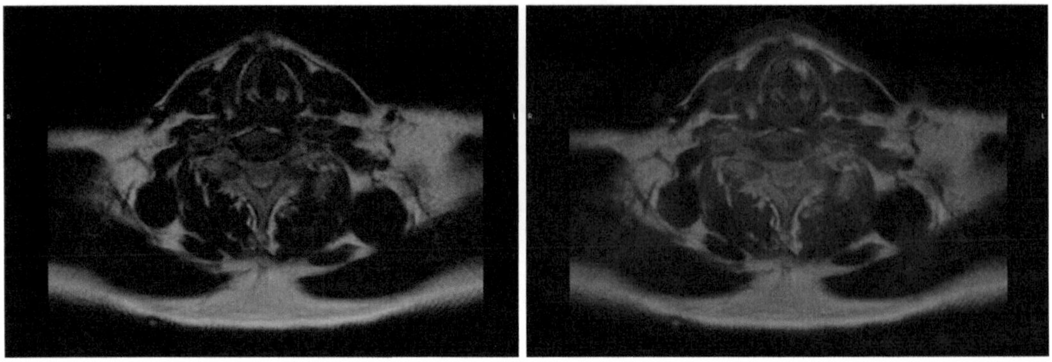

**Fig. 4.1** Fused PET–MRI images in a 50-year-old heavy smoker with newly diagnosed (positive biopsy) laryngeal cancer referred for primary staging with $^{18}$F-FDG-PET/CT. Images show a small lesion with high FDG uptake located in the left part of the larynx. No regional lymph nodes or distant metastases were depicted. *CT* computed tomography, *FDG* fluoro-deoxy-glucose, *MRI* magnetic resonance imaging, *PET* positron emission tomography

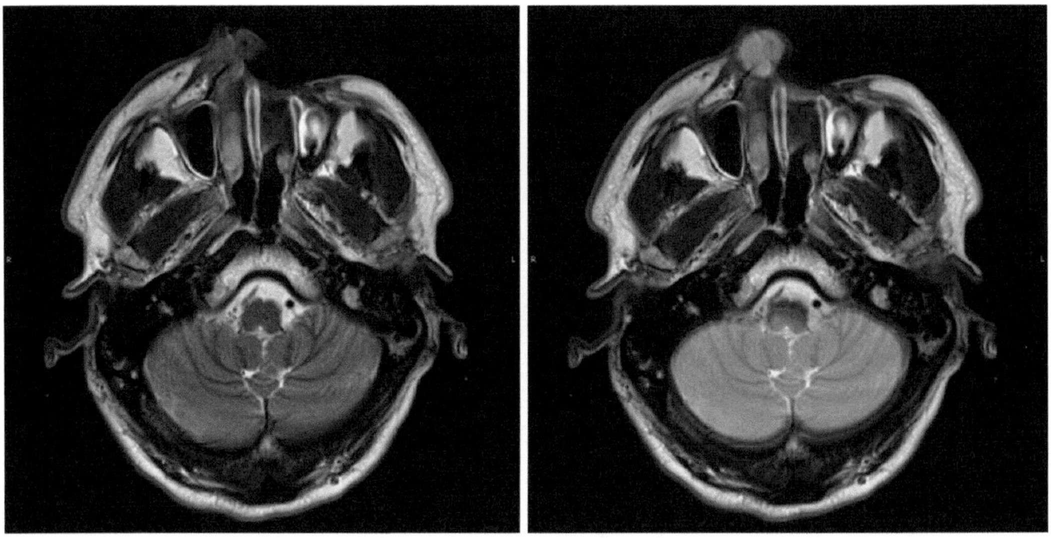

**Fig. 4.2** Fused PET–MRI images in a 65-year-old male patient with known nasal carcinoma referred for restaging—evaluation with $^{18}$F-FDG-PET/CT 6 months after surgery, due to equivocal findings on MRI. Images show intense FDG uptake in the area, compatible with local recurrence. No regional lymph nodes or distant metastases were depicted. PET–MRI method has high diagnostic accuracy in Head and Neck cancers combining metabolic activity data and high resolution anatomic imaging information. *CT* computed tomography, *FDG* fluoro-deoxy-glucose, *MRI* magnetic resonance imaging, *PET* positron emission tomography

## 4.2 Artificial Intelligence: Performing Tasks Requiring Human Intelligence

Artificial intelligence (AI) can be defined as the theoretical basis and the development of computer systems which are able to perform tasks normally requiring human intelligence, such as visual recognition and decision-making [4]. Nowadays, AI includes applications in various fields of science, which mimic human intelligence using logic, decision tress, and machine learning (ML). In oncology, AI represents a promising tool that may contribute to the clinical decision-making, particularly in complex cases. Nevertheless, over the last seven decades, there have been periods of great promise, as well as serious disappointment, in the field of AI.

The first step towards AI implementation was the article entitled "A logical calculus of the ideas immanent in nervous activity" [4]. In their model, McCulloch and Pitts provided a demonstration of the computational power that can be obtained using simple elements connected in a neural network. Later, based on the "McCulloch-Pitts neuron," Hebbian proposed a model for neural networks learning and, in 1950, Minsky and Edmonds built the first analogue neural net machine. In parallel, the initial development of AI was significantly influenced by the studies of Turing. His computing machine could perform any mathematical computation, provided that it could be represented as an algorithm.

The term AI was coined by McCarthy, during a two-month workshop at Dartmouth College in 1956 [4]. The results of the Dartmouth Conference were strongly related to the work of Newell and Simon, demonstrating a mathematics-based system for proving symbolic logic theories. During the same period, Samuel's work is regarded as the first reinforcement learning-based AI programme, a type of AI algorithm in which an AI agent learns to fulfil its scope through a reward system. In 1957, Rosenblatt presented an analogue neural network with the ability to learn via trial and error. One year later, McCarthy introduced the first AI-specific programming language (LISP), while Freidberg conducted the first experimental work involving evolutionary algorithms in AI. Furthermore, in 1962, Widrow and Rosenblatt enhanced the Hebbian learning method in their networks (Adaline and Perceptrons, respectively). Interestingly, in 1966, Weizenbaum presented ELIZA which was developed to serve as a virtual therapist. ELIZA was able to ask questions and provide follow-ups in response to the patients. Several other research projects were also developed and presented to the media, causing high expectations to the public [4].

Mainstream AI research efforts had a general purpose approach, aiming to provide general solutions [4]. A main drawback of this approach (weak AI) was the lack of scalability to larger or more complex domains. In the early 1980s, another research strategy was developed using domain-specific information for stronger reasoning, albeit in narrower areas of expertise (expert systems) [4]. DENDRAL was the first effective knowledge-intensive system, successfully inferring molecular structure from mass spectrometry data. Another system, MYCIN, could identify bacteria causing sepsis and recommend antibiotic dosage according to patient weight. Moreover, in 1980, Fukushima proposed the first convolutional neural network architecture (neocognitron) and his work is currently regarded as the origin of the present-day convolutional neural networks.

In the late 1980s and the 1990s, a conservative shift was observed in the field of AI research, towards more established theories, such as statistics-based methods (e.g. Markov models) [4]. Another important parameter was the development of public benchmark datasets during the 1990s, such as breast or lung cancer datasets and liver or thyroid disorders datasets. The availability of these public datasets permitted a thorough evaluation of AI research advancements [4]. Apart from statistics, additional tools, like control theory and operational analysis, were included in AI research in the 1990s. Moreover, decision theory and probabilistic reasoning were introduced in the field, while uncertainty was represented more efficiently by adopting Bayesian networks. In the late 1990s, it became obvious that massive amount of data would be generated, given the significant developments of microchip manufacturing technologies and the concurrent growth of global Internet. The emerging era of big data, including electronic medical records, led to a new beginning of wide interest in AI.

## 4.3 Artificial Intelligence in Medicine

In 2012, convolutional neural networks came back to the forefront. Hinton's research group at the University of Toronto, Canada, demonstrated a deep convolutional neural network (AlexNet) which was able to train more layers of neurons. Since then, deep learning-based methods have been used in several applications, including medical image diagnosis, with promising results [4].

In general, deep learning (DL) is a subset of ML that is composed of algorithms. The implementation of these algorithms aims to train the software to perform tasks, like image recognition, by exposing multi-layered neural networks to vast amount of data. On the other hand, ML is the subset of AI that enables machines to improve at tasks with experience, using abstruse statistical methods. Radiomics include ML techniques for the analysis of image features. Combined with AI approaches, radiomics could extract valuable information that is not perceivable by the human eye, or cannot be comprehended by the human brain. These advanced techniques can facilitate pattern recognition in images, analysis of biomarker data, and integration with non-imaging parameters [5].

Depending on the predicted outcome, medical ML can be classified as focused on regression (e.g. linear regression, polynomial, and support vector regression) or classification tasks (e.g. logistic regression and random forest) [5]. Regression methods are used for the prediction of continuous values, like biomarker levels and tumour volume reduction, while classification methods aim to predict a binary/categorical value, such as tumour recurrence and toxicity development. Additionally, Cox hazard regression incorporates the time-to-event together with a binary event (e.g. death).

## 4.4 Artificial Intelligence in Oncology: Head and Neck Cancer

In oncology, risk prediction of overall survival and tumour control after therapy represents the most evident example of AI in treatment decision-making, based on imaging data. Using model-based personalized strategies, cancer therapy could be tailored to the anticipated risk of failure before treatment. Toxicity development after chemo−/radiotherapy may represent another application of AI in oncology. On the other hand, auto-segmentation of tumour or organ at risk is a voxel-based classification task that has already contributed in organ and tumour definition, decreasing delineation times [5]. Moreover, AI is being deployed for magnetic resonance imaging (MRI) deformation, improved image reconstruction, and MRI to pseudo-CT [5].

In HNC, the analysis of functional imaging data can contribute significantly not only to the diagnostic investigation but also to the evaluation of treatment response and the follow-up of the patients. Novel diagnostic and prognostic biomarkers could be developed through the extraction of high-dimensional sets of quantitative descriptors (radiomic features) from medical images, including PET images. These high-dimensional data can be analysed using ML algorithms and AI methods, offering information complementary to the conventional clinical predictors. Notably, radiomics features commonly refer to shape, intensity (histogram), and texture characteristics. Previous studies demonstrated correlations between diagnostic or outcome variables and radiomics features since they represent biological characteristics of the tissues, such as cellularity, heterogeneity, and necrosis [6]. Moreover, radiomics features have been also correlated to genomic and molecular characteristics of malignant tumours (radiogenomics).

Based on the analysis of such relationships, a more personalized form of cancer care could be implemented, using ML and AI approaches. The value of radiomics data is expected to be higher when combined with clinical variables, serum markers, and additional conventional biomarkers. Given their significant statistical power, ML methods can offer efficient analysis and development of predictive models, using high-dimensional data. Recently, several classification and regression models have been applied in the field of HNC, aiming at the prediction of molecular markers, genomic identification, diagnostic differentiation of suspected tissue, survival prognostication, and prediction of treatment response [6]. PET studies aiming at the investigation of outcome prediction using radiomics are presented in Table 4.1 [7–18].

**Table 4.1** PET studies for outcome prediction using radiomics

| Outcome prediction | Imaging | Ref |
|---|---|---|
| Locoregional recurrence, treatment response, survival | 3-month post-treatment FDG-PET | [7] |
| | Pre-treatment FDG-PET | [8] |
| | Pre-treatment FDG-PET | [9] |
| | Pre-treatment FDG-PET | [10] |
| | Pre-treatment FDG-PET | [11] |
| | Pre-treatment FDG-PET | [12] |
| | Pre-treatment FDG-PET | [13] |
| | Pre-treatment FDG-PET | [14] |
| | Pre-treatment FDG-PET | [15] |
| | Pre-treatment FDG-PET | [16] |
| | Pre-treatment FLT-PET | [17] |
| Xerostomia (based on salivary gland radiomics features | Pre-treatment FDG-PET | [18] |

*FDG* fluoro-deoxy-glucose, *FLT* fluoro-thymidine, *PET* positron emission tomography

## 4.5 Conclusions

The development of novel multivariate diagnostic and prognostic biomarkers is now more feasible, given the increasing numbers of publicly available mega-data and open-source ML algorithms. These tools could integrate radiomics features and clinical parameters for risk stratification, outcome prediction, and personalized treatment planning in HNC patients. In the future, radiomics analysis may provide a fast, low-cost, and comprehensive tumour and tissue characterization, in combination with the conventional clinical testing and prognostication. However, despite the exponential growth of radiomics and AI research studies in medicine, most of the prediction models have not reached a level of clinical usability. Effective interpretability to the end user seems to be of great importance for clinical implementation. Therefore, apart from the fact that models must be reliable, results should be presented in a manner adequately interpreted by the clinicians who are responsible for therapy decision-making.

## References


1. Wong WL. PET-CT for staging and detection of recurrence of head and neck cancer. Semin Nucl Med. 2021;51(1):13–25.
2. Marcus C, Subramaniam RM. Role of non-FDG-PET/CT in head and neck cancer. Semin Nucl Med. 2021;51(1):68–78.
3. Huellner MW. PET/MR in head and neck cancer—an update. Semin Nucl Med. 2021;51(1):26–38.
4. Toosi A, Bottino AG, Saboury B, et al. A brief history of AI: how to prevent another winter (a critical review). PET Clin. 2021;16(4):449–69.
5. Van Dijk LV, Fuller CD. Artificial intelligence and radiomics in head and neck cancer care: opportunities, mechanics, and challenges. Am Soc Clin Oncol Educ Book. 2021;41:1–11.
6. Haider SP, Burtness B, Yarbrough WG, Payabvash S. Applications of radiomics in precision diagnosis, prognostication and treatment planning of head and neck squamous cell carcinomas. Cancers Head Neck. 2020;5:6.
7. Bogowicz M, Leijenaar RTH, Tanadini-Lang S, et al. Post-radiochemotherapy PET radiomics in head and neck cancer–the influence of radiomics implementation on the reproducibility of local control tumor models. Radiother Oncol. 2017;125(3):385–91.
8. Bogowicz M, Riesterer O, Stark LS, et al. Comparison of PET and CT radiomics for prediction of local tumor control in head and neck squamous cell carcinoma. Acta Oncol. 2017;56(11):1531–6.
9. Cheng NM, Fang YH, Chang JT, et al. Textural features of pretreatment 18F-FDG PET/CT images: prognostic significance in patients with advanced T-stage oropharyngeal squamous cell carcinoma. J Nucl Med. 2013;54(10):1703–9.
10. Cheng NM, Fang YH, Lee LY, et al. Zone-size nonuniformity of 18F-FDG PET regional textural features predicts survival in patients with oropharyngeal cancer. Eur J Nucl Med Mol Imaging. 2015;42(3):419–28.
11. Feliciani G, Fioroni F, Grassi E, et al. Radiomic profiling of head and neck cancer: (18)F-FDG PET texture analysis as predictor of patient survival. Contrast Media Mol Imaging. 2018;2018:3574310.
12. Folkert MR, Setton J, Apte AP, et al. Predictive modeling of outcomes following definitive chemoradiotherapy for oropharyngeal cancer based on FDG-PET image characteristics. Phys Med Biol. 2017;62(13):5327–43.

13. Ger RB, Zhou S, Elgohari B, et al. Radiomics features of the primary tumor fail to improve prediction of overall survival in large cohorts of CT- and PET-imaged head and neck cancer patients. PLoS One. 2019;14(9):e0222509.
14. Lv W, Ashrafinia S, Ma J, et al. Multi-level multi-modality fusion radiomics: application to PET and CT imaging for prognostication of head and neck cancer. IEEE J Biomed Health Inform. 2019;24(8): 2268–77.
15. Lv W, Yuan Q, Wang Q, et al. Radiomics analysis of PET and CT components of PET/CT imaging integrated with clinical parameters: application to prognosis for nasopharyngeal carcinoma. Mol Imaging Biol. 2019;21(5):954–64.
16. Vallieres M, Kay-Rivest E, Perrin LJ, et al. Radiomics strategies for risk assessment of tumour failure in head-and-neck cancer. Sci Rep. 2017;7(1):10117.
17. Ulrich EJ, Menda Y, Boles Ponto LL, et al. FLT PET Radiomics for response prediction to chemoradiation therapy in head and neck squamous cell cancer. Tomography. 2019;5(1):161–9.
18. van Dijk LV, Noordzij W, Brouwer CL, et al. (18) F-FDG PET image biomarkers improve prediction of late radiation-induced xerostomia. Radiother Oncol. 2018;126(1):89–95.

# PET-CT in Lung Cancer

# 5

Roxani D. Efthymiadou

An appropriate staging of lung cancer is of great value for patient's management and prognosis. The evaluation includes, except the detailed clinical examination, a variety of laboratory tests and imaging methods. PET-CT has much promise as an aid to the noninvasive evaluation of lung cancer. In fact, lung cancer is one of the main and well-established indications of the method [1].

As a product of the advanced technology in imaging, PET-CT combines in one single method the detailed anatomic information provided by CT with the functional data provided by PET. PET-CT has many applications but is widely used in lung cancer because of its superiority, compared to other imaging modalities, in the detection of nodal and metastatic disease. The radiotracer used for PET is $^{18}$F-FGD, which is a glucose labeled with $^{18}$F, a radionuclide with relatively long half-life—of almost 110 min—and small photonic energy of 0.64 MeV. $^{18}$F-FDG is the most widely used in oncology radiotracer because cancer cells have increased metabolic activity and exclusively use glucose as a source of energy [2]. After an appropriate preparation, the scan is performed following well-predefined instructions. One hour after the $^{18}$F-FDG injection, both a PET and a CT are obtained. The procedure covers the whole body and lasts about 40 min. The amount of radiotracer trapped in cancer sites can be quantified by using methods such as the SUV (the standardized uptake value). The PET, CT, and fused PET-CT images are studied by specialists (radiologists and nuclear medicine doctors) in order to combine all the provided data.

$^{18}$F-FDG PET-CT currently is indicated for the characterization of lung lesions, staging of non-small cell lung carcinoma (NSCLC), detection of distant metastases, diagnosis of recurrent disease, planning radiotherapy, and for treatment monitoring [3].

One of the main indications of PET-CT is the evaluation of the solitary pulmonary nodule (SPN). SPN is an opacity in the lung parenchyma that measures up to 3 cm and that has no associated mediastinal adenopathy or atelectasis. CT is considered an excellent tool for the evaluation of the nodule but is characterized by poor specificity (58%). $^{18}$F-FDG PET-CT provides complementary information about the metabolic activity of a nodule that cannot be obtained by radiographic methods. The development of $^{18}$F-FDG PET-CT has taken the evaluation of solitary pulmonary nodules beyond anatomic and predictive analyses to functional and metabolic analyses of disease. PET alone has been described as a better predictor of malignancy than clinical and morphologic criteria combined. A study showed that when an SUV equal to or greater than 2.5 was used for detecting malignancy, the sensitivity, specificity,

R. D. Efthymiadou (✉)
CT, MRI and PET-CT Department, Hygeia Hospital, Attiki, Greece


J. A. Andreou et al. (eds.), *Artificial Intelligence in PET/CT Oncologic Imaging*,
https://doi.org/10.1007/978-3-031-10090-1_5

and accuracy of PET-CT were 97%, 82%, and 92%, respectively [4]. The negative predictive value of the method is high enough to avoid a biopsy. However, PET-CT may be false negative in small nodules with a diameter less than 8–10 mm. It may also be negative in malignancies with low metabolic activity such as focal bronchioalveolar cell carcinoma or carcinoid. A hypermetabolic nodule needs further investigation as increased $^{18}$F-FDG is not specific and may represent a malignant as well as an inflammatory lesion [4].

Conventional chest radiography, computed tomography (CT), magnetic resonance imaging, radionuclide scintigraphy, and positron emission tomography (PET) all have been used for NSCLC staging. TNM staging is of great importance for determining the therapeutic strategy [5].

Although CT, until now, has been widely used for the evaluation of tumor size and infiltration of adjacent structures, PET-CT is much more accurate in determination of T staging, as the accuracy of the method is 82% while the accuracy of CT is 68%. One of the main advantages of PET-CT is the ability to differentiate the hypermetabolic central neoplasm from the non-metabolic postobstructive atelectasis. PET-CT may also reveal subtle areas of invasion which are not occult on CT.

Lymph node status (N staging) is of great importance in determining the resectability of a tumor; PET-CT has been shown to be substantially more sensitive and specific in the detection and characterization of metastases to mediastinal lymph nodes: PET has a sensitivity of 83% and a specificity of 94%, while CT has 63% and 73%, respectively. By combining anatomic and functional data in a one single imaging method, dual-modality PET-CT represents the most efficient and accurate approach to NSCLC staging, with a profound influence on therapeutic management and patient prognosis [6]. The use of PET-CT results in further improved N staging compared with the use of CT. The limitations of size-based node characterization system in CT studies are well documented. In CT a lymph node is considered to be abnormal if its short-axis diameter is more than 1 cm. However, a large percentage (44% according to one study) of small lymph nodes (measured less than 1 cm) is metastatic, whereas an even larger percentage (77% according to the same study) of enlarged nodes (measured more than 1 cm in the short axis) is proved to be nonmetastatic. PET-CT reveals not only the presence and morphology but also the metabolic activity even of small nodes (<1 cm) [1]. The method is characterized by 78% accuracy and 94% negative predictive value in the detection of mediastinal lymph nodes. Although mediastinoscopy remains the gold standard, PET-CT is the best noninvasive imaging procedure for N staging in NSCLC. The high negative predictive value of PET-CT in the evaluation of mediastinal lymph node involvement led to the avoidance of invasive methods, such as mediastinoscopy, in most of the PET-CT negative patients.

M status defines the presence or absence of a tumor spread to distant lymph nodes or organs. Lung cancer may metastasize to almost every organ of the body but mainly to the brain, the adrenals, the bone, the liver, and the contralateral lung. Thirty percent of patients with NSCLC have occult distant secondary deposits at the time of presentation of the disease. Detection of distant metastasis (M staging) is another critical step in determining the resectability of the lung tumor. During the past few decades, CT has been used as the method of choice for the detection of metastatic disease in NSCLC. The addition of PET in the evaluation of NSCLC reveals metastatic sites in more patients [7]. PET-CT has a high sensitivity in the detection of adrenal metastases. Increased $^{18}$F-FDG uptake in an adrenal enlargement can differentiate a metastatic from a benign lesion. PET-CT has also been shown as a sensitive method for the detection of bone and pleural metastases. Although CT may reveal focal thickening at the pleura or the pericardium, PET-CT can confirm the diagnosis of malignancy showing increased FDG uptake at the suspicious sites. As a whole-body study, PET-CT may reveal distant unexpected metastases not found in conventional staging. Previous studies demonstrated the high accuracy of PET-CT in the detection of unsuspected extrathoracic metastases in up to 17% of patients. The preoperative use of PET has led to avoid unnecessary thoracotomies in patients considered to be operable on the basis of CT and clinical criteria. Although PET-CT is superior to conventional imaging methods in detection of metastatic disease in the body, MRI of the brain remains the method of choice for detecting metastatic disease.

The ability of PET-CT to detect both intra- and extrathoracic metastatic sites in one single examination with a better accuracy than conventional procedures has a potential impact on patient's management. The PET in Lung Cancer Staging (PLUS) trial and the American College of Surgeons Oncology Group trial confirmed that PET-CT—when added to the standard work-up of patients with NSCLC—led to upstage up to 25% of them and to improve selection of patients who can benefit from curative surgical resection.

PET-CT is an excellent tool for radiotherapy planning. PET-CT-guided planning devices will further refine three-dimensional conformal radiotherapy. PET-CT can demonstrate more accurately the sites of active tumor, which may probably have an impact on radiation therapy volume delineation in NSCLC. PET-CT provides safe delivery of high dose of radiation to the neoplasmatic site protecting the normal tissues, as it can differentiate tumor from nontumor lesions such as atelectasis, consolidation, or scar tissue. According to a study of 26 patients with stages I through III of NSCLC, Bradley et al. found changes in radiation therapy planning in over 40% of patients after integrated PET-CT in comparison with CT-guided treatment [8].

Although PET-CT is the best noninvasive imaging method for the evaluation of NSCLC, numerous pitfalls exist. The most frequently observed false-positive findings are due to brown fat, foci of infection, benign tumors like adenomas, post-therapeutic thymic hyperplasia, attenuation-related artifacts, recent trauma, surgery, or radiotherapy but also to sites with physiologically increased $^{18}$F-FDG uptake such as the brain, the myocardium, the vasculature, the bowel, and the collecting urinary system [5]. False-negative findings can be found in tumors with low metabolic activity such as the bronchioalveolar cell carcinoma and the carcinoid, in cases of hyperglycemia but also in very small pulmonary nodules (with a short-axis diameter less than 8 mm).

Many studies have established the role of $^{18}$F-FDG PET-CT in lung cancer restaging, concerning the detection of residual or recurrent tumor and the response to first-line therapy. With the use of $^{18}$F-FDG PET-CT, residual or recurrent disease should, when possible, be differentiated from therapy-related changes in the lungs. $^{18}$F-FDG PET-CT has prognostic value and correlates strongly with rates of survival of patients with treated NSCLC meaning that patients with positive $^{18}$F-FDG PET-CT results have a significantly worse prognosis than patients with negative results [6, 9]. It was found that a reduction in metabolic activity correlated closely with the final outcome of the therapy. An early metabolic response (drop in SUV more than 50%) predicted better survival while as poor response predicted progression of the disease.

Despite its high cost, PET-CT—when properly used—has proved to be a cost-effective method in the evaluation of lung cancer [10]. In about 35% of cases first staged with CT, the stage of the disease has changed—in most cases the disease is upstaged—after subsequent PET-CT, with resultant changes in patient's management.

According to NCCN practice guidelines, PET-CT is recommended in NSCLC for:

(a) Diagnosis in patients with one or two pulmonary nodules.
(b) Initial staging except if multiple distant metastases exist.
(c) Restaging stage III or IV after 2–3 months after treatment or before surgery.
(d) Restaging in patients with symptoms suggestive of recurrence.
(e) Radiation therapy.

Small cell lung cancer accounts for 15% of all lung cancers and is characterized by rapid growth and early spread to regional lymph nodes and to distant sites. The role of PET-CT in the evaluation of SCLC is still under study [3, 11]. SCLC is $^{18}$F-FDG avid at the primary site and at metastatic sites. PET-CT may be used in staging patients with SCLC in order to select potential candidates for the addition of thoracic radiation therapy to chemotherapy. PET-CT may also lead to upstaging or downstaging of patients and to alteration of radiation fields due to the detection of additional sites of nodal involvement.

By combining anatomic and functional data in a single imaging method, dual-modality PET-CT represents the most efficient and accurate approach to NSCLC staging, with a profound influence on therapeutic strategy and patient prognosis. It also represents a useful and promising method for SCLC management (Figs. 5.1, 5.2, 5.3, 5.4, and 5.5).

Artificial intelligence (AI) is an expanding era of research promising valuable aid in the diagnosis and the management of oncologic patients [12]. On the other hand $^{18}$F-FDG PET-CT is a noninvasive functional imaging method with an established important role in routine imaging work-up of lung cancer. Many published studies, most of them related to lung cancer, discussed the possible applications of AI in $^{18}$F-FDG PET-CT imaging, regarding the diagnosis, the staging, the restaging, the response to therapy, and determination of prognosis [13].

Artificial intelligence techniques such as machine learning (ML) and deep learning can

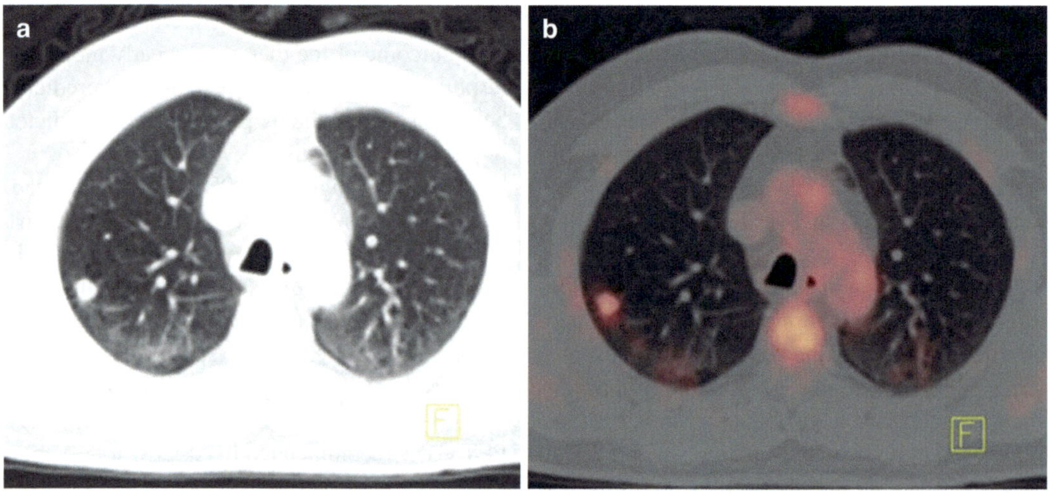


**Fig. 5.1** Hypermetabolic SPN at the right lung on CT (**a**) and PET-CT images (**b**) proved—on biopsy—to represent primary lung cancer

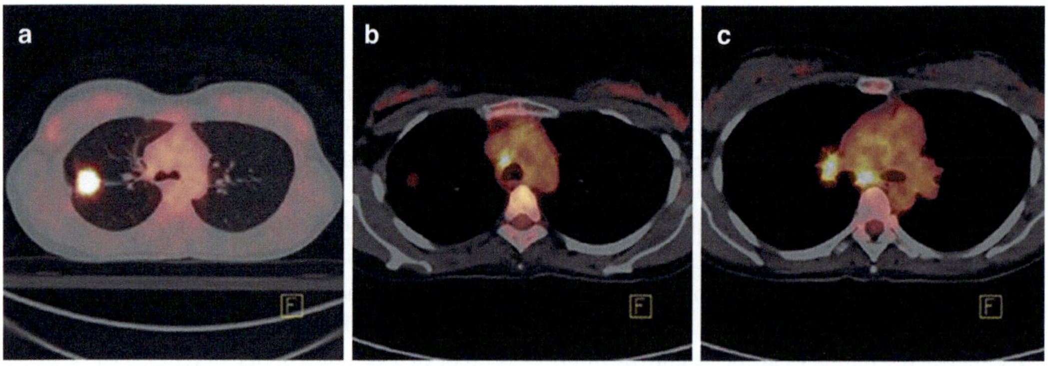


**Fig. 5.2** Fused PET-CT images: primary tumor at the right lung (**a**) with hypermetabolic lymph nodes at the mediastinum (**b**, **c**)

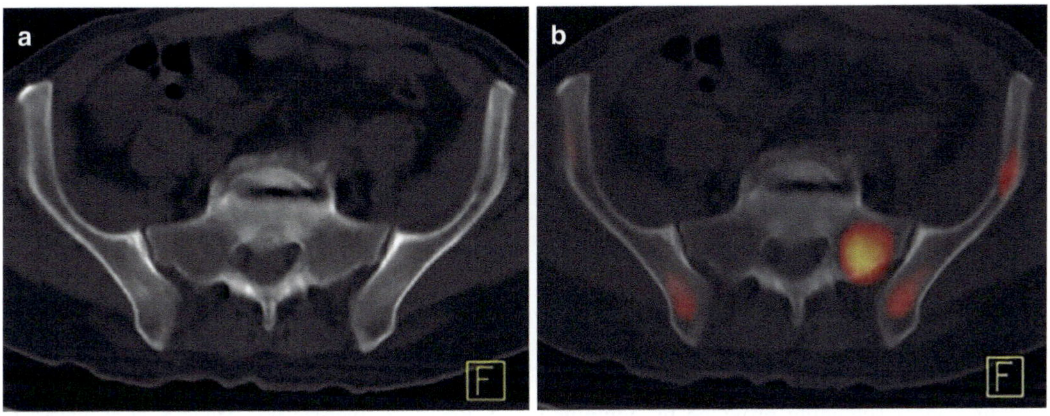


**Fig. 5.3** Hypermetabolic metastasis at the iliac bones and the sacrum (**b**) which are not obvious or have subtle appearance on CT images (**a**) in NSCLC restaging

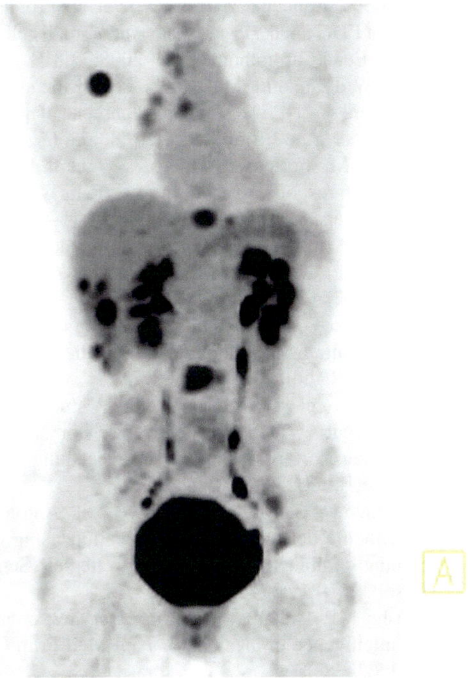


**Fig. 5.4** Whole-body PET image: widespread metastatic NSCLC

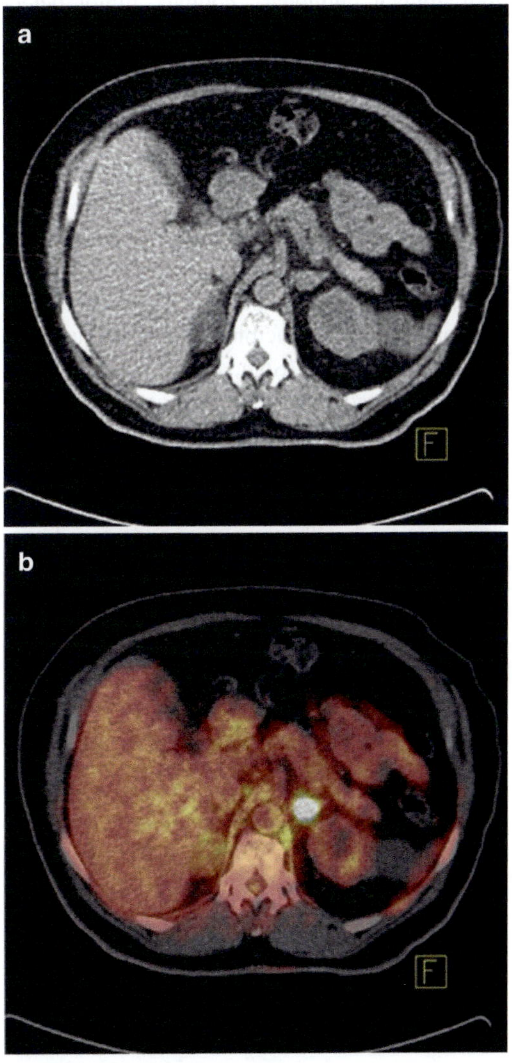


**Fig. 5.5** Secondary deposit at the left adrenal on CT (**a**) and PET-CT images (**b**) in an NSCLC patient

provide efficient analysis of the huge amount of information pertaining to the lung conditions [14]. The automated analysis allows better characterization of pulmonary lesions, such as pulmonary nodules as well as earlier detection of lung cancer [15].

Early detection is important in all types of cancer. Among the cancer-related deaths worldwide, lung cancer is the most frequent cause. A noninvasive and high performing method should be ideal to screen lung cancer in early stage.

Artificial Intelligence emerges as a promising advancement [16]. Almost all the related studies show that the incorporation of AI in imaging can improve patient care by earlier and accurate detection of the disease, which is related with a good prognosis. Due to the better evaluation of the majority of lung nodules, undiagnosed cancers can be reduced [13, 15].

Artificial intelligence provides radiologists the ability to manage in an efficient way the data load of lung cancer screening provided by computed tomography. AI techniques target different aspects of lung cancer imaging including characterization of malignant pulmonary nodules, tumor detection, differentiation of lung cancer subtypes, lung cancer staging, and response assessment. In addition, AI-based models promise added value in predicting tumor behavior, response to therapies, and estimation of patients' survival [17].

Despite the potential benefits of AI in cancer imaging, the routine application of AI-based models according $^{18}$F-FDG PET-CT in clinical practice is limited at least partially due to lack of standardized, reproducible, generalizable, precise techniques [18]. Standardization of imaging data is required for the clinical and widespread use of computer-based automated examinations. More studies are needed regarding validation of AI models in the future, so that they can be incorporated in the healthcare system and proved beneficial in daily practice [12, 18].

## References

1. Bunyaviroch T, Coleman R. PET evaluation of lung cancer. J Nucl Med. 2006;47(3):451–69.
2. Fanti S, Franchi R, Batista G, et al. PET and PET-CT. State of the art and future prospects. Radiol Med. 2005;110:1–15.
3. Ambrosini V, Nicolini S, Caroli P, et al. PET/CT imaging in different types of lung cancer: an overview. Eur J Radiol. 2012;81(5):988–1001.
4. Vahid R, Dabbagh K. Positron emission tomography (PET) in the management of lung cancer. Rev Pneumon. 2007;20(1):43–8.
5. UyBico SJ, Wu C, Suh R, et al. Lung cancer staging essentials: the new TNM staging system and potential imaging pitfalls. Radiographics. 2010;30:1163–81.
6. Kligerman S, Digumarthy S. Staging of non–small cell lung cancer using integrated PET/CT. Am J Roentgenol. 2009;193(5):1203–11.
7. Czernin J, Schelbert H. PET/CT imaging: facts, opinions, hopes, and questions. J Nucl Med. 2004;45(Supp l):1S.
8. Bradley J, Thorstad WL, Mutic S, et al. Impact of FDG-PET on radiation therapy volume delineation in non-small-cell lung cancer. Int J Radiat Oncol Biol Phys. 2007;59:4–5.
9. Hanin FX, Lonneux M, Cornet J, et al. Prognostic value of FDG uptake in early stage non-small cell lung cancer. Eur J Cardiothorac Surg. 2008;33:819–23.
10. Saif MW, Tzannou I, Makrilia N, et al. Role and cost effectiveness of PET/CT in management of patients with cancer. Yale J Biol Med. 2010;83:53–65.
11. Fischer BM, Mortensen J, Langer SW, et al. PET/CT imaging in response evaluation of patients with small cell lung cancer. Lung Cancer. 2006;54:41–9.
12. Miller DD, Brown EW. Artificial intelligence in medical practice: the question to the answer? Am J Med. 2018;131(2):129.
13. Chassagnon G, Vakalopoulou M, Paragios N, et al. Artificial intelligence applications for thoracic imaging. Eur J Radiol. 2020;123:108774.
14. Huang CH, Zeng C, Wang YC, et al. A study of diagnostic accuracy using a chemical sensor array and a machine learning technique to detect lung cancer. Sensors (Basel). 2018;18:2845.
15. Nasrullah N, Sang J, Alam MS, et al. Automated lung nodule detection and classification using deep learning combined with multiple strategies. Sensors (Basel). 2019;19:3722.
16. Amisha MP, Pathania M, et al. Overview of artificial intelligence in medicine. J Fam Med Prim Care. 2019;8:2328–31.
17. Miller DD, Brown EW. How cognitive machines can augment medical imaging. AJR Am J Roentgenol. 2019;212(1):9–14.
18. Jacobs C, van Ginneken B. Google's lung cancer AI: a promising tool that needs further validation. Nat Rev Clin Oncol. 2019;16:532–3.

# Breast Cancer: PET/CT Imaging

# 6

Vasiliki P. Filippi

PET/CT is a hybrid method that combines anatomical imaging with metabolic information in a single examination. The combination of these two methods has the advantage of precise localization of foci of pathologically increased metabolic activity. Pathological metabolic activity in malignant tissue often precedes anatomical changes, and in some cases, due to previous surgery or radiotherapy, anatomical findings alone are not specific for recurrence or dissemination of disease.

Fluorodeoxyglucose (FDG) is a tracer, analog to glucose, that is mainly used, currently, for PET and PET/CT imaging. FDG uptake by metabolically active tissue is related to the fact that malignant cells have proportionally increased demand for glucose [1].

FDG PET has a limited role in the detection of primary breast cancer (Fig. 6.1). The overall sensitivity of the method is 64–96% and specificity is 73–100%. The reported accuracy is 70–97%, the positive predictive value is 81–100%, and the negative predictive value is 52–89% [2].

The limitations of the method are due to the low sensitivity of the method in detection of small lesions (<1 cm) and to low FDG uptake in specific histological types (such as lobular carcinomas and ductal carcinoma in situ) and well-differentiated tumors. Taking into account these limitations, as well as the low availability and the high cost, FDG PET is not currently indicated as a screening test for breast cancer [3].

In order to improve the efficacy of the method, the development of dedicated breast positron emission mammography (PEM) units seems promising. Possible applications of PEM are detection of small primary breast tumors, local staging and restaging, and evaluation of tumor response to therapy. So far, the method is not validated in large trials [4].

Accurate locoregional staging of the disease is very useful in patient management, as it is related to patient prognosis. For early-stage breast cancer patients, FDG PET has relatively low sensitivity in axillary staging and is not recommended by the literature for this purpose. However, in patients with advanced disease, FDG PET may provide additional information such as distant occult metastases or pathological internal mammary lymph nodes [4].

FDG PET may be useful in assessment of tumor response to therapy, since metabolic changes precede morphological regression. A decrease in the level of FDG uptake—compared to the baseline scan—following even the first or second cycle of chemotherapy, can predict response to chemotherapy treatment (accuracy 64–91%). Nonresponders are obviously benefited by avoiding useless, toxic treatment [5].

V. P. Filippi (✉)
MRI, CT and PET/CT Departments, Hygeia and Mitera Hospitals, Maroussi, Greece



J. A. Andreou et al. (eds.), *Artificial Intelligence in PET/CT Oncologic Imaging*,
https://doi.org/10.1007/978-3-031-10090-1_6

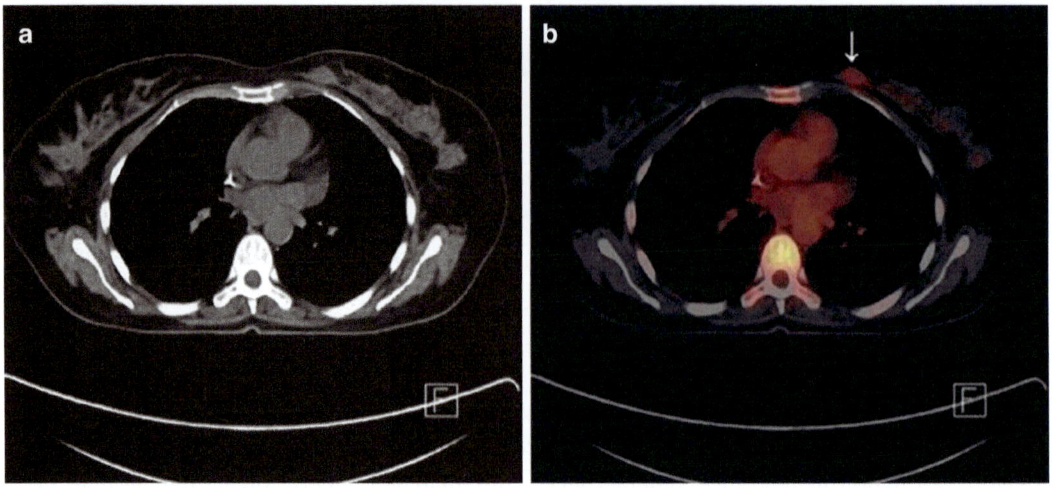


**Fig. 6.1** (**a**) CT image within normal limits. (**b**) PET/CT image shows an area with increased metabolic activity in the left breast (*arrow*), finding suspicious for malignancy, as an incidental finding

On the basis of scientific results obtained to date, there is not enough evidence to substitute anatomical imaging methods with molecular imaging modalities. However, FDG PET may play a complementary role in assessment of possible disease progression [6].

Recurrence of disease is frequent in patients with breast cancer, after completion of initial treatment. Early detection of tumor recurrences is beneficial for breast cancer patients and is associated both with prognosis and appropriate treatment choice. Estimation of the true extent may sometimes be quite challenging, due to occult recurrences. This may be correlated to the small size of a lesion that is considered normal with anatomical–morphological criteria, e.g., a lymph node, or inconclusive findings in areas that coexist with posttreatment findings, e.g., scar tissue post-radiotherapy (Fig. 6.2).

FDG PET has been shown to be effective in early accurate restaging of patients with breast cancer, as it detects pathologic metabolic activity of tumors, which usually can be detected earlier than anatomic–morphologic alterations. FDG PET is considered an effective diagnostic tool and is recommended in the follow-up of breast cancer patients. Isasi et al. estimated the diagnostic performance of FDG PET using meta-analysis. Among the studies with patient-based data, median sensitivity was 92.7%, and median specificity was 81.6% [7].

The higher sensitivity of the method, compared to computed tomography, especially in detecting lymphatic dissemination of the disease is the main advantage of the method [8].

FDG PET/CT has an even greater diagnostic accuracy compared to PET alone, since lesions are better localized and false-positive findings, attributed to physiological FDG uptake, are avoided.

Moreover, FDG PET/CT is of great importance in patients with elevated tumor markers and negative or equivocal findings on conventional imaging techniques, as it provides information about the disease status in terms of localization of recurrence. In these patients it seems that although tumor marker levels may strongly indicate that there is occult tumor recurrence, conventional imaging methods cannot always estimate the true extent of the disease. FDG PET/CT in this population has a sensitivity of 86.8%, specificity of 87.5%, and accuracy of 86.9% (Figs. 6.3 and 6.4). The positive prognostic value is 97% and the negative prognostic value 58.3% [9].

Bone metastases are very common in breast cancer patients. FDG PET and bone scintigraphy are methods complementary to each other, since

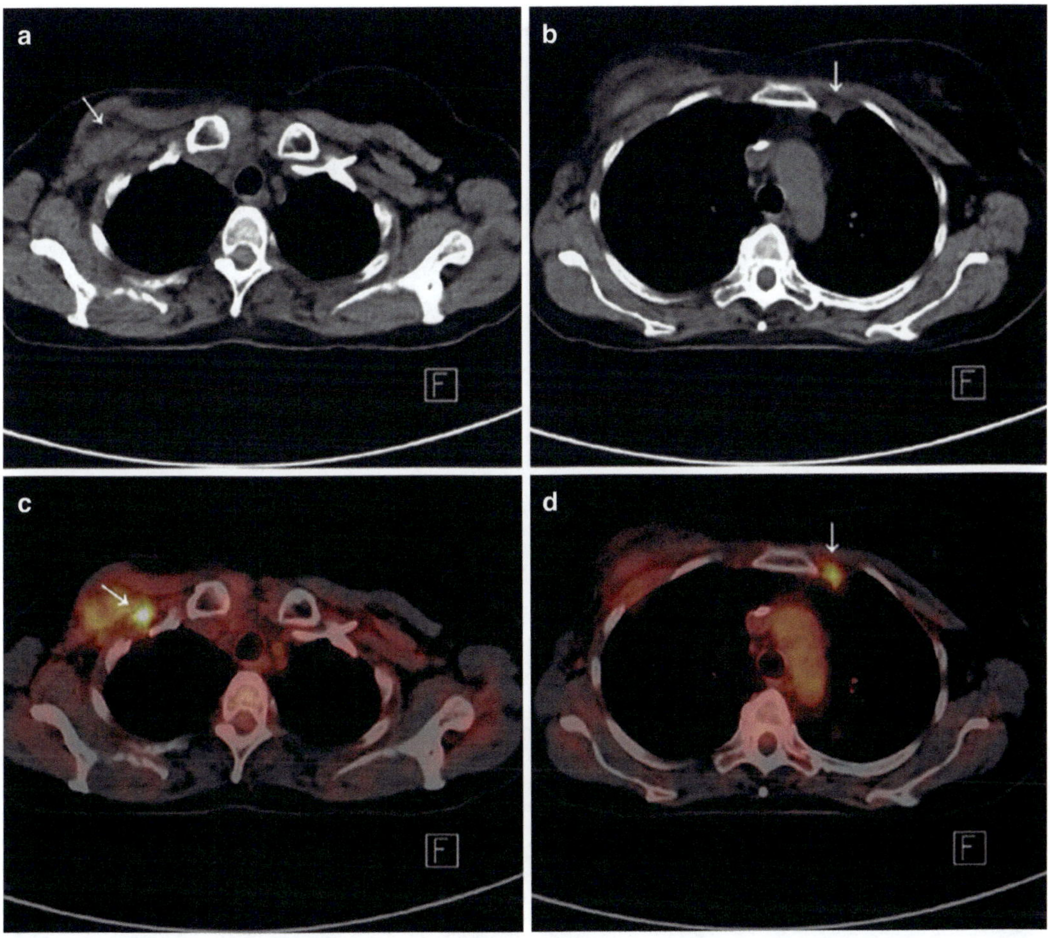


**Fig. 6.2** Patient with suspicious recurrence in the right breast after surgery. CT images show abnormal soft tissue at the surgical region (**a**, *arrow*) and a borderline left internal mammary lymph node (**b**, *arrow*). PET/CT images confirm the local recurrence (**c**, *arrow*) and additionally show increased uptake in the left internal mammary lymph node (**d**, *arrow*)

FDG PET is more sensitive in detection of lytic and intramedullary secondary deposits and bone scintigraphy is superior in detection of osteoblastic lesions [10].

FDG PET has an important clinical impact in the management of breast cancer patients. By altering, which is more often upgrading, the stage of the disease, clinical management decisions are usually influenced. FDG PET has been shown to change the clinical stage of the patients examined in 36%. Even if the stage of the disease is not changed by FDG PET results, information about the true extent of the disease provided may result in differentiation in treatment options. Physicians seem to rely on FDG PET results, thus altering clinical management in 58% of cases. This fact is of proof that FDG PET is already considered as an important diagnostic tool among physicians [11].

Currently, FDG is the radiopharmaceutical in clinical use. New tracers like fluorothymidine (FLT), fluoroestradiol, methionine, and choline seem promising, especially in the field of monitoring tumor response to therapy [12].

In conclusion, the role of FDG PET/CT is complementary to conventional imaging methods and should not replace them. The main indication currently is to provide additional

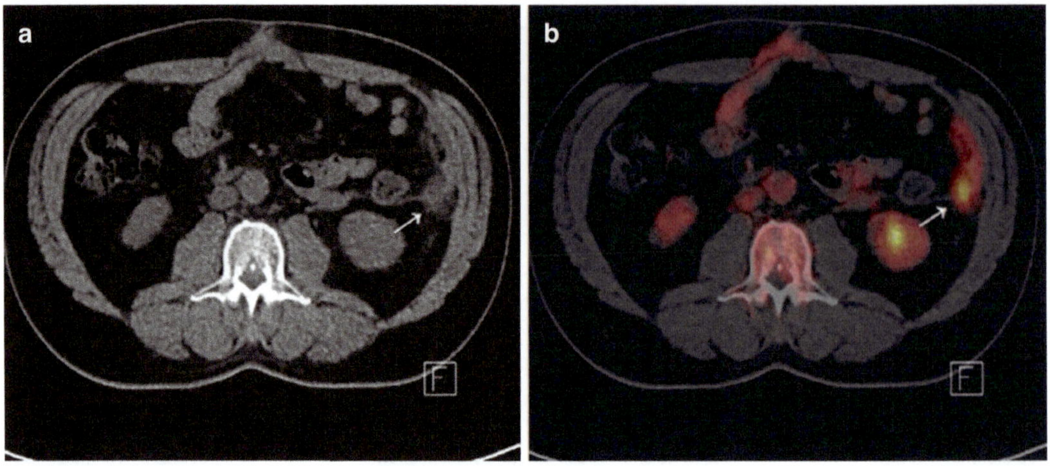


**Fig. 6.3** (**a**) Equivocal findings on CT (obliteration of the left paracolic fat, *arrow*) in a patient with breast cancer history and elevated tumor markers. (**b**) PET/CT image shows a focus of increased metabolic activity (*arrow*), suspicious for peritoneal implantation

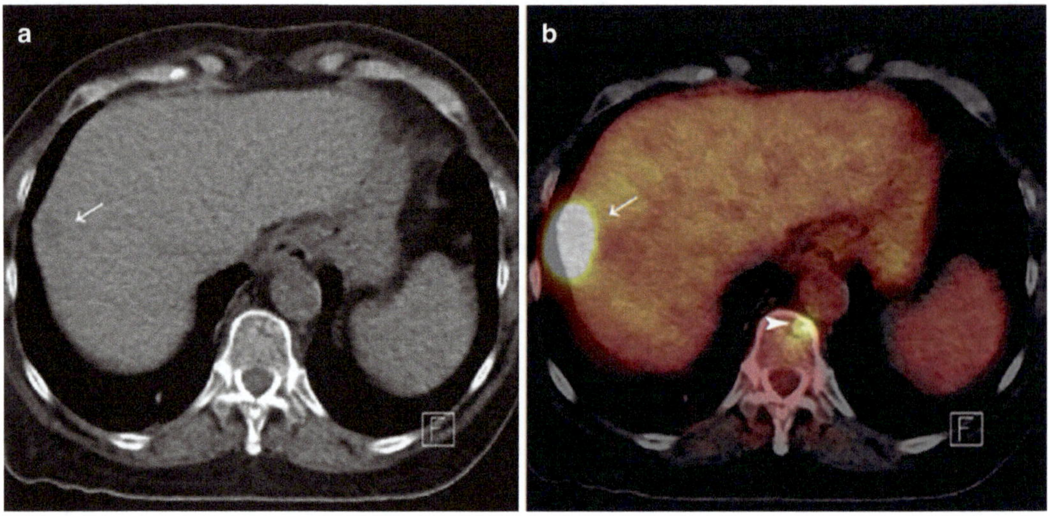


**Fig. 6.4** On CT image (**a**) a small hypodense lesion in the liver (*arrow*) is hardly detected. PET/CT image (**b**) shows that the finding (*arrow*) has intensive hypermetabolic activity and is compatible with secondary deposit. Additionally, in the same image (**b**), a hypermetabolic focus (*arrowhead*) is seen in the anterior aspect of the 11th thoracic vertebra

information in selected cases in the restaging of breast cancer patients and in evaluation of response to treatment (Fig. 6.5).

Nowadays, a new era has been introduced in medical imaging. Artificial intelligence is a growing and promising tool in early and accurate detection and precise and personalized management of patients with cancer. A possible application of AI in $^{18}$F-FDG PET imaging is the management of breast cancer patients in terms of early detection, differentiation malignant from benign lesions, accurate staging, early response to treatment assessment, and prognosis determination [13].

However, there are not enough data yet, to introduce the method in clinical practice.

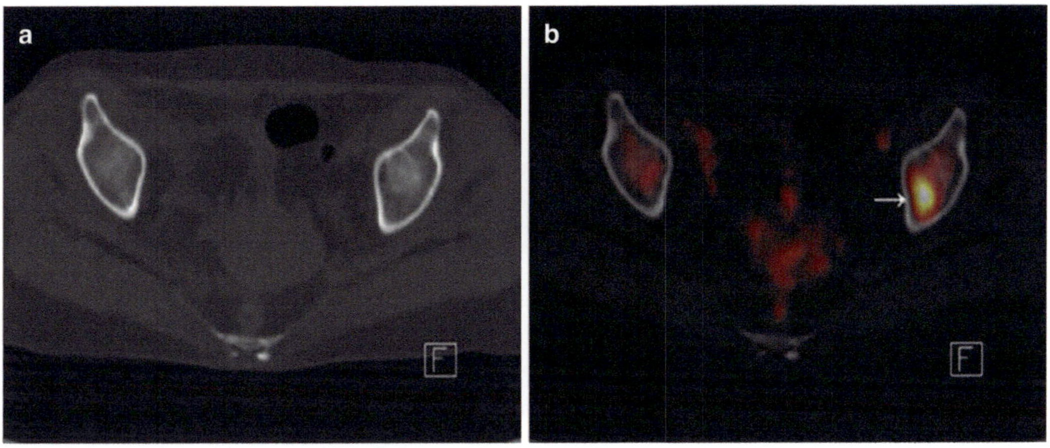


**Fig. 6.5** CT image (**a**) shows no abnormal findings. PET/CT image (**b**) shows a lesion of increased uptake in the left ilium (*arrow*), consistent with bone metastases

## References

1. Kapoor K, McCook B, Torok FS. An introduction to PET-CT imaging. Radiographics. 2004;24:523–43.
2. Scheidhauer K, Walter C, Seemann MD. FDG PET and other imaging modalities in the primary diagnosis of suspicious breast lesions. Eur J Nucl Med Mol Imaging. 2004;31(1):70–9.
3. Kumar R, Chauhan A, Zhuang H, Chandra P, Schnall M, Alavi A. Clinicopathologic factors associated with false negative FDG-PET in primary breast cancer. Breast Cancer Res Treat. 2006;98(3):267–74.
4. Rosen E, Eubank W, Mankoff D. FDG PET, PET/CT and breast cancer imaging. Radiographics. 2007;27:S215–29.
5. Avril N, Sassen S, Roylance R. Response to therapy in breast cancer. J Nucl Med. 2009;50:55S–63S.
6. Eisenhauera EA, Therasseb P, Bogaertsc J, Schwartzd LH, Sargente D, Fordf R, Danceyg J, Arbuckh S, Gwytheri S, Mooneyg M, Rubinsteing L, Shankarg L, Doddg L, Kaplanj R, Lacombec D, Verweijk J. New response evaluation criteria in solid tumours: revised RECIST guideline (version 1.1). Eur J Cancer. 2009;45:228–47.
7. Isasi C, Moadel R, Blaufox M. A meta-analysis of FDG-PET for the evaluation of breast cancer recurrence and metastases. Breast Cancer Res Treat. 2005;90:105–12.
8. Eubank W, Mankoff D, Vessele H, Eary J, Schubert E, Dunnwald L, Lindsley S, Grallow J, Austin-Seymour M, Ellis G, Livingston R. Detection of locoregional and distant recurrences in breast cancer patients by using FDG PET. Radiographics. 2002;22:5.
9. Filippi V, Malamitsi J, Vlachou F, Laspas F, Georgiou E, Prassopoulos V, Andreou J. The impact of FDG-PET/CT on the management of breast cancer patients with elevated tumor markers and negative or equivocal conventional imaging modalities. Nucl Med Commun. 2011;32(2):85–90.
10. Lee J, Rosen E, Maankoff D. The role of radiotracer imaging in the diagnosis and management of patients with breast cancer: part 1-overview detection, and staging. J Nucl Med. 2009;50(4):569–81.
11. Yap S, Seltze M, Schiepers C, Gambhir S, Rao J, Phelps M, Valk P, Czernin J. Impact of whole body 18F-FDG PET on staging and managing patients with breast cancer: the referring physician's perspective. J Nucl Med. 2001;42(9):1334–7.
12. Kenny L, Al-Nahhas A, Aboagye E. Novel PET biomarkers for breast cancer imaging. Nucl Med Commun. 2011;32:333–5.
13. Sadaghiani MS, Rowe SP, Sheikhbahaei S. Applications of artificial intelligence in oncologic 18F-FDG PET/CT imaging: a systematic review. Ann Transl Med. 2021;9(9):823.

# 7 PET/CT in Gynecologic Cancer

Evangelia V. Skoura and Ioannis E. Datseris

## 7.1 PET/CT with [$^{18}$F]FDG in Cervical Cancer

### 7.1.1 Initial Diagnosis and Prognosis

Imaging with [$^{18}$F]FDG-PET/CT is not routinely used for the initial diagnosis of cervical cancer although the primary tumor is generally [$^{18}$F]FDG avid, because of the lack of precise anatomic information which limits its clinical utility.

[$^{18}$F]FDG uptake of the primary cervical tumor, as measured by SUVmax, provides valuable prognostic information for predicting lymph node involvement, treatment response, and overall survival. Although there is no standard SUVmax cutoff value defining the prognosis in patients with cervical cancer, cervical tumors with a higher SUVmax are more likely to be poorly differentiated and have an increased risk of lymph node involvement. Median preoperative SUVmax values in the primary tumors were significantly higher in patients with higher FIGO stages ($p = 0.0149$), pelvic lymph node metastasis ($p = 0.0068$), parametrial involvement ($p = 0.0002$), large (>4 cm) tumor size ($p = 0.0022$), presence of lymphovascular space invasion ($p = 0.0055$), and deep cervical stromal invasion ($p < 0.0001$) [1].

A recent study that classified cervical cancer into two major histological types, squamous cell and non-squamous cell carcinoma, such as adenocarcinoma and adenosquamous carcinoma, showed that pretreatment [$^{18}$F]FDG-PET provided different prognostic implications between histological subtypes [2]. Metabolic tumor burden (metabolic tumor volume (MTV) and total lesion glycolysis (TLG)) could be beneficial for the prognostic prediction of patients with squamous cell carcinoma, whereas metabolic intensity (SUVmax) could be beneficial for non-squamous cell carcinoma [2].

Radiomics allows a high-throughput extraction of multiple features from images with artificial intelligence (AI) approaches and develops rapidly worldwide [3]. They are statistical or model-based metrics to quantify tumor intensity, shape, and heterogeneity, which have been shown to reflect intratumoral histopathological properties and provide prognostic information in several malignancies [4, 5].

Radiomics on pretreatment PET/CT have been shown to predict response to therapy and risk of pelvic recurrence. Studies have shown that radiomics features on $^{18}$F-FDG-PET/CT have significantly higher prognostic power than clinical parameters with accuracy of 94% for predicting recurrence and 100% for predicting lack of

E. V. Skoura · I. E. Datseris (✉)
Nuclear Medicine Department, Evangelismos General Hospital, Athens, Greece
e-mail: datseris@otenet.gr


J. A. Andreou et al. (eds.), *Artificial Intelligence in PET/CT Oncologic Imaging*,
https://doi.org/10.1007/978-3-031-10090-1_7

loco-regional control (versus ~50–60% for clinical parameters) [4].

### 7.1.2 Initial Staging

Most primary tumors over 1 cm are easily detectable with [$^{18}$F]FDG-PET/CT, but due to the relatively poor spatial resolution of this modality, it is not considered suitable for T staging. However, [$^{18}$F]FDG-PET/CT is quite helpful in delineating the margins in cases that an invasive tumor extends superiorly into the uterine cavity and inferiorly into the vaginal cuffs.

[$^{18}$F]FDG-PET/CT has an important role in staging cervical cancer, and it aids particularly in identifying the involvement of lymph nodes and distant metastases. Although the assessment of lymph nodes is not a part of the FIGO staging, it is generally performed during the initial workup of patients with cervical cancer as an important component of treatment planning, since the survival rates for patients with nodal metastases are significantly lower than those without. Recently, PET/CT scan has been increasingly used for staging workup [6–8]. [$^{18}$F]FDG-PET/CT shows a significant benefit to assess the metabolic activities of the tumor, especially for distant metastases, taking advantage from the whole-body cross-sectional images. [$^{18}$F]FDG-PET/CT demonstrates a specific benefit to assess the pelvic and paraaortic lymph node involvement with equivocal size and morphology on CT or MRI.

In studies where [$^{18}$F]FDG-PET/CT was evaluated in patients with negative CT/MR, the sensitivity and specificity of [$^{18}$F]FDG-PET/CT for detection of metastases have been found 83.3–85.7% and 94.4–96.7%, respectively [9, 10]. In recent meta-analyses, [$^{18}$F]FDG-PET or [$^{18}$F]FDG-PET/CT showed the highest pooled sensitivity (79–84%) and specificity (95–99%), compared with 47–50% and 92–97%, respectively, for CT and 56–72% and 90–96%, respectively, for MR imaging [11–16]. [$^{18}$F]FDG-PET/CT positivity for lymph node metastases correlates well with survival and is highly predictive of progression-free survival. A multivariate analysis demonstrated that the most significant prognostic factor for progression-free survival was the presence of positive paraaortic lymph nodes as detected by PET imaging ($p$ = 0.025) [12]. Concerning paraaortal nodal disease, [$^{18}$F]FDG-PET/CT demonstrated a sensitivity of 100% and specificity of 99% despite another study that demonstrated lower values (50% and 83.3%, respectively) [17, 18].

According to American College of Radiology appropriateness criteria, [$^{18}$F]FDG-PET/CT with concurrent abdominopelvic CT is considered highly appropriate in assessing nodal disease at stage II or higher and in patients with suspected tumor recurrence [19]. Also, for detecting distant metastases, [$^{18}$F]FDG-PET/CT demonstrated a sensitivity of 100% and specificity of 94% [18].

### 7.1.3 Radiotherapy Planning

[$^{18}$F]FDG-PET/CT has been shown to impact external-beam radiotherapy planning by modifying the treatment field and customizing the radiation dose. This particularly applies to detection of previously uncovered paraaortic and inguinal nodal metastases.

[$^{18}$F]FDG-PET/CT-based brachytherapy optimization allows improved tumor volume dose distribution and detailed 3D dosimetric evaluation of risk organs.

Furthermore, [$^{18}$F]FDG-PET/CT-guided intensity-modulated radiation therapy (IMRT) allows delivery of higher doses of radiation to the primary tumor and to grossly involved nodal disease while minimizing treatment-related toxicity. IMRT use in cervical cancer has been demonstrated to produce equivalent or better results [20].

### 7.1.4 Restaging after Treatment

The current literature supports the use of [$^{18}$F]FDG-PET/CT for evaluating response after chemoradiation for locally advanced carcinoma of the cervix. The optimal timing to obtain $^{18}$F-FDG-PET/CT to assess for treatment response is at least 6 weeks after surgery and 3 months after completion of concurrent chemoradiation therapy. The posttreatment metabolic response seems to be predictive of both cause-specific and progression-free survival after chemoradiation for cervical cancer.

A study showed that the ratio of SUVmax at posttherapy to SUVmax at pretherapy of <0.33 correlated with tumor pathologic response ($P < 0.001$) and a 35% improvement of 6-month progression-free survival (PFS) ($P = 0.004$) in advanced-stage IB2-IVA patients [21]. A prospective cohort study demonstrated that [$^{18}$F]FDG-PET/CT can provide reliable long-term prognostic information and may be used to guide early interventions for patients with less than a complete metabolic response [22].

[$^{18}$F]FDG-PET/CT can be used to monitor treatment response during treatment as the change in [$^{18}$F]FDG uptake during chemoradiation therapy is associated with response to treatment [21]. $^{18}$F-FDG-PET/CT seems to be superior to MRI for posttherapy evaluation in patients with advanced cervical cancer 2–3 months after definitive concurrent chemoradiotherapy. A study showed that the sensitivity, specificity, and accuracy of PET/CT were 60%, 100%, and 89% versus those of MRI 27%, 100%, and 80%, respectively [23].

Abnormal [$^{18}$F]FDG uptake in the cervix or lymph nodes after completion of radiotherapy is associated with poor survival outcomes. The optimal timing to obtain [$^{18}$F]FDG-PET/CT scans during RT for cervical cancer is unclear. FDG activity tends to show an initial increase followed by a steady decline after treatment. Early elevation of FDG activity may be associated with acute inflammation in normal tissue or elevated metabolic activity within the tumor cells; the later reduction in FDG uptake is a reflection of a decrease in the number of viable tumor cells or a reduction in tumor metabolic activity.

### 7.1.5 Tumor Recurrence

[$^{18}$F]FDG-PET/CT appears to have an acceptable diagnostic performance in suspected recurrent cervical cancer, and it may affect patient management. Furthermore, FDG avidity may predict the prognosis of recurrent cervical cancer (Figs. 7.1 and 7.2).

For the detection of combined local and metastatic recurrence of cervical cancer, according to several studies, the sensitivity of [$^{18}$F]FDG-PET/CT ranges from 92% to 93%, the specificity from 81 to 100%, and the accuracy from 87 to 96% [24–27]. [$^{18}$F]FDG-PET/CT was strongly predictive of overall survival [24]. Patients with negative [$^{18}$F]FDG-PET/CT for recurrence had a significantly better 2-year disease-free survival (DFS) rate compared to patients with positive PET/CT (85.0% vs. 10.9%, respectively, $P = 0.002$) [28]. The results of another study were in accordance with the above, and [$^{18}$F]FDG-PET/CT for the evaluation of local recurrence showed sensitivity, specificity, positive predictive value, and negative predictive value of 93%, 93%, 86%, and 96%, respectively, and for metastatic disease showed sensitivity, specificity, positive predictive value, and negative predictive value of 96%, 95%, 96%, and 95%, respectively [29].

The low rate of false-positive results and high prognostic value suggest that [$^{18}$F]FDG-PET/CT is an important diagnostic tool for detecting recurrent cervical cancer in clinically equivocal patients. For treatment planning, it is reported that [$^{18}$F]FDG-PET/CT may change management in 23.1–48% of cases in suspected recurrent cervical cancer [24, 25]. Because of its high sensitivity and positive predictive value, [$^{18}$F]FDG-PET/CT should be the imaging technique of choice for evaluating extra-pelvic disease prior to performing pelvic exenteration. It seems to be useful in identifying recurrent cervical cancer in both asymptomatic and symptomatic patients with elevated tumor markers and negative imaging findings (squamous cell carcinoma antigen >1.5 ng/mL) [30].

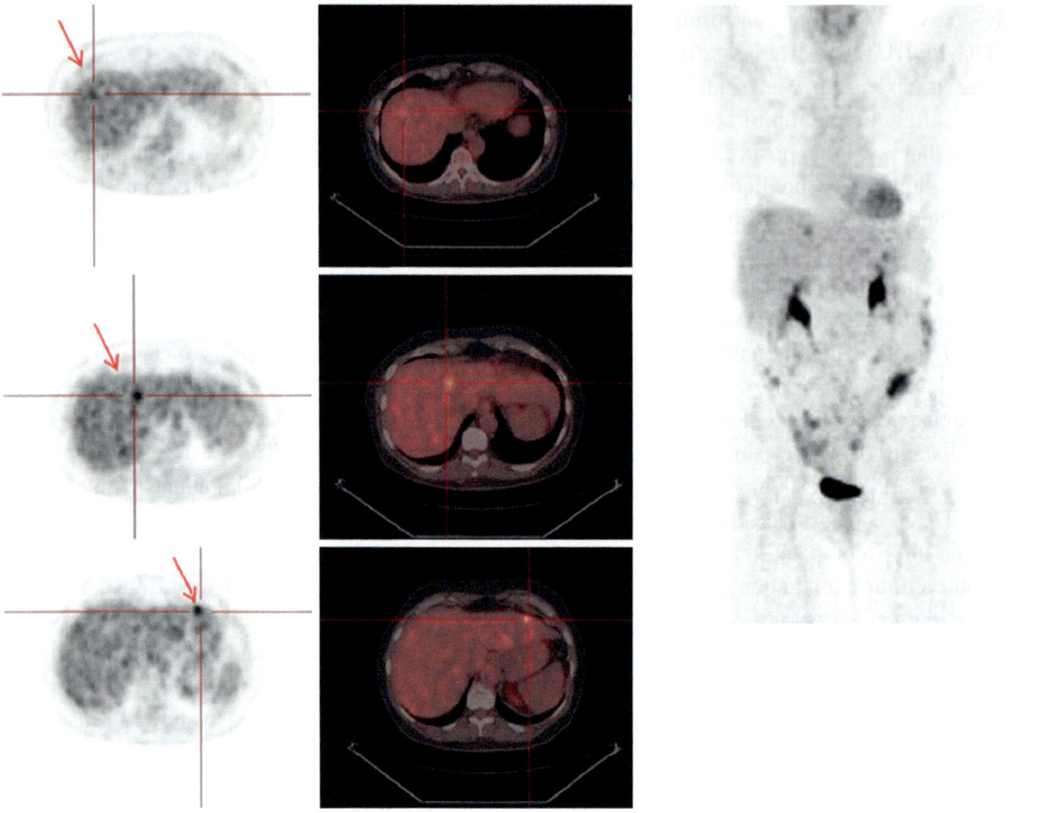

**Fig. 7.1** A 56-year-old woman, with previously treated cervical cancer, presenting with increased serum tumor markers and equivocal findings in conventional imaging. [18F]FDG-PET/CT showed increased [18F]FDG uptake in multiple lesions in the liver

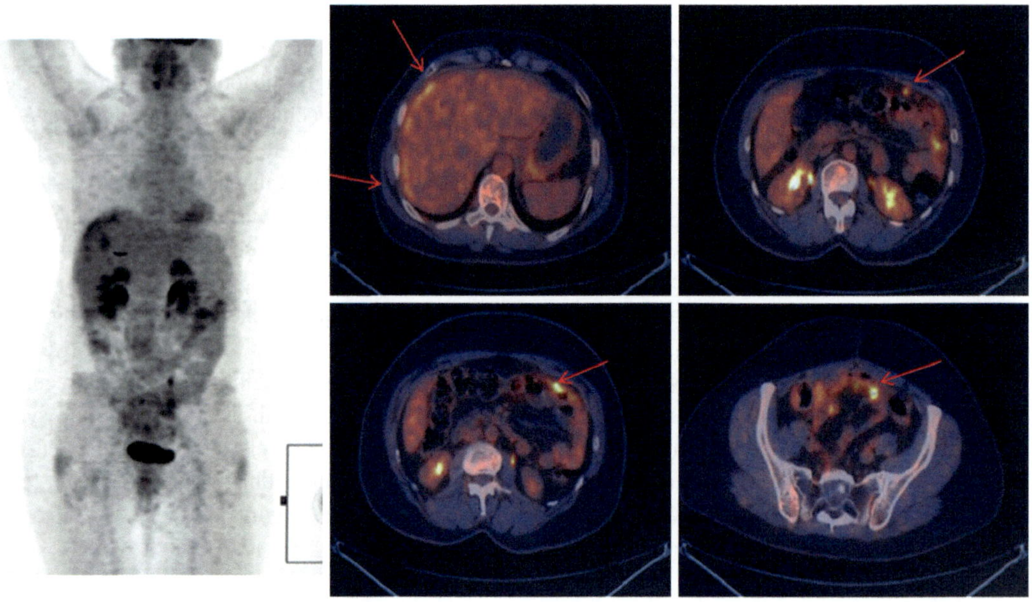

**Fig. 7.2** A 51-year-old woman, with previously treated cervical cancer presenting with elevated CEA serum levels and negative findings on CT and MRI imaging. [18F] FDG-PET/CT showed several areas of increased metabolic activity in the peritoneum (peritoneal implants)

### 7.1.6 Conclusion

[18F]FDG-PET/CT provides pretreatment prognostic information concerning the aggressiveness of cervical tumors which may contribute to optimizing and individualizing patient therapy. Although [18F]FDG-PET/CT is not considered suitable for T staging, it has an important role in staging cervical cancer, and it aids particularly in identifying the involvement of lymph nodes and distant metastases. In this context, it is helpful in targeted radiotherapy planning. Finally, [18F]FDG-PET/CT is an important diagnostic tool for detecting recurrent cervical cancer in clinically equivocal patients.

## 7.2 PET/CT with [18F]FDG in Endometrial Cancer

### 7.2.1 Initial Diagnosis and Prognosis

Like most neoplasms, endometrial carcinoma does demonstrate an increased rate of glycolysis and takes up [18F]FDG. Imaging with [18F]FDG-PET/CT may play a role as a prognostic factor in endometrium cancer. Several studies have shown that there is a statistically significant correlation between SUVmax and FIGO stage, histological grade, depth of myometrial invasion, lymph node metastasis, lymphovascular space involvement, and tumor size. Also, they have demonstrated that high SUVmax was an independent prognostic factor for both disease-free survival (DFS) and overall survival (OS), $p < 0.05$ [31–33]. The analysis of survival ROC curve revealed SUVmax cutoff value of 17.7 to predict high risk of recurrence. Endometrial cancer patients with SUVmax higher than 17.7 were characterized by worse prognosis and lower overall survival [34].

### 7.2.2 Initial Staging

There have been several reports demonstrating the accuracy of [18F]FDG-PET/CT for detecting lymph node metastasis in endometrial cancer. The referred sensitivity and specificity of [18F]FDG-PET/CT on region-specific analyses are 36–72% and 88–99%, respectively, and that corresponding values for patient-based analyses were 41–100% and 56–100%, respectively [35–43]. It seems that [18F]FDG-PET/CT tends to show low sensitivity and higher specificity. Studies have shown that the negative predictive value of [18F]FDG-PET/CT is very high (96–98%) [44, 45]. So, the combined high specificity and high negative predictive value confirm that [18F]FDG-PET/CT is presently the most promising imaging method to potentially exclude lymph node metastases and thus help avoid potentially harmful lymphadenectomy for staging.

But there is still a major limitation, the inability of the method to detect microscopic metastasis. As tiny lymph nodes tend to show smaller SUV than real values due to the partial volume effect, it is difficult to use the usual cutoff point (2.5–3.0) for differentiating malignant from benign lymph nodes [46]. A study has shown that in metastatic lymph nodes with a short axis diameter of 4 mm or less, [18F]FDG-PET/CT had a detection sensitivity of 12.5%; with a diameter between 5 and 9 mm, the sensitivity was 66.7%; and with a diameter of 10 mm or greater, it was 100.0% [36].

A recent study that compared the diagnostic performance of [18F]FDG-PET/CT, MRI and two-dimensional ultrasound (2DUS) found that all three methods were comparable in predicting myometrial invasion [44]. For cervical invasion and lymph node metastases, however, [18F]FDG-PET/CT was more accurate [44]. It seems that compared to MRI, [18F]FDG-PET/CT has a limited role for local staging of primary cancer, whereas it is a useful technique for assessing distant metastases throughout the whole body in a single examination in patients with advanced-stage disease [47].

### 7.2.3 Tumor Recurrence

Unlike conventional imaging modalities which provide morphological information, PET with [18F]FDG is able to identify viable tumor lesions based on the increased glucose metabolism of malignant tissue. [$^{18}$F]FDG-PET/CT can detect recurrent lesions otherwise missed or misinterpreted on conventional imaging studies and several studies support this.

A recent meta-analysis of the literature and several studies demonstrated that the patient-based sensitivity and specificity for detection of endometrial cancer recurrence were 91–100% and 83–100%, respectively [27, 36, 46, 48–50]. A previous study showed that the overall lesion site-based sensitivity and specificity of [$^{18}$F]FDG-PET/CT were 94.7% and 99.5%, respectively [27]. The lesion site-based sensitivity and specificity of [$^{18}$F]FDG-PET/CT for the detection of pelvic recurrence were 92.3% and 97.3%, while for the detection of extrapelvic recurrence, the indices were all 100% [27].

### 7.2.4 Conclusion

[$^{18}$F]FDG-PET/CT has a limited role for local staging of primary cancer, whereas it is a useful technique for assessing lymph node and distant metastases throughout the whole body in a single examination in patients with advanced-stage disease. Its main role is in detecting recurrent lesions otherwise missed or misinterpreted on conventional imaging studies.

## 7.3 PET/CT with [$^{18}$F]FDG in Ovarian Cancer

### 7.3.1 Initial Diagnosis: Differentiation Between Malignant and Benign Ovarian Tumors and Prognosis

The role of [$^{18}$F]FDG-PET/CT for differentiating between malignant and benign ovarian tumors remains controversial, and false-negative and false-positive cases have been reported. Concerning the prognostic value of [$^{18}$F]FDG-PET/CT, there have been reports that a high (>13.15) pretreatment SUVmax of the primary tumor in patients with ovarian cancer was associated with a poor prognosis [51]. The SUVmax of the primary tumor had a statistically significant association with stage ($p = 0.010$) and histology ($p = 0.001$) [51].

Intratumoral heterogeneity of PET/CT has been proved to be a prognostic predictor for many malignancies and the radiomics features extracted from PET/CT images allow the assessment of intratumoral and metabolic heterogeneity quantitatively [52, 53].

Radiomics signatures of PET seem that can improve the diagnostic accuracy and provide complementary prognostic information compared with the use of clinical factors alone or combined with CT components [52].

### 7.3.2 Initial Staging

In ovarian cancer [$^{18}$F]FDG-PET/CT has an effective role in staging patients with advanced disease, providing useful information about extrapelvic sites, such as supraclavicular and paraaortic nodular involvement, peritoneum and omentum implants, and bone and muscle metastases. A recent meta-analysis, including data from 882 patients with ovarian cancer, showed that [$^{18}$F]FDG-PET or [$^{18}$F]FDG-PET/CT was a more accurate modality for detecting metastatic lymph nodes [54]. Approximately 70% of metastatic lymph nodes and 97% of negative lymph nodes could be correctly diagnosed by [$^{18}$F]FDG-PET or [$^{18}$F]FDG-PET/CT. Though significantly better than those of CT and MR imaging, the sensitivity of [$^{18}$F]FDG-PET or [$^{18}$F]FDG-PET/CT was moderate [54]. A possible explanation is that this method can only detect lesions with sufficient malignant cells to change the glucose metabolism and that FDG uptake may not be increased in low-grade tumors.

The main effect of [$^{18}$F]FDG-PET/CT seems to be the detection of metastases outside the pelvis as it may detect distant metastasis in the liver, pleura, mediastinum, and supraclavicular lymph nodes that had been missed on CT imaging. It has been shown that [F]FDG-PET/CT may increase the pretreatment staging accuracy to 69–87% compared with 53–55% with CT alone [55, 56]. [$^{18}$F]FDG-PET/CT is particularly useful in distinguishing patients with stages IIIC–IV cancer from those with stages I–IIIB. For this classification, the specificity, sensitivity, and accuracy of [18F]FDG-PET/CT was 91%, 100%, and 98%, respectively, in comparison with 64%, 97%, and 88% for CT [57].

Although fusion PET/CT shows higher staging accuracy, mostly by identifying extra-abdominopelvic disease, it has not been widely adopted, as evidence that this capability alters treatment is lacking [58].

### 7.3.3 Radiotherapy Planning

In the literature, there is only one report about the role of [18F]FDG-PET/CT on intensity-modulated radiation therapy (IMRT) planning that showed that [18F]FDG-PET/CT information seems to change gross tumor volume (GTV) delineation in 35% of cases. In these patients, the average increase in GTV was 21.6%, due to the incorporation of additional lymph node metastases, minimal recurrent nodularity, and extension of the metastatic tumor beyond the frame defined by CT [59].

### 7.3.4 Restaging After Treatment

Several studies have demonstrated that [18F]FDG-PET/CT-derived parameters, including SUV and percentage change, have the potential to predict response to therapy in patients with ovarian cancer (Fig. 7.3).

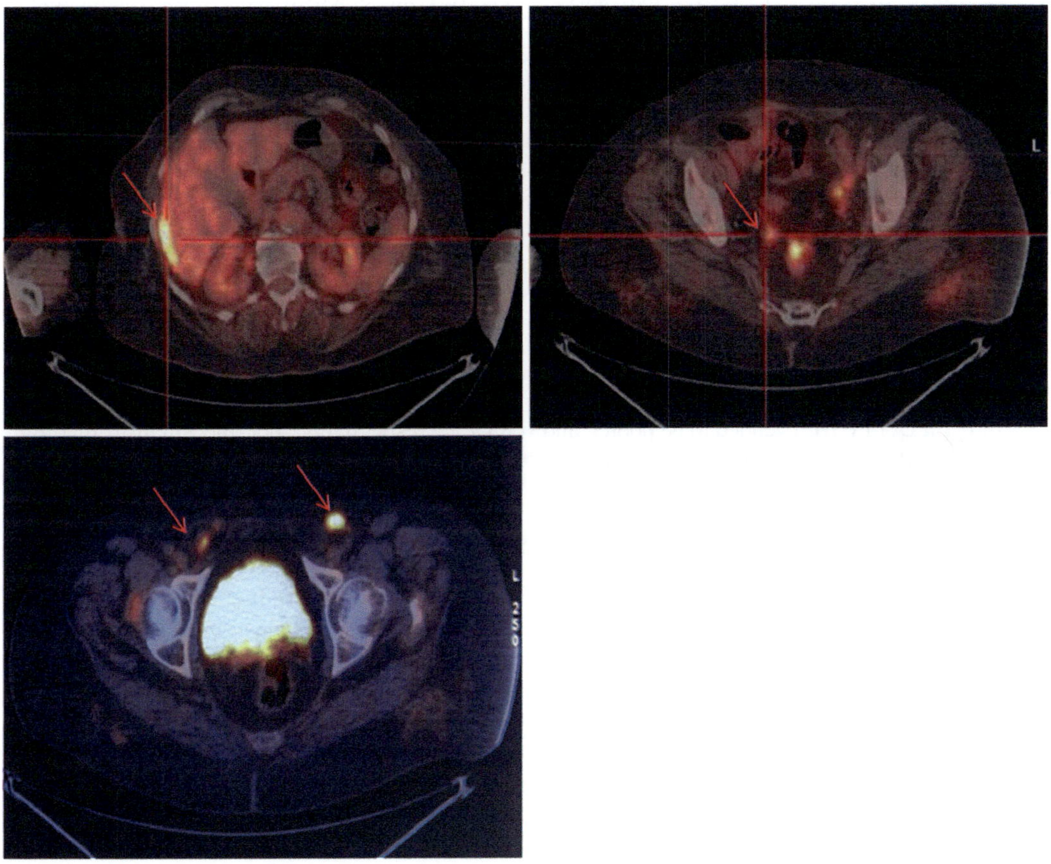


**Fig. 7.3** A 78-year-old woman posttreatment for ovarian carcinoma, presenting with rising tumor serum markers and negative findings on recent CT imaging. [18F]FDG-PET/CT revealed increased [18F]FDG uptake in the peritoneum and in bilateral inguinal lymph nodes

When an arbitrary SUV of 3.8 was taken as the cutoff for differentiating between responders and nonresponders after therapy, [$^{18}$F]FDG-PET/CT showed a sensitivity of 90% and specificity of 63.6%. When an arbitrary percentage change of 65% was taken as the cutoff, the sensitivity was 90% and specificity 81.8% [60].

### 7.3.5 Tumor Recurrence

Potential advantages of the use of integrated [$^{18}$F]FDG-PET/CT for evaluation of recurrent ovarian cancer include increased lesion detection with the use of a metabolic tracer, simultaneous acquisition of anatomic reference points to determine the exact location of lesions, and, in most cases, differentiation of disease processes from physiologic processes. Moreover, [$^{18}$F]FDG_PET/CT may survey the entire body in one examination. These superior qualities may help identify which patients are eligible for secondary surgical cytoreduction. There have been many reports discussing the usefulness of [$^{18}$F]FDG-PET/CT for detecting ovarian cancer recurrence. When the gold standard was clinical follow-up including radiological imaging, the diagnostic accuracy of [$^{18}$F]FDG-PET/CT was very high with 73–100% sensitivity, 71–100% specificity, and 83–100% accuracy in patient-based analysis [57, 61–71]. However, when the gold standard was histopathology by surgery, the diagnostic accuracy of [$^{18}$F]FDG-PET/CT tended to be poorer, and it was reported that the sensitivity, specificity, and accuracy of patient-based analysis were 53–83%, 40–86%, and 63–82%, respectively [72–74]. The discrepancies in these values between the clinical follow-up and the surgical histopathology as a gold standard may partly depend on the resolution of the [$^{18}$F]FDG-PET/CT systems used and partly on the size of microscopically small lesions. The spatial resolution of PET is approximately 6–10 mm; therefore, its sensitivity for depicting lesions smaller than 1 cm is lower than that for larger lesions [75] (Figs. 7.4 and 7.5).

Several studies and a meta-analysis have compared techniques for detection of recurrence and demonstrated that [$^{18}$F]FDG-PET/CT was better (sensitivity 91% and specificity 88%) than CT (sensitivity 79%, specificity 84%) or MRI (sensitivity 75%, specificity 78%) [57, 62, 68, 76, 77]. In addition, [$^{18}$F]FDG-PET/CT had the highest positive predictive value (89–98%) for recurrence of ovarian cancer when compared with other modalities [78, 79].

A major indication for [$^{18}$F]FDG-PET/CT is the evaluation of ovarian cancer recurrence after first-line therapy in patients in which CA-125 levels are rising and conventional imaging studies show negative or equivocal findings [61, 80]. Investigators have reported that [$^{18}$F]FDG-PET or PET/CT has a sensitivity of 96% for localizing recurrent disease in patients with rising CA-125 levels and that PET evidence of recurrent ovarian cancer preceded CT findings by 6 months, allowing earlier reintroduction of therapy [81, 82]. In accordance with the results of recent studies, [$^{18}$F]FDG-PET/CT has a higher predictive value than the CA125 serum marker in the detection of disease recurrence [83].

Concerning the detection of peritoneal implants in a recent study, the sensitivity and specificity of [$^{18}$F]FDG-PET/CT were 97.5% and 100%, whereas those of MRI were 95% and 85.7%, respectively. For the small-to-medium-sized (0.5–2 cm) peritoneal implants, diagnostic accuracy values of [$^{18}$F]FDG-PET/CT were significantly better than those of MRI ($p < 0.05$) [84].

As reported in the literature, the change in management of patients with ovarian cancer recurrence who have undergone [$^{18}$F]FDG-PET/CT ranges between 25% and 58% [57, 64, 65, 83, 85].

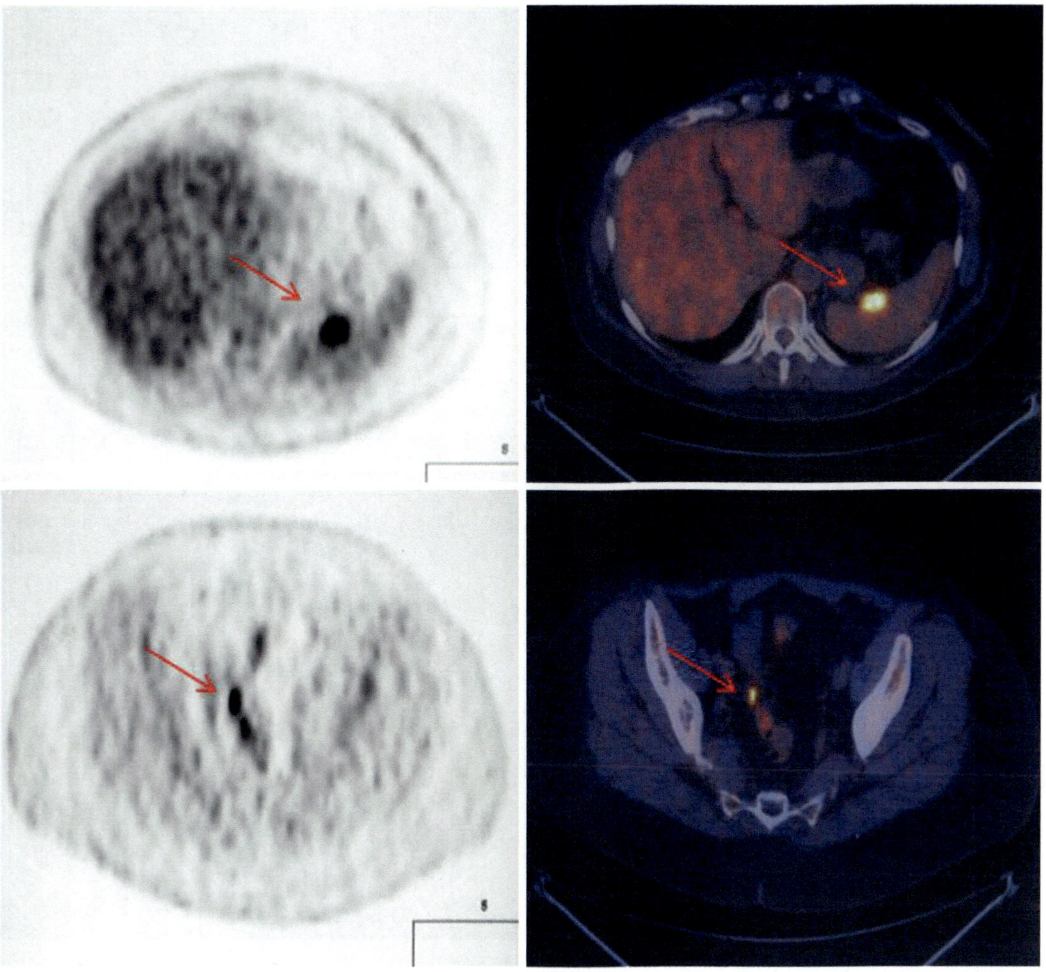

**Fig. 7.4** A 52-year-old woman with a history of bilateral ovarian carcinoma presenting with slight but persistent elevation of tumor marker serum levels and negative findings on MRI imaging. [$^{18}$F]FDG-PET/CT revealed two [$^{18}$F]FDG avid lesions in the peritoneum

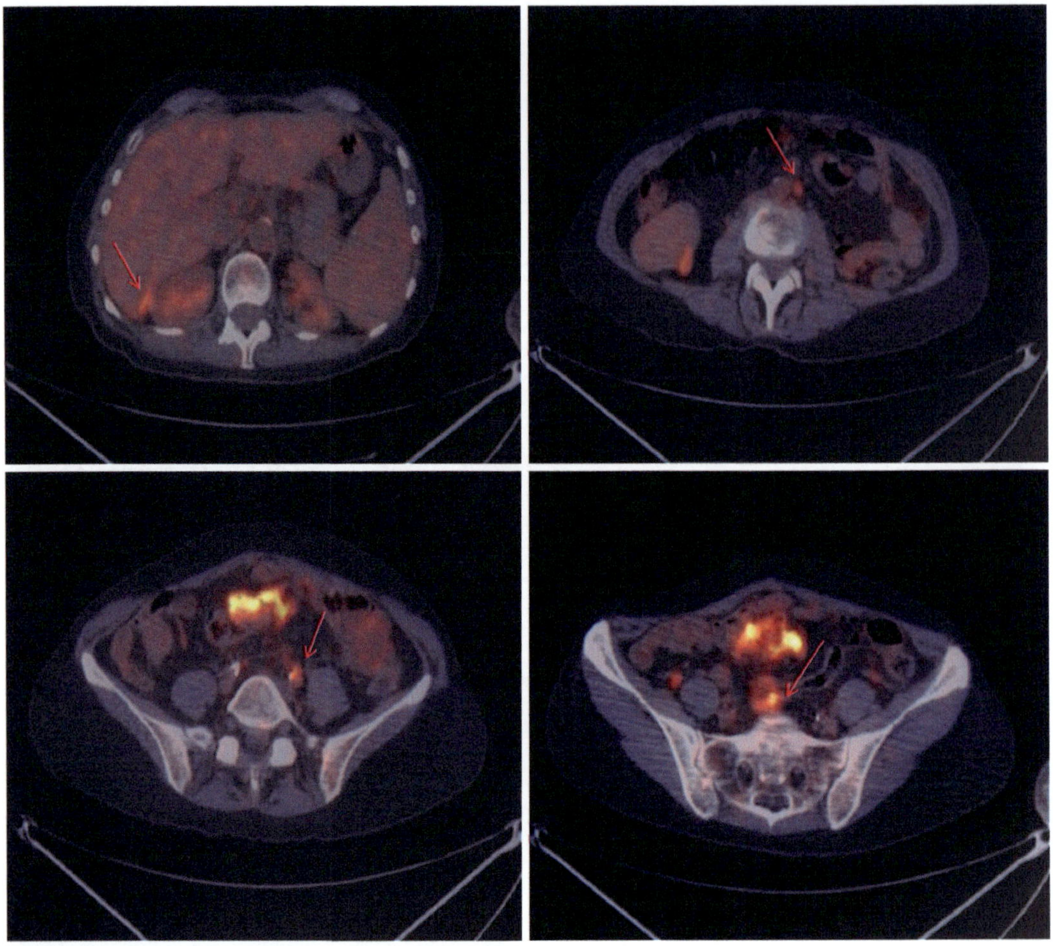

**Fig. 7.5** A 66-year-old woman, status posttreatment for ovarian carcinoma, presenting with progressively elevated CA-125 antigen and negative conventional imaging evaluation. [18F]FDG-PET/CT revealed several foci of increased [18F]FDG uptake in the peritoneum. Abnormal metabolic activity was also present in a small left paraaortic and a small left common iliac lymph node

### 7.3.6 Conclusion

[18F]FDG-PET/CT has an effective role in the detection of metastases outside the pelvis as it may detect distant metastasis in the liver, pleura, mediastinum, and supraclavicular lymph nodes that may be missed on CT imaging. Another major indication of the modality is the evaluation of ovarian cancer recurrence after first-line therapy in patients in which CA-125 levels are rising, and conventional imaging studies show negative or equivocal findings.

## References


1. Chung HH, Nam BH, Kim JW, Kang KW, Park NH, Song YS, Chung JK, Kang SB. Preoperative [18F] FDG PET/CT maximum standardized uptake value predicts recurrence of uterine cervical cancer. Eur J Nucl Med Mol Imaging. 2010;37:1467–73.
2. Rahman T, Tsujikawa T, Yamamoto M, et al. Different prognostic implications of 18F-FDG PET between histological subtypes in patients with cervical cancer. Medicine (Baltimore). 2016;95:e3017.
3. Li W, Liu H, Cheng F, et al. Artificial intelligence applications for oncological positron emission tomography imaging. Eur J Radiol. 2021;134:109448.

4. Lucia F, Visvikis D, Desseroit MC, et al. Prediction of outcome using pretreatment (18)F-FDG PET/CT and MRI radiomics in locally advanced cervical cancer treated with chemoradiotherapy. Eur J Nucl Med Mol Imaging. 2018;45:768–86.
5. Ho KC, Fang YH, Chung HW, et al. A preliminary investigation into textural features of intratumoral metabolic heterogeneity in (18)F-FDG PET for overall survival prognosis in patients with bulky cervical cancer treated with definitive concurrent chemoradiotherapy. Am J Nucl Med Mol Imaging. 2016;6:166–75. eCollection 2016
6. Haie-Meder C, Mazeron R, Magne N. Clinical evidence on PET-CT for radiation therapy planning in cervix and endometrial cancers. Radiother Oncol. 2010;96:351–5.
7. Petsuksiri J, Jaishuen A, Pattaranutaporn P, Chansilpa Y. Advanced imaging applications for locally advanced cervical cancer. Asian Pac J Cancer Prev. 2012;13:1713–8.
8. Yoon MS, Ahn SJ, Nah BS, Chung WK, Song HC, Yoo SW, Song JY, Jeong JU, Nam TK. Metabolic response of lymph nodes immediately after RT is related with survival outcome of patients with pelvic node-positive cervical cancer using consecutive [($^{18}$)F]fluorodeoxyglucose-positron emission tomography/computed tomography. Int J Radiat Oncol Biol Phys. 2012;84:e491–7.
9. Lin WC, Hung YC, Yeh LS, Kao CH, Yen RF, Shen YY. Usefulness of ($^{18}$)F-fluorodeoxyglucose positron emission tomography to detect para-aortic lymph nodal metastasis in advanced cervical cancer with negative computed tomography findings. Gynecol Oncol. 2003;89:73–6.
10. Yeh LS, Hung YC, Shen YY, Kao CH, Lin CC, Lee CC. Detecting para-aortic lymph nodal metastasis by positron emission tomography of $^{18}$F-fluorodeoxyglucose in advanced cervical cancer with negative magnetic resonance imaging findings. Oncol Rep. 2002;9:1289–92.
11. Grigsby PW. 4th international cervical cancer conference: update on PET and cervical cancer. Gynecol Oncol. 2005;99(3 suppl 1):S173–5.
12. Sugawara Y, Eisbruch A, Kosuda S, Recker BE, Kison PV, Wahl RL. Evaluation of FDG PET in patients with cervical cancer. J Nucl Med. 1999;40:1125–31.
13. Choi HJ, Roh JW, Seo SS, et al. Comparison of the accuracy of magnetic resonance imaging and positron emission tomography/computed tomography in the presurgical detection of lymph node metastases in patients with uterine cervical carcinoma: a prospective study. Cancer. 2006;106:914–22.
14. Havrilesky LJ, Kulasingam SL, Matchar DB, Myers ER. FDG-PET for management of cervical and ovarian cancer. Gynecol Oncol. 2005;97:183–91.
15. Kim SK, Choi HJ, Park SY, et al. Additional value of MR/PET fusion compared with PET/CT in the detection of lymph node metastases in cervical cancer patients. Eur J Cancer. 2009;45:2103–9.
16. Choi HJ, Ju W, Myung SK, Kim Y. Diagnostic performance of computer tomography, magnetic resonance imaging, and positron emission tomography or positron emission tomography/computer tomography for detection of metastatic lymph nodes in patients with cervical cancer: meta-analysis. Cancer Sci. 2010;101:1471–9.
17. Loft A, Berthelsen AK, Roed H, Ottosen C, Lundvall L, Knudsen J, Nedergaard L, Højgaard L, Engelholm SA. The diagnostic value of PET/CT scanning in patients with cervical cancer: a prospective study. Gynecol Oncol. 2007;106:29–34.
18. Yildirim Y, Sehirali S, Avci ME, Yilmaz C, Ertopcu K, Tinar S, Duman Y, Sayhan S. Integrated PET/CT for the evaluation of para-aortic nodal metastasis in locally advanced cervical cancer patients with negative conventional CT findings. Gynecol Oncol. 2008;108:154–9.
19. American College of Radiology. ACR appropriateness criteria. Women's imaging: staging of invasive cancer of the cervix. 2010; http://www.acr.org/. Accessed 20 Mar 2010.
20. Kizer NT, Zighelboim I, Case AS, Dewdney SB, Thaker PH, Massad LS. The role of PET/CT in the management of patients with cervical cancer: practice patterns of the members of the society of gynecologic oncologists. Gynecol Oncol. 2009;114:310–4.
21. Kunos C, Radivoyevitch T, Abdul-Karim FW, Faulhaber P. 18F-fluoro-2-deoxy-D-glucose positron emission tomography standard uptake value ratio as an indicator of cervical cancer chemoradiation therapeutic response. Int J Gynecol Cancer. 2011;21:117–23.
22. Antoch G, Freudenberg LS, Beyer T, Bockisch A, Debatin JF. To enhance or not to enhance? $^{18}$F-FDG and CT contrast agents in dual-modality $^{18}$F-FDG PET/CT. J Nucl Med. 2004;45(suppl 1):56S–65S.
23. Su TP, Lin G, Huang YT, et al. Comparison of positron emission tomography/computed tomography and magnetic resonance imaging for posttherapy evaluation in patients with advanced cervical cancer receiving definitive concurrent chemoradiotherapy. Eur J Nucl Med Mol Imaging. 2018;45:727–34.
24. van der Veldt AA, Buist MR, van Baal MW, Comans EF, Hoekstra OS, Molthoff CF. Clarifying the diagnosis of clinically suspected recurrence of cervical cancer: impact of $^{18}$F-FDG PET. J Nucl Med. 2008;49:1936–43.
25. Chung HH, Jo H, Kang WJ, et al. Clinical impact of integrated PET/CT on the management of suspected cervical cancer recurrence. Gynecol Oncol. 2007;104:529–34.
26. Kitajima K, Murakami K, Yamasaki E, Domeki Y, Kaji Y, Sugimura K. Performance of FDG- PET/CT for diagnosis of recurrent uterine cervical cancer. Eur Radiol. 2008;18:2040–7.
27. Sironi S, Picchio M, Landoni C, Galimberti S, Signorelli M, Bettinardi V, et al. Post-therapy surveillance of patients with uterine cancers: value of integrated FDG PET/CT in the detection of recurrence. Eur J Nucl Med Mol Imaging. 2007;34:472–9.

28. Kidd EA, Thomas M, Siegel BA, et al. Changes in cervical cancer FDG uptake during chemoradiation and association with response. Int J Radiat Oncol Biol Phys. 2013;85:116–22.
29. Mittra E, El-Maghraby T, Rodriguez CA, Quon A, McDougall IR, Gambhir SS, Iagaru A. Efficacy of $^{18}$F-FDG PET/CT in the evaluation of patients with recurrent cervical carcinoma. Eur J Nucl Med Mol Imaging. 2009;36:1952–9.
30. Jover R, Lourido D, Gonzalez C, Rojo A, Gorospe L, Alfonso JM. Role of PET/CT in the evaluation of cervical cancer. Gynecol Oncol. 2008;110(3 suppl 2):S55–9.
31. Nakamura K, Joja I, Fukushima C, Haruma T, Hayashi C, Kusumoto T, Seki N, Hongo A, Hiramatsu Y. The preoperative SUVmax is superior to ADCmin of the primary tumour as a predictor of disease recurrence and survival in patients with endometrial cancer. Eur J Nucl Med Mol Imaging. 2013;40:52–60.
32. Kitajima K, Kita M, Suzuki K, Senda M, Nakamoto Y, Sugimura K. Prognostic significance of SUVmax (maximum standardized uptake value)measured by [$^{18}$F]FDG PET/CT in endometrial cancer. Eur J Nucl Med Mol Imaging. 2012;39:840–5.
33. Nakamura K, Hongo A, Kodama J, Hiramatsu Y. The measurement of SUVmax of the primary tumor is predictive of prognosis for patients with endometrial cancer. Gynecol Oncol. 2011;123:82–7.
34. Walentowicz-Sadlecka M, Malkowski B, Walentowicz P, et al. The preoperative maximum standardized uptake value measured by 18F-FDG PET/CT as an independent prognostic factor of overall survival in endometrial cancer patients. Biomed Res Int. 2014;2014:234813.
35. Kitajima K, Murakami K, Yamasaki E, et al. Accuracy of FDG PET/CT in detecting pelvic and paraortic lymph node metastasis in patients with endometrial cancer. AJR Am J Roentgenol. 2008;190:1652–8.
36. Kitajima K, Murakami K, Yamasaki E, Kaji Y, Sugimura K. Accuracy of integrated FDG-PET/contrast-enhanced CT in detecting pelvic and para aortic lymph node metastasis in patients with uterine cancer. Eur Radiol. 2009;19:1529–36.
37. Kitajima K, Yamasaki E, Kaji Y, Murakami K, Sugimura K. Comparison of DWI and PET/CT in evaluation of lymph node metastasis in uterine cancer. World J Radiol. 2012;4:207–14.
38. Sironi S, Buda A, Picchio M, Perego P, Moreni R, Pellegrino A, Colombo M, Mangioni C, Messa C, Fazio F. Lymph node metastasis in patients with clinical early-stage cervical cancer: detection with integrated FDG PET/CT. Radiology. 2006;238:272–9.
39. Park JY, Kim EN, Kim DY, Suh DS, Kim JH, Kim YM, Kim YT, Nam JH. Comparison of the validity of magnetic resonance imaging and positron emission tomography/computed tomography in the preoperative evaluation of patients with uterine corpus cancer. Gynecol Oncol. 2008;108:486–92.
40. Chung HH, Park NH, Kim JW, Song YS, Chung JK, Kang SB. Role of integrated PET-CT in pelvic lymph node staging of cervical cancer before radical hysterectomy. Gynecol Obstet Investig. 2009;67:61–6.
41. Signorelli M, Guerra L, Buda A, Picchio M, Mangili G, Dell'Anna T, Sironi S, Messa C. Role of the integrated FDG PET/CT in the surgical management of patients with high risk clinical early stage endometrial cancer: detection of pelvic nodal metastases. Gynecol Oncol. 2009;115:231–5.
42. Picchio M, Mangili G, Samanes Gajate AM, et al. High-grade endometrial cancer: value of 18F- FDG PET/CT in preoperative staging. Nucl Med Commun. 2010;31:506–12.
43. Nayot D, Kwon JS, Carey MS, et al. Does preoperative positron emission tomography with computed tomography predict nodal status in endometrial cancer? A pilot study. Curr Oncol. 2008;15:123–5.
44. Antonsen SL, Jensen LN, Loft A, Berthelsen AK, Costa J, Tabor A, et al. MRI, PET/CT and ultrasound in the preoperative staging of endometrial cancer—a multicenter prospective comparative study. Gynecol Oncol. 2013;128:300–8.
45. Husby JA, Reitan BC, Biermann M, et al. Metabolic tumor volume on 18F-FDG PET/CT improves preoperative identification of high-risk endometrial carcinoma patients. J Nucl Med. 2015;56:1191–8.
46. Kitajima K, Murakami K, Yamasaki E, et al. Performance of FDG-PET/CT in the diagnosis of recurrent endometrial cancer. Ann Nucl Med. 2008;22:103–9.
47. Kitajima K, Murakami K, Kaji Y, Sugimura K. Spectrum of FDG PET/CT findings of uterine tumors. AJR Am J Roentgenol. 2010;195:737–43.
48. Chung HH, Kang WJ, Kim JW, et al. The clinical impact of [18F]FDG PET/CT for the management of recurrent endometrial cancer: correlation with clinical and histological findings. Eur J Nucl Med Mol Imaging. 2008;35:1081–8.
49. Park JY, Kim EN, Kim DY, et al. Clinical impact of positron emission tomography or positron emission tomography/computed tomography in the post therapy surveillance of endometrial carcinoma: evaluation of 88 patients. Int J Gynecol Cancer. 2008;18:1332–8.
50. Kadkhodayan S, Shahriari S, Treglia G, Yousefi Z, Sadeghi R. Accuracy of 18-F-FDG PET imaging in the follow up of endometrial cancer patients: systematic review and meta-analysis of the literature. Gynecol Oncol. 2013;128:397–404.
51. Nakamura K, Hongo A, Kodama J, Hiramatsu Y. The pretreatment of maximum standardized uptake values (SUVmax) of the primary tumor is predictor for poor prognosis for patients with epithelial ovarian cancer. Acta Med Okayama. 2012;66:53–60.
52. Wang X, Lu Z. Radiomics analysis of PET and CT components of 18F-FDG PET/CT imaging for prediction of progression-free survival in advanced high-grade serous ovarian cancer. Front Oncol. 2021;11:638124.
53. Yang B, Zhong J, Zhong J, et al. Development and validation of a radiomics nomogram based on 18F-Fluorodeoxyglucose positron emission tomog-

raphy/computed tomography and clinicopathological factors to predict the survival outcomes of patients with non-small cell lung cancer. Front Oncol. 2020;17(10):10422.
54. Yuan Y, Gu ZX, Tao XF, Liu SY. Computer tomography, magnetic resonance imaging, and positron emission tomography or positron emission tomography/computer tomography for detection of metastatic lymph nodes in patients with ovarian cancer: a meta-analysis. Eur J Radiol. 2012;81:1002–6.
55. Castelluci P, Perrone AM, Picchio M, Ghi T, Farsad M, Nanni C, et al. Diagnostic accuracy of 18F-FDG PET/CT in characterizing ovarian lesions and staging ovarian cancer: correlation with transvaginal ultrasonography, computed tomography, and histology. Nucl Med Commun. 2007;28:589–95.
56. Yoshida Y, Kurokawa T, Kawahara K, Tsuchida T, Okazawa H, Fujibayashi Y, Yonekura Y, Kotsuji F. Incremental benefits of FDG positron emission tomography over CT alone for the preoperative staging of ovarian cancer. AJR Am J Roentgenol. 2004;182:227–33.
57. Kitajima K, Murakami K, Yamasaki E. Diagnostic accuracy of integrated FDG-PET/ contrast-enhanced CT in staging ovarian cancer: comparison with enhanced CT. Eur J Nucl Med Mol Imaging. 2008;35:1912–20.
58. Lee SI, Catalano OA, Dehdashti F. Evaluation of gynecologic cancer with MR imaging, 18F-FDG PET/CT, and PET/MR imaging. J Nucl Med. 2015;56:436–43.
59. Du XL, Jiang T, Sheng XG, Li QS, Wang C, Yu H. PET/CT scanning guided intensity-modulated radiotherapy in treatment of recurrent ovarian cancer. Eur J Radiol. 2012;81:3551–6.
60. Nishiyama Y, Yamamoto Y, Kaneishi K, Ohno M, Hata T, Kushida Y, et al. Monitoring the neoadjuvant therapy response in gynecological cancer patients using FDG PET. Eur J Nucl Med Mol Imaging. 2008;35:287–95.
61. Chung HH, Kang WJ, Kim JW, Park NH, Song YS, Chung JK, Kang SB, Lee HP. Role of [18F]FDG PET/ CT in the assessment of suspected recurrent ovarian cancer: correlation with clinical or histological findings. Eur J Nucl Med Mol Imaging. 2007;34:480–6.
62. Hauth EA, Antoch G, Stattaus J, Kuehl H, Veit P, Bosckisch A, et al. Evaluation of integrated whole-body PET/CT in the detection of recurrent ovarian cancer. Eur J Radiol. 2005;56:263–8.
63. Nanni C, Rubello D, Farsad M, De Iaco P, Sansovini M, Erba P, et al. 18F-FDG PET/CT in the evaluation of recurrent ovarian cancer: a prospective study on forty-one patients. Eur J Surg Oncol. 2005;31:792–7.
64. Simcock B, Neesham D, Quinn M, Drummond E, Milner A, Hicks RJ. The impact of PET/CT in the management of recurrent ovarian cancer. Gynecol Oncol. 2006;103:271–6.
65. Mangili G, Picchio M, Sironi S, Vigano R, Rabaiotti E, Bornaghi D, et al. Integrated PET/CT as a first-line re-staging modality in patients with suspected recurrence of ovarian cancer. Eur J Nucl Med Mol Imaging. 2007;34:658–66.
66. Thrall MM, DeLoia JA, Gallion H, Avril N. Clinical use of combined positron emission tomography and computed tomography (FDG-PET/CT) in recurrent ovarian cancer. Gynecol Oncol. 2007;105:17–22.
67. Kim CK, Park BK, Choi JY, Kim BG, Han H. Detection of recurrent ovarian cancer at MRI: comparison with integrated PET/CT. J Comput Assist Tomogr. 2007;31:868–75.
68. Sebastian S, Lee SI, Horowitz NS, Scott JA, Fischman AJ, Simeone JF, et al. PET-CT vs. CT alone in ovarian cancer recurrence. Abdom Imaging. 2008;33:112–8.
69. Iagaru AH, Mittra ES, McDougall IR, Quon A, Gambhir SS. 18FFDG PET/CT evaluation of patients with ovarian carcinoma. Nucl Med Commun. 2008;29:1046–51.
70. Soussan M, Wartski M, Cherel P, Fourme E, Goupil A, Le Stanc E, et al. Impact of FDG PET/CT imaging on the decision making in the biologic suspicion of ovarian carcinoma recurrence. Gynecol Oncol. 2008;108:160–5.
71. Fulham MJ, Carter J, Baldey A, Hicks RJ, Ramshaw JE, Gibson M. The impact of PET/CT in suspected recurrent ovarian cancer: a prospective multi-Centre study as part of the Australian PET data collection project. Gynecol Oncol. 2009;112:462–8.
72. Makhija S, Howden N, Edwards R, Kelley J, Townsend DW, Meltzer CC. Positron emission tomography/ computed tomography imaging for the detection of recurrent ovarian and fallopian tube carcinoma: a retrospective review. Gynecol Oncol. 2002;85:53–8.
73. Bristow RE, DelCarmen MG, Pannu HK, Cohade C, Zahurak ML, Fishman EK, et al. Clinically occult recurrent ovarian cancer: patient selection for secondary cytoreductive surgery using combined PET/ CT. Gynecol Oncol. 2003;90:519–28.
74. Sironi S, Messa C, Mangili G, Zangheri B, Aletti G, Garevaglia E, et al. Integrated FDG-PET/CT in patients with persistent ovarian cancer: correlation with histologic findings. Radiology. 2004;233:433–40.
75. Torizuka T, Nobezawa S, Kanno T, et al. Ovarian cancer recurrence: role of whole-body positron emission tomography using 2-[fluorine-18]-fluoro-2-deoxy-D-glucose. Eur J Nucl Med Mol Imaging. 2002;29:797–803.
76. Gu P, Pan LL, Wu SQ, Sun L, Huang G. CA125, PET alone, PET-CT, CT and MRI in diagnosing recurrent ovarian carcinoma: a systematic review and meta-analysis. Eur J Radiol. 2009;71:164–74.
77. Nakamoto Y, Saga T, Ishimori T, et al. Clinical value of positron emission tomography with FDG for recurrent ovarian cancer. Am J Roentgenol. 2001;176:1449–54.
78. Prakash P, Cronin CG, Blake MA. Role of PET/ CT in ovarian cancer. AJR Am J Roentgenol. 2010;194:W464–70.
79. Antunovic L, Cimitan M, Borsatti E, et al. Revisiting the clinical value of 18F-FDG PET/CT in detection of recurrent epithelial ovarian carcinomas: correlation with histology, serum CA-125 assay, and conventional radiological modalities. Clin Nucl Med. 2012;37:e184–8.

80. Kitajima K, Murakami K, Sakamoto S, Kaji Y, Sugimura K. Present and future of FDG-PET/CT in ovarian cancer. Ann Nucl Med. 2011;25:155–64.
81. Son H, Khan SM, Rahaman J, Cameron KL, Prasad-Hayes M, Chuang L, Machac J, Heiba S, Kostakoglu L. Role of FDG PET/CT in staging of recurrent ovarian cancer. Radiographics. 2011;31:569–83.
82. Zimny M, Siggelkow W, Schruder W, et al. 2-[Fluorine-18]-fluoro-2-deoxy-D-glucose positron emission tomography in the diagnosis of recurrent ovarian cancer. Gynecol Oncol. 2001;83:310–5.
83. Evangelista L, Palma MD, Gregianin M, et al. Diagnostic and prognostic evaluation of fluoro deoxy glucose positron emission tomography/computed tomography and its correlation with serum cancer antigen-125 (CA125) in a large cohort of ovarian cancer patients. J Turk Ger Gynecol Assoc. 2015;16:137–44.
84. Sanli Y, Turkmen C, Bakir B, Iyibozkurt C, Ozel S, Has D, Yilmaz E, Topuz S, Yavuz E, Unal SN, Mudun A. Diagnostic value of PET/CT is similar to that of conventional MRI and even better for detecting small peritoneal implants in patients with recurrent ovarian cancer. Nucl Med Commun. 2012;33:509–15.
85. Chung HH, Kwon HW, Kang KW, et al. Prognostic value of preoperative metabolic tumor volume and total lesion glycolysis in patients with epithelial ovarian cancer. Ann Surg Oncol. 2012;19:1966–72.

# 8 PET-CT Staging of Rectal Carcinoma

Maria G. Skilakaki

## 8.1 Introduction

Rectal cancer comprises over 1/3 of cases of all colorectal cancers and is one of the most frequent causes of cancer-related mortality in Western countries. The expectation of cure strongly depends on the local extent of initial tumor, infiltration of lymph nodes, and presence of distant metastatic disease. Accurate initial staging, early recognition of recurrence, and assessment of residual masses after treatment are mandatory for optimal management of patients with rectal cancer. Although contrast-enhanced multi-detector CT of the chest, abdomen, and pelvis and pelvic MRI are the modalities of choice for preoperative staging of rectal cancers, appropriate imaging for the diagnosis and management of these tumors remains a topic of current investigation.

Fusion imaging with combined positron emission tomography (PET) and computed tomography (CT) has been introduced in clinical practice since 2001. The glucose analog, $^{18}$F-fluorodeoxyglucose ($^{18}$F-FDG), due to its ability to accumulate in highly metabolic lesions, is the most widely used radiotracer for PET tumor imaging. As a noninvasive whole-body imaging modality able to provide metabolic and anatomic information, $^{18}$F-FDG-PET/CT has been extensively used in the evaluation of patients with rectal carcinoma [1–3].

In recent years AI has emerged as a very promising tool in improving many aspects of medicine, including cancer imaging and management. Radiomics, a new field in imaging of clinical oncology, use AI methods to extract and analyze a large number of features from radiographic images to optimize technical factors, improve tumor characterization, quantification and staging, assess treatment response, and predict survival. Limited, preliminary data show that PET/CT-derived radiomics can increase method's accuracy and be of potential value in the evaluation of patients with rectal cancer [4–6].

## 8.2 Diagnosis and Initial Staging

Although most rectal tumors are FDG avid, PET/CT is not generally recommended for the initial diagnosis and staging of rectal cancer because it has a low sensitivity for locoregional staging due to its limited spatial resolution combined with the intense FDG uptake by the primary tumor and its inability to detect microscopic lymph nodal disease.

However, several studies in the literature that have investigated the specific impact of PET/CT on management of patients with locally advanced and low rectal tumors found FDG-PET/CT to be superior to contrast-enhanced multi-detector CT

M. G. Skilakaki (✉)
Evangelismos General Hospital, Athens, Greece
e-mail: skmaria@otenet.gr


J. A. Andreou et al. (eds.), *Artificial Intelligence in PET/CT Oncologic Imaging*,
https://doi.org/10.1007/978-3-031-10090-1_8

in identifying both intrahepatic and extrahepatic metastatic disease with a high (>90%) sensitivity and specificity. Additionally, these studies reported a change in treatment strategy in 12–31% of cases. This is mainly due to more accurate tumor volume delineation for preoperative radiation treatment planning, discrimination of responders from nonresponders to chemoradiotherapy, and detection of abnormal metabolic activity in inguinal lymph nodes, a common place of metastasis in patients with low rectal cancer (Fig. 8.1) [2, 7, 8].

Moreover, an intense FDG uptake before therapy seems to be a bad prognostic factor related to reduced overall survival. It is therefore currently widely acceptable the use of FDG-PET/CT in the initial staging of patients with locally advanced rectal carcinomas who will receive chemoradiation preoperatively [9–11].

In recent years, whole-body FDG-PET/MRI has been reported as a promising tool for the evaluation of advanced rectal cancer. Hybrid PET/MRI combines the high soft tissue contrast and functional information of MRI and the metabolic information provided by PET. The current evidence suggests that PET/MRI is superior to PET/CT in T staging, whereas in N staging both modalities have similar diagnostic accuracy [12, 13].

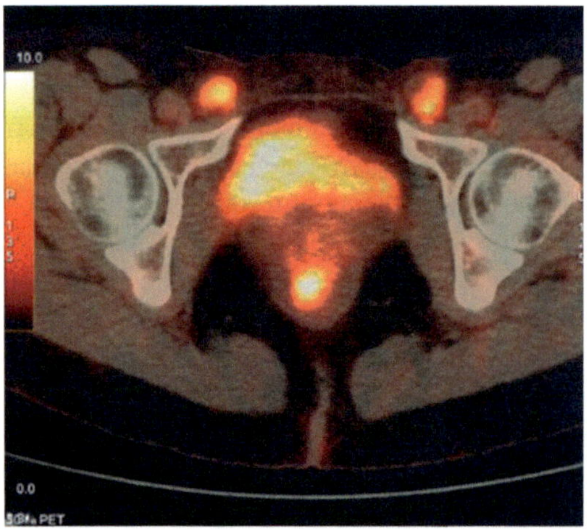


**Fig. 8.1** A 58-year-old male with low rectal cancer. Axial fused PET/CT at the level of the pelvis shows abnormal metabolic activity in the primary tumor and in inguinal lymph nodes

## 8.3 Detection and Staging of Recurrent Disease

Locoregional recurrence and hepatic metastatic disease are the most common sites of relapse in patients with rectal carcinoma and usually occur in the first two years after resection of the primary tumor. Early diagnosis of local recurrence at the level of the anastomosis and identification of liver metastases are very important for patient care because surgery is the only curable option. One of the most challenging matters in post-therapy patients with locally advanced primary tumors is differentiation of surgical scarring and radiation fibrosis from viable tumor. PET/CT performed 3–6 months after radiotherapy is able to diagnose tumor recurrence by detecting abnormal metabolic activity in the presacral surgical bed and has been noted to have a sensitivity of 84–100%, specificity of 80–100%, positive predictive value of 76–88%, and negative predictive value of 92–100%. Thus, on this aspect PET/CT is superior to multi-detector CT and MRI [10, 14–16] (Figs. 8.2, and 8.3.).

Moreover, FDG-PET/CT with its whole-body imaging capabilities has a significantly higher sensitivity (92%) for detection of extrahepatic metastatic disease than does CT or MRI and can play a crucial role in determining whether patients are suitable candidates for curative surgery. It seems that incorporation of PET/CT into the preoperative investigation of patients with recurrent disease and potential resectable local or hepatic lesions leads to reduced morbidity due to futile surgery and probably also to a considerable cost saving [14, 15, 17].

Another situation in which PET/CT is very helpful is the evaluation of patients with progressively elevated carcinoembryonic antigen (CEA) and no identifiable lesions on conventional imaging modalities (Figs. 8.4, and 8.5). In this patient population FDG-PET and PET/CT have reported sensitivity, specificity, positive and negative predictive values for detection of recurrence 79–100%, 50–83%, 89–95%, and 85–100%, respectively [15–17].

Additionally, several studies have shown that PET/CT may also be useful for detecting recur-

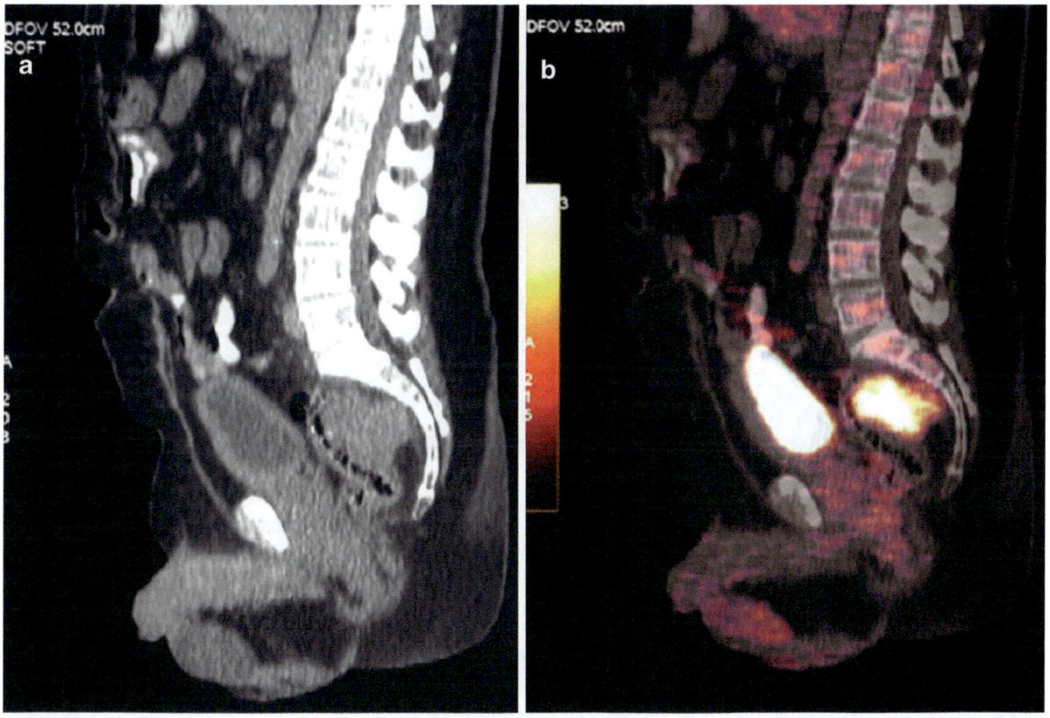


**Fig. 8.2** (**a**), (**b**) A 62-year-old patient with rectal carcinoma, status post-surgery, and chemoradiotherapy. Sagittal CT and fused PET/CT images reveal increased FDG uptake in a presacral mass representing local recurrence

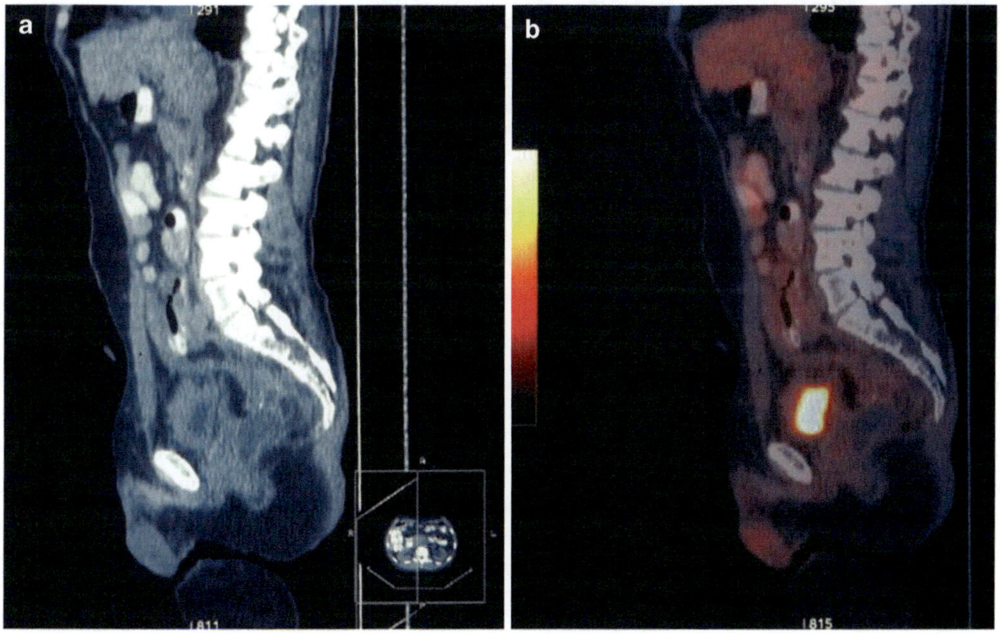


**Fig. 8.3** (**a**), (**b**) A 72-year-old patient with rectal carcinoma, status post-surgery, and chemoradiotherapy. Sagittal CT and fused PET/CT images reveal no FDG uptake in presacral soft tissue representing post-radiation fibrosis

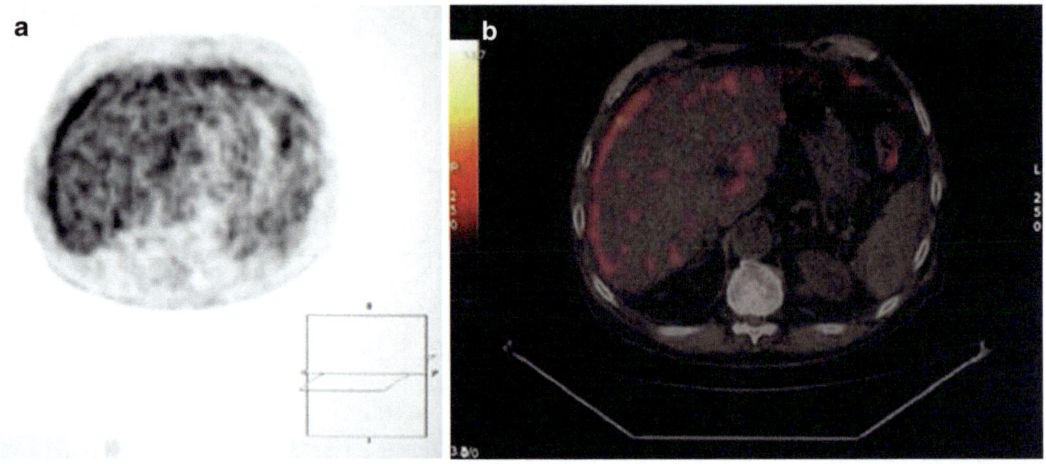


**Fig. 8.4** (**a**), (**b**) A 68-year-old man status post-treatment for rectal cancer presenting with rising CEA serum levels and negative results on CT imaging. Axial PET and corresponding fused PET/CT image of the abdomen show diffuse infiltration of the anterolateral peritoneum

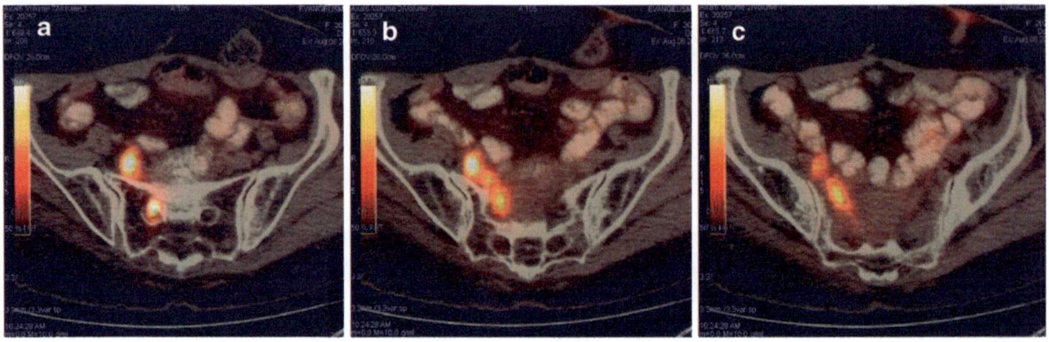


**Fig. 8.5** (**a**), (**b**), (**c**) A 63-year-old patient with rectal carcinoma, status post-surgery, and chemoradiotherapy, with rising CEA serum levels and negative results on CT imaging. Axial fused PET/CT images of the pelvis show infiltration of the right sciatic nerve

rence in patients with suspicious clinical findings and/or radiologic features regardless of the CEA level [8].

## 8.4 Monitoring Treatment Response and Planning of Radiation Therapy

Although the gold standard for assessing the tumoral response to therapy is histopathological analysis, interest in imaging for post-treatment response assessment is growing. Traditionally, cancer response to therapy is based on comparison of tumor sizes visualized on conventional imaging modalities (most commonly CT) before and after treatment. According to response evaluation criteria in solid tumors (RECIST) a tumor is considered responding when there is at least a 30% decrease of its largest diameter. Although the RECIST criteria are widely accepted in current clinical practice, there is a weak correlation between changes in tumor size and patient outcome. Moreover, biologic response to therapy may precede morphologic changes and residual masses may lack any malignant activity. Several recent studies and meta-analyses show that the combined functional and anatomical information provided by FDG-PET/CT seems to be very helpful in monitoring therapeutic activity [1, 8, 14, 15, 18–21].

Preoperative chemoradiotherapy in locally advanced rectal tumors has been noted to downstage the disease and allow sphincter preserving surgery in selected cases. Furthermore, it has been reported to increase the rate of complete surgical resection and reduce the risk of local recurrence, compared with postoperative treatment [1, 15, 22, 23]. The tumoral response to this neoadjuvant chemoradiotherapy is very heterogeneous and ranges from complete response, seen in 8–31% of the patients, to no response at all, while most patients (54–75%) achieve a partial response. Discrimination of responders from nonresponders with FDG-PET/CT has based on several predictive parameters including visual response, standardized uptake value (SUV), percentage SUV reduction (Response Index = RI), total lesion glycolysis (TLG), and metabolic tumor volume (MTV). The most studied PET parameter in therapy response prediction is the RI, which expresses the relative change in SUV measured before and after treatment and reflects a semiquantitative estimation of FDG activity within a selected lesion [8, 18–21].

However, there is a substantial variability among different studies in selecting optimal time for imaging and defining a minimum post-therapeutic SUV reduction indicative of response. In addition, hypermetabolic inflammatory changes that may be present after radiation therapy can cause issues with image interpretation and limit the accuracy of FDG-PET/CT in assessing tumor response [10]. Thus, although the available data suggest that $^{18}$F-FDG-PET/CT may be a very useful contribution to the conventional imaging modalities in the assessment of treatment response, the international guidelines still state that PET/CT should not be used to monitor progress of neoadjuvant therapy [18]. Further investigation with multicenter studies is needed to define the role of $^{18}$F-FDG-PET/CT imaging for predicting response to neoadjuvant therapy in patients with rectal cancer.

Another field, in which FDG-PET/CT can provide additional information, is the early detection of residual malignancy after targeted therapies in patients with unresectable liver metastases. Treatment choices for these patients include local radiofrequency ablation, selective internal radiation therapy, and transcatheter arterial chemoembolization. Identification of increased focal metabolic activity in the area of a treated lesion is considered as persistent disease. The reported negative predictive value of PET/CT scans performed at 1–4 weeks and at 3–11 months after targeted therapy is 100%, whereas the positive predictive value ranges from 80 to 88% [8, 10, 15]. Moreover, because the aim of many locoregional therapies is to stabilize disease rather than reduce tumor size, measuring both metabolic and anatomic response by PET/CT is preferable to measuring anatomic response alone by CT or MRI [8].

There are limited data in the literature supporting the use of FDG-PET/CT in radiotherapy planning for rectal cancer. PET/CT is reported to provide useful information for identification of more aggressive tumor subvolumes that should receive higher doses of radiation leading to accurate delineation of tumor volume, more effective local tumor control, and decreased toxicity [8, 11]. Although the NCCN is increasingly recognizing the effectiveness of PET/CT on tumor delineation for radiotherapy planning, the impact of PET on patient outcomes has yet to be established [8].

## 8.5 PET/CT Radiomics in Rectal Cancer

PET/CT-based radiomics literature in rectal cancer is rather limited with most of the studies analyzing colorectal cancer patients in general and, thus, mixing different kind of malignancies. There are only a few publications mainly targeted to the prediction of tumor response to neoadjuvant treatment in patients with locally advanced rectal cancer [5, 24–26].

Intratumoral heterogeneity and tumor genetic mutational status are the parameters that have mostly been investigated with controversial results [27–29]. Bang et al., [28] in their study of 74 patients, that investigated 50 textural parameters for predicting tumor responses to neoadjuvant chemoradiotherapy failed to show significant associations between any of these features and treatment response, whereas Shen et al., [29] in their study of 169 patients with newly diagnosed, locally advanced rectal cancer, that evaluated 68 textural features using a different AI technique reported high accuracy in prediction of pathological complete response. Obviously, multicenter, larger, prospective, clinical studies and independent validation of existing artificial intelligence techniques are needed before clinical use in personalized treatment planning.

## 8.6 Conclusions

FDG-PET/CT can be reliably used in the evaluation of patients with rectal carcinoma, particularly for the assessment of residual presacral masses after treatment, the localization and staging of recurrent disease before surgery, and the investigation of cases with progressive elevation of serum CEA and negative findings on conventional imaging techniques. The available data suggest that PET/CT is very useful in assessing neoadjuvant therapy response in patients with locally advanced rectal cancer and targeted therapies in patients with unresectable liver metastases. There may also be a potential role of PET/CT in planning of radiation therapy, but NCCN has not yet officially recommended it. Finally, PET/CT-based radiomics is a new, increasingly explored and promising field in modern oncologic imaging but its implementation in every day clinical practice is limited mainly due to lack of standardization and reproducibility of AI techniques.

## References

1. De Geus-Oei LF, Vriens D, van Laarhoven HWM, et al. Monitoring and predicting response to therapy with 18F-FDG PET in colorectal cancer: a systematic review. J Nucl Med. 2009;50:43S–54S.
2. Raman SP, Chen Y, Fishman EK. Evolution of imaging in rectal cancer: multimodality imaging with MDCT, MRI and PET. J Gastrointest Oncol. 2015;6(2):172–84.
3. Network, N.C.C. NCCN clinical practice guidelines in oncology: rectal cancer, version 1.2016. J Natl Compr Canc Netw. 2015;7(8):838–81.
4. Lee JW, Lee SM. Radiomics in oncological PET/CT: clinical applications. Nucl Med Mol Imaging. 2018;52:170–89.
5. Li W, Liu H, Cheng F, Li Y, Li S, Yan J. Artificial intelligence applications for oncological positron emission tomography imaging. Eur J Radiol. 2021;134:109448.
6. Yakar M, Etiz D. Artificial intelligence in rectal cancer. Artif Intell Gastroenterol. 2021;2(2):10–68.
7. Agarwal A, Marcus C, Xiao J, et al. FDG PET/CT in the management of colorectal and anal cancers. Am J Roentgenol. 2014;203:1109–19.
8. Ozis SE, Soydal C, Akyol C, et al. The role of 18F-fluorodeoxyglucose positron emission tomography/computed tomography in the primary staging of rectal cancer. World J Surg Oncol. 2014;12:26–32.
9. Lonneux M. FDG-PET and PET/CT in colorectal cancer. PET Clin. 2008;3:147–53.
10. O'Connor OJ, McDermott S, Slattery J, et al. The use of PET-CT in the assessment of patients with colorectal carcinoma. Int J Surg Oncol. 2011;14:846512.
11. Patel DA, Chang ST, Goodman KA, et al. Impact of integrated PET/CT on variability of target volume delineation in rectal cancer. Technol Cancer Res Treat. 2007;6(1):31–6.
12. Cerny M, Dunet V, Prior JO, et al. Initial staging of locally advanced rectal cancer and regional lymph nodes. Comparison of diffusion-Weighted MRI with 18F-FDG-PET/CT. Clin Nucl Med. 2016;41:289–95.
13. Jeong JH, Cho IH, ChuN KA, et al. Correlation between apparent diffusion coefficients and standardized uptake values in hybrid 18F-FDG PET/MR: preliminary results in rectal cancer. Nucl Med Mol Imaging. 2016;50:150–6.
14. Hebertson RA, Lee ST, Tebbutt N, et al. The expanding role of PET technology in the management of patients with colorectal cancer. Ann Oncol. 2007;18:1774–81.
15. De Geus-Oei LF, Ruers TJM, Punt CJA, et al. FDG-PET in colorectal cancer. Cancer Imaging. 2006;6:S71–81.
16. Delbeke D, Martin WH. FDG PET and PET/ CT for colorectal cancer. Methods Mol Biol. 2011;727:77–103.
17. Mosley CK, Schuster DM. Practical PET/CT of the abdomen. In: Wani RL, editor. RSNA categorical course in diagnostic radiology—clinical PET and PET/CT imaging; 2007. p. 71–81.
18. Maffione AM, Marzola MC, Caprici C, Calletti PM, Rubello D. Value of 18F-FDG PET for predicting response to neoadjuvant therapy in rectal cancer: systematic review and meta-analysis. Am J Roentgenol. 2015;204:1261–8.
19. Joye I, Deroose CM, Vandecaveye V, Haustermans K. The role of diffusion-weighted MRI and 18F-FDG PET/CT in the prediction of pathologic complete response after radiochemotherapy for rectal

cancer: a systematic review. Radiother Oncol. 2014;113:158–65.
20. Rymer B, Curtis NJ, Siddiqui MR, Chand M. FDG PET/CT can assess the response of locally advanced rectal cancer to neoadjuvant chemoradiotherapy: evidence from meta-analysis and systematic review. Clin Nucl Med. 2016;41(5):371–5.
21. Koo PJ, Kim SJ, Chang S, Kwak JJ. Interim fluorine-18 fluorodeoxyglucose positron emission tomography/computed tomography to predict pathologic response to preoperative chemoradiotherapy and prognosis in patients with locally advanced rectal cancer. Clin Colorectal Cancer. 2016;15(4):e213–9.
22. Guerra L, Niespolo R, Di Pisa G, et al. Change in glucose metabolism measured by 18F-FDG PET/ CT as a predictor of histopathologic response to neoadjuvant treatment in rectal cancer. Abdom Imaging. 2011;36:38–45.
23. Gascini GL, Avallone A, Delrio P, et al. 18F FDG PET is an early predictor of pathologic tumor response to preoperative radiochemotherapy in locally advanced rectal cancer. J Nucl Med. 2006;47:1241–8.
24. Sadaghiani MS, Rowe SP, Sheikhbahaei S. Applications of artificial intelligence in oncologic 18F-FDG PET/CT imaging: a systematic review. Ann Transl Med. 2021;9(9):823–35.
25. Dinapoli N, Casa C, Barbaro B, et al. Radiomics for rectal cancer. Transl Cancer Res. 2016;5(4):424–31.
26. Badic B, Tixier F, Cheze Le Reste C, Hatt M, Visvikis D. Radiogenomics in colorectal cancer, (review). Cancers (Basel). 2021;13:973–92.
27. Lovinfosse P, Koopmansch B, Lambert F, Jodogne S, Kustermans G, Hatt M, et al. (18)F-FDG PET/CT imaging in rectal cancer: relationship with the RAS mutational status. Br J Radiol. 2016;89:20160212.
28. Bang JI, Ha S, Kang SB, Lee KW, Lee HS, Kim JS, et al. Prediction of neoadjuvant radiation chemotherapy response and survival using pretreatment [(18)F] FDG PET/CT scans in locally advanced rectal cancer. Eur J Nucl Med Mol Imaging. 2016;43:422–31.
29. Shen W-C, Chen S-W, Wu K-C, et al. Prediction pathological complete response in rectal cancer after chemoradiotherapy with a random forest using 18F-fluorodeoxyglucose positron emission tomography and computed tomography radiomics. Ann Transl Med. 2020;8(5):207–18.

# Advances in Neuroendocrine Tumor Imaging, Including PET and Artificial Intelligence (AI)

9

Dimitrios Fotopoulos, Kapil Shirodkar, and Himansu Shekhar Mohanty

## 9.1 Introduction

Although neuroendocrine tumors (NET) can arise from various neuroendocrine cells containing tissues, in clinical practice, they arise majorly from the gastroenteropancreatic (GEP) sites and the lungs.

Gastrointestinal neuroendocrine tumors (NET) range over a broad spectrum of aggressiveness and differentiation, including well-differentiated tumors and poorly differentiated carcinomas. They are classified according to WHO based on cell proliferation, Ki index, and the number of mitoses, assigned designation from G1 to G3.

The inherent limitations of conventional cross-sectional imaging techniques like CT and MRI in detecting lesions smaller than 2 cm and tumors without discernible arterial phase enhancement (Up to 20%) are prone to false negatives. Hence, hybrid imaging with PET-CT has overtaken CT and MRI in identification and staging.

D. Fotopoulos (✉) · K. Shirodkar
Royal Lancaster Infirmary, University Hospitals Morecambe Bay NHS Foundation Trust, Lancaster, UK
e-mail: d.fotopoulos@mbht.nhs.uk

H. S. Mohanty
Yashoda Super Specialty and Cancer Hospital, Ghaziabad, Delhi NCR, India

Recent advances in computer technology, improved computational power of chipsets, along the acquisition of large radiology datasets have provided opportunities for machine learning and optimization of diagnostics using deep and machine learning algorithms and deep neural networks to unlock the true potential of imaging data into meaningful insights aimed at better lesion detection, optimization of image acquisition, and better targeting of therapy. These improved insights or "consensus-derived experience" from machine learning can then be used for further deep learning to design neural networks with the ultimate goal of improving diagnostic and treatment techniques.

Currently, various research studies are published in the public domain, which aids in detection, segmentation, classification (radiophenomics), characterization (radiomics), and statistical classification (prediction/prognosis).

## 9.2 SSTR-Based Imaging

Conventional CT is better at detecting lung lesions. Diffusion-weighted imaging (DWI) allows better lesion detection in the liver and pancreas than CT. PET/CT and PET/MR combined metabolic and structural imaging to further improve imaging studies' diagnostic accuracy.



J. A. Andreou et al. (eds.), *Artificial Intelligence in PET/CT Oncologic Imaging*,
https://doi.org/10.1007/978-3-031-10090-1_9

Somatostatin receptors (SSTR) are expressed in a majority of NETs and are responsible for the shift from conventional image acquisition to molecular imaging for both diagnostic and targeted therapy.

SSTR imaging gives up to 50% improved sensitivity and up to 30% improved specificity in primary tumor detection compared to multiphasic contrast CT.

SSTR imaging with gallium has revolutionized the diagnostic approach to neuroendocrine tumors. The agents currently used are Ga-68 1,4,7,10-tetraazacyclododecane-1,4,7,10-tetraacetic acid (DOTA)-Phe1-Tyr3-Octreotide (TOC)/Tyr3-Octreotide (TATE)/NaI3-Octreotide (NOC)/lanreotide PET/CT or 99mTc-hydrazinonicotinyl (HYNIC)-TOC/111InDOTA-TOC/lanreotide scintigraphy, 4,14–17 among others—referred to onwards as Ga-68 SSTR [1].

The agents used for SSTR imaging (SRI) can be either agonists or antagonists. The majority of the clinically used tracers are somatostatin agonists (68 Ga-DOTATE, 69 Ga-DOTATOC, and 68Ga-DOTANOC); however, antagonists (68Ga-NODAGA-JR11) have shown higher tumor uptakes, improved lesion detection, better image contrast, and overall higher sensitivity in preclinical settings. However, further research is required to ascertain whether antagonist tracers could be used instead of traditional agonists in the clinical diagnostic setting (Fig. 9.1).

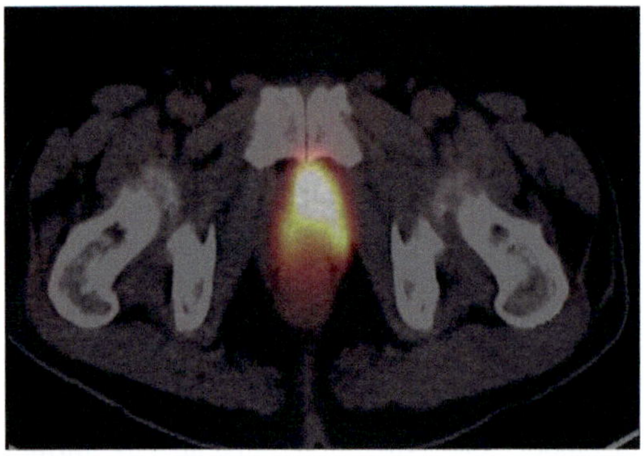

**Fig. 9.1** Axial fused image of Gallium-68 DOTATOC scan showing uptake in NET of prostate

Gallium has shown 4–8 times more affinity for SST2 receptors than yttrium or indium derivatives. Although 68Galium has been traditionally used due to its wider availability, its limited availability from a generator source and higher half-life (68 min) has always been a technical limitation. 64 Copper has recently challenged this with a half-life of 12.7 h and better spatial resolution. 64 Cu-DOTATATE has been recently approved by the US-FDA for clinical use and has shown some promising results by detecting more additional true positive lesions and greater SUVmax in tumors and the background organs. However, higher beta-radiation and limited physical availability, limits the use of 64Cu in the current settings.

The hallmark of the well-differentiated (G1) and intermediate differentiated group (G2) is the lower expression of SSTR. The higher the SSTR expression in NET, the lower the tumor's grade and vice versa. These receptors can be targeted by modifying a small portion of the somatostatin peptides for artificially increasing the affinity for specific receptor subtypes.

Ga 68 SSTR imaging comes into its own in identifying tumors with SSTRs—generally, higher tumor differentiation is associated with lower SSTR detection. SST2a is the most expressed receptor subtype, followed by SST3 and SST1. Different octreotide chelator complexes have different affinities for the receptors, and the clinically relevant SSTR-based imaging targets these receptors.

The Krenning scoring system is a visual assessment of Ga-68 SSTR uptake on a 0–4 scale using liver uptake (up to 2) and splenic uptake (up to 4) as reference points. Most probably, Ga-68 TATE is the agent of choice when a primary neuroendocrine tumor is suspected, based on a combination of clinical symptoms pointing to an underlying gastroenteropancreatic neuroendocrine tumor with a relevant biochemical profile.

The superiority of PET NET imaging compared to gamma scintigraphy techniques has been well documented in previous research

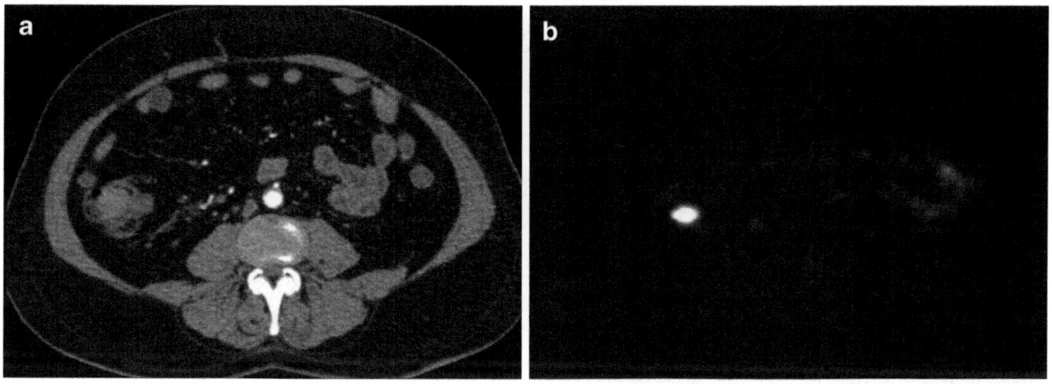


**Fig. 9.2** (**a**) Axial fused image of CECT Abdomen showing enhancing mass in the cecum. (**b**) Corresponding Gallium-68 DOTATOC scan showing uptake in the cecal mass

papers, and they provide higher sensitivity and have the most significant impact on clinical decision-making. Lower radiation dose than CT is another advantage; however, longer acquisition times are a strong deterrent (Fig. 9.2).

Also, false positives of Ga-68 PET/CT can arise due to many causes. These include the (1) uncinate process of the pancreas (well-established area of false-positive uptake); (2) intra-abdominal splenosis-related pseudo-nodules in Post-Splenectomy states (as splenectomy is frequently employed in the therapeutic operative regimen of NET tumors and residual splenic parenchyma in the splenosis manifests Ga-68 uptake); (3) osteophytes, because of SSTR2 expression in osteoclasts; (4) pituitary, thyroid, kidneys, and adrenals; and (5) sites of inflammation [2].

## 9.3 Ga-68 SSTR-vs. F18-FDG

In comparison between the two, Ga-68 SSTR PET/CT outperforms F18-FDG PET in disease sensitivity, although they have similar specificity; however, the combination of both maximizes the detection rate.

F-18 PET-FDG is more sensitive to high-grade tumors and less likely to express SSTRs. As high-grade tumors are more metabolically active, they are more likely to engage glycolytic energy-generating metabolic pathway which FDG-PET/CT better detects.

In comparison, Ga-68 TATE is more efficacious for highly differentiated tumors, retaining their original ability to express SSTRs, prone to selective Ga-68 uptake, albeit metabolically less active.

The arrival of SSTR-specific PET imaging has not rendered F-18 PET/CT imaging obsolete; on the contrary, a study by Binderup et al. showed that low sensitivity of F-18 FDG-PET studies is associated with a prolonged survival rate [Binderup et al.] (Fig. 9.3).

F-18 FDG/PET remains a highly reliable study for the prognostication of disease progression [Garin et al., Rodrigues et al.].

Additional value of F-18 FDG/PET is that it is an excellent prognosticator of survival when negative in a patient with SSTR expression—in particular, high values correlate with decreased overall survival.

A particular group (Binderup et al.) went so far as to define a cut-off value of SUV 9 as a prognosticator of greater mortality.

These studies render the use of F18-FDG-PET/CT and Ga-68 SSTR PET/CT not mutually exclusive but rather complementary. They serve to identify different populations of cells, depicting different identities, including levels of cell differentiation, thereby facilitating guided biopsy targeting different phenotypes. Therefore, it is self-evident that this would directly impact both proper tumor grading and tumor prognostication, as blind biopsies might miss a tumor subsite har-

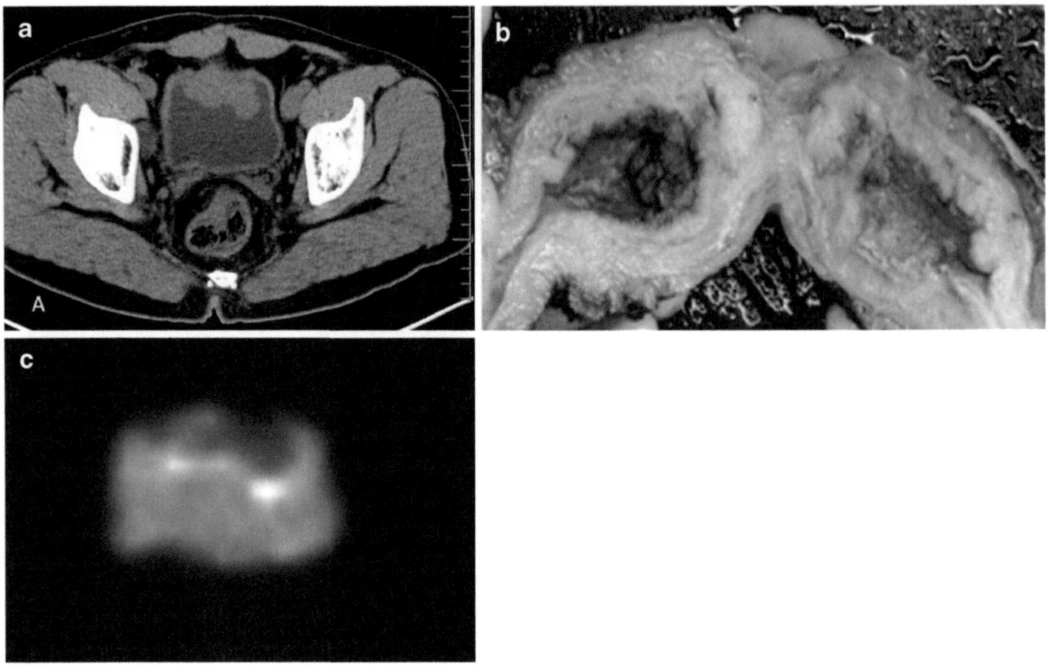


**Fig. 9.3** (**a**) Axial NCCT images of pelvis showing mass in the urinary bladder. Histopathology photograph showing high-grade NET. (**b**) Postoperative gross specimen image showing the NET. (**c**) Insignificant uptake on corresponding PET images

boring different cell populations, hence underestimating tumor grade, directly affecting its therapy and patient prognosis.

One additional advantage of Ga-68 SSTR PET/CT compared to F-18 FDG/PET CT is that the former can identify subcentimeter lesions thanks to its high target-to-background contrast, a property especially true of GaTate (exemplified by the fact that SUV of GaTate is significantly higher than FDG). Ga-68 outperforms FDG PET for the identification of bony secondary deposits.

It is advised to perform F-18 FDG/PET initially and in cases where Ga-68 SSTR PET/CT shows progression.

Furthermore, it should be reminded that since the introduction of checkpoint inhibitors, the mere application of RECIST criteria does not apply to accurate follow-up, as size reduction is not applicable for tumor response assessment. Instead, iRECIST criteria should be employed. Identifying this tumor subgroup with a high concentration of SSRs has been paramount since introducing peptide receptor radionuclide therapy.

## 9.4 Theragnostics in Neuroendocrine Tumors

Theragnostics (hybrid of the two Greek words Therapeutics and Diagnostics) is the principle of tailoring a specific therapeutic regimen to a patient deemed suitable for this therapy through diagnostics.

The principle of PRRT (peptide receptor radionuclide therapy) exploits the hypothesis that targeted high doses of radiation, mediated by agents specifically attached at high-affinity sites with an abundance of somatostatin receptors, allow for locally administered higher radiation dose. PRRT is far more efficacious than an external radiotherapy beam, on the condition that the concentration of SSTR receptors is high and is accomplished by specifically binding beta-emitting particles with a peptide that attach to SSTR.

Radiolabeled somatostatin analogs can be used for therapy in patients with refractory disease, provided the tumors express SSTRs on their surface. Yttrium-90 (90Y) and Lutetium-177 (177Lu) are the most frequently used radionuclides, with different emitted particles, energies, and tissue penetration.

If therapy-related systemic complications, particularly hematologic, are factored in, it is inferred that careful selection of patients is mandated, based not only on identification of somatostatin receptors expression but also on imaging-related quantified parameters.

However, no uniform agreement has been reached so far in the current literature to set a specific SUV cut-off value.

The introduction of PRRT has necessitated the principle of somatostatin analog dosimetry, in the interest of both patient safety and therapeutic efficacy, particularly by evaluating quantitative parameters about tumor texture, known as radiomics, to create an individualized tumor profile that might prognosticate potential tumor response. However, no imaging study currently has validated this attempt in neuroendocrine tumors.

This is further compounded by the fact that efficacy of PRRT treatment cannot be relied upon RECIST criteria, as tumor size does not correlate well with overall survival prolongation—in up to almost one-third of PRRT therapy, the overall tumor size might even increase (without adverse implications for patient prognosis). This further exemplifies the fact that conventional imaging alone is not sufficient for response assessment [3].

## 9.5 Tentative Approach to AI in PET/CT Regarding Neuroendocrine Tumors

Artificial intelligence (AI) is a computer-based entity that tries to emulate and even surpass human intelligence with pinpoint accuracy based on algorithmic computational models, deep learning (DL), machine learning (ML), and deep neural networks (DNNs) to facilitate clinical decisions and treatment. Using complex algorithms to post-process complex multiparametric morphological and functional imaging data, AI has enormous potential to facilitate improved image acquisition, improved lesion detection, overall improved diagnostic accuracy, improved imaging workflows, and improved targeted therapy, making it a hot commodity in the field of oncology.

It also allows new opportunities for treatment response assessment and survival prognostication using complex algorithms for automated post-processing of images acquired in routine clinical practice to extract standard quantitative parameters (currently done manually like size, percentage contrast enhancement, and SUV values) as well as analyze information beyond standard parameters to generate more insights into tumor burden assessment, disease response patterns as well as dose reduction and attenuation correction.

However, the literature regarding Artificial Intelligence in neuroendocrine tumor imaging is either sparse, not clinically validated, or not yet out in the public domain.

A study by Huejiao Han et al. [4] concerned itself with AI application in differentiation between pancreatic cystadenoma and pancreatic neuroendocrine tumors, but without reference to PET-CT.

The latest meta-analysis study by Ephraim Partouche et al. [5] conducted to standardize imaging practices in pancreatic neuroendocrine tumors identified a host of factors that constitute barriers towards effective integration of AI in neuroendocrine imaging studies. These include discrepancies between clinical and radiologic studies, geographic non-uniformity of studies, non-conformity to the proposed guidelines (e.g., ENETS 2017), and under-representation in the available literature of novel PET/CT imaging methods when compared to their conventional CT (and MRI) counterparts. This inhomogeneity will have to be addressed to achieve standardization of data towards ensuring pooled data use.

Ignat et al. [6] tried to preoperatively grade pancreatic NETs based on CECT imaging and validation of deep learning using convoluted neural networks. The challenges they raised include the complexity of data, difficulties with mathematical interpretation, signal differentiation from noise, and the complexity of the bio-mathematical models. They suggested mathematical integration of functional imaging, circulating transcriptomics, and "omic" clustering amalgamated with master regulator tumor interrogation to provide the basis for a new discipline of neuroendocrine Oncotheranomics.

Zimmerman et al. [7] tried to use machine learning techniques to provide better decision support/decision trees to reduce NET misdiagnosis using a combination of factors (e.g., abdominal pain, and endoscopic/biopsy procedure, vomiting) or longer times to diagnosis (e.g., asthma diagnosis with visits to >6 providers) to increase the probability of NET detection.

Schwyzer et al. [8] explored the possibility of using machine learning algorithms to analyze PET CT imaging data to allow automated lung cancer detection using very low radiation doses to improve the specificity of lung cancer screening tests.

Koong et al. [9] described how machine learning could detect and predict treatment outcomes of pituitary neuroendocrine and other sellar tumors by utilizing machine learning of MRI radiomic data of the sellar region.

Wei et al. discussed in their review paper the various application of sophisticated image processing and machine learning algorithms to PET/CT imaging in several applications, including segmentation, reconstruction, and outcome modeling, with a special focus on the oncological radiotherapy domain areas and image-based prediction of treatment outcomes.

Zheng Q et al. [10] published a paper about utilizing AI algorithms for radiology imaging to provide equivalent or improved NET tumor metastasis detection than healthcare professionals.

Niazi et al. [11] developed deep learning methods to reduce pathologists' workload by identifying tumor boundaries in images of Ki67-stained NETs using transfer learning techniques.

Hirai et al. [12] used deep learning AI to classify subepithelial lesions on EUS images with higher diagnostic performance than expert endoscopists leading to an improved clinical diagnosis.

Trebeschi et al. [13] explored the possibility of using AI algorithms to auto-quantify noninvasive radiomic biomarkers to assess response to immunotherapy in both neoadjuvant and palliative oncology settings for improved patient stratification.

Partouche et al. [14] advocated standardization of PNETs imaging to accumulate extensive homogenous imaging pooled data to enable AI data mining to identify new imaging biomarkers for treatment effectiveness, ultimately leading to better PNET treatment optimization.

Other potential application examples of AI in NET imaging which are currently being researched include:

1. Hyperplane or decision boundary separation to better classify imaging data
2. Decision support tool giving decision algorithms based on machine learning
3. Automated image detection and segmentation
4. Pattern recognition for classification of benign from malignant masses
5. Better 3D extrapolation of 2D imaging volume data
6. Pre-processing of imaging data for artifact reduction and automatic imaging protocol selection
7. 3D and 4D segmentation of dynamic contrast MR data

The hurdles of various AI studies for integration into daily clinical practice include (1) standardization of results, (2) robust validation by regulatory authorities, (3) reproducibility, (4) lack of gold reference standards, (5) absence of consensus of results or cross-study comparisons, (6) availability of abundant anonymized open clinical and imaging data sharing for research purposes due to strict patient safety and confidentiality issues, and (7) lack of harmonization between various AI guidelines [15].

However, AI is continuing to gain traction in the last decade and hopefully will overcome the various discovered and undiscovered digital, physical, financial, statistical, human, and mental limitations to become better integrated into the healthcare systems with the ultimate goal of better patient care. However, for AI to reach its full potential, high-quality data, including outcome information, is mandatory to train the sophisticated AI algorithms on large prospective trials using standardized examinations.

## References

1. Margarida Rodrigues MD, Svirydenka H, Virgolini I. Theragnostics in neuroendocrine tumors. PET Clin. 2021;16(3):365–73.
2. Hofman MS, et al. Somatostatin receptor Imaging with Ga-68 DOTATATE PET/CT: clinical utility, normal patterns, pearls and pitfalls in interpretation. Radiographics. 2013;35(2):500–16.
3. Wong RKS, Metser U, Veit-Haibach P. Neuroendocrine tumors imaging perspective. PET Clin. 2021;16(3):353–64.
4. Han X, Yang J, Luo J, Chen P, Zhang Z, Alu A, Xiao Y, Ma X. Application of CT-based radiomics in discriminating pancreatic cystadenomas from pancreatic neuroendocrine tumours using machine learning methods. Front Oncol. 2021;11:606677.
5. Partouche E, Yeh R, Eche T, Rozenblum L, Carrere N, Guimbaud R, Dierickx LO, Rousseau H, Dercle L, Mokrane F-Z. Updated trends in imaging practices for pancreatic neuroendocrine tumors (PNETs): a systematic review and meta-analysis to pave the way for standardization in the new era of big data and artificial intelligence. Front Oncol. 2021;11:628408.
6. Ignat IM, Bodeic AD. The use of deep learning and neural networks in imaging: welcome to the new mathematical milieu of medicine. Neuroendocrinology. 2020;110(5):322–7.
7. Zimmerman NM, Ray D, Princic N, Moynihan M, Clarke C, Phan A. Exploration of machine learning techniques to examine the journey to neuroendocrine tumor diagnosis with real-world data. Future Oncol. 2021;17(24):3217–30.
8. Schwyzer M, Ferraro DA, Muehlematter UJ, Curioni-Fontecedro A, Huellner MW, Von Schulthess GK, Kaufmann PA, Burger IA, Messerli M. Automated detection of lung cancer at ultralow dose PET/CT by deep neural networks–initial results. Lung Cancer. 2018;126:170–3.
9. Koong K, Preda V, Jian A, Liquet-Weiland B, Di Ieva A. Application of artificial intelligence and radiomics in pituitary neuroendocrine and sellar tumors: a quantitative and qualitative synthesis. Neuroradiology. 2021;64(4):647–68.
10. Zheng Q, Yang L, Zeng B, Li J, Guo K, Liang Y, Liao G. Artificial intelligence performance in detecting tumor metastasis from medical radiology imaging: a systematic review and meta-analysis. EClinicalMedicine. 2021;31:100669.
11. Niazi MK, Tavolara TE, Arole V, Hartman DJ, Pantanowitz L, Gurcan MN. Identifying tumor in pancreatic neuroendocrine neoplasms from Ki67 images using transfer learning. PLoS One. 2018;13(4):e0195621.
12. Hirai K, Kuwahara T, Furukawa K, Kakushima N, Furune S, Yamamoto H, Marukawa T, Asai H, Matsui K, Sasaki Y, Sakai D. Artificial intelligence-based diagnosis of upper gastrointestinal subepithelial lesions on endoscopic ultrasonography images. Gastric Cancer. 2021;25(2):382–91.
13. Trebeschi S, Drago SG, Birkbak NJ, Kurilova I, Călin AM, Pizzi AD, Lalezari F, Lambregts DM, Rohaan MW, Parmar C, Rozeman EA. Predicting response to cancer immunotherapy using noninvasive radiomic biomarkers. Ann Oncol. 2019;30(6):998–1004.
14. Partouche E, Yeh R, Eche T, Rozenblum L, Carrere N, Guimbaud R, Dierickx LO, Rousseau H, Dercle L, Mokrane FZ. Updated trends in imaging practices for pancreatic neuroendocrine tumors (PNETs): a systematic review and meta-analysis to pave the way for standardization in the new era of big data and artificial intelligence. Front Oncol. 2021;11:628408.
15. Thomasian NM, Kamel IR, Bai HX. Machine intelligence in non-invasive endocrine cancer diagnostics. Nat Rev Endocrinol. 2021;18(2):81–95.

# PET/CT in the Evaluation of Adrenal Gland Mass

# 10

Alexandra V. Nikaki

## 10.1 Introduction

Adrenal glands serve as potential sites for secondary infiltration of various cancers. Moreover, primary tumors can arise, either from the cortex or from the medulla of the glands. Single-photon emitters with g-camera procedures have long been used for the evaluation of primary tumors with high sensitivity and specificity. F-18-FDG-PET/CT has mostly been evaluated as a diagnostic tool in detection of adrenal metastasis, while other positron radiopharmaceuticals have been used for the identification and evaluation of disease extent in primary adrenal tumors.

## 10.2 PET/CT in Evaluation of Adrenal Masses in Cancer and Noncancer Patients

Although adrenal masses incidentally discovered in general population are usually benign and diagnosis is usually achieved by CT and MRI, they are common cause of differential diagnostic problems when conventional imaging is indeterminate in noncancer patients or when they consist of the only site of potential metastasis in cancer patients [1–5]. In the first case scenario, with sensitivity and negative predictive value of up to 100% [1], PET/CT may be helpful and should be considered [6].

Common primary tumors that metastasize in adrenal glands are from non-small cell lung cancer, gastrointestinal tract cancer, and melanoma. Sensitivity, specificity, and accuracy of FDG-PET/CT in identification and characterization of adrenal masses in cancer patients have been demonstrated to be high (Figs. 10.1 and 10.2). Qualitative analyses, using liver [2] or aorta uptake [7] as a reference standard, quantitative measurements using SUVmax cutoff values [2] or target to adjacent tissues' and organs' ratios, and a variety of interpretive criteria and scanning protocols have been proposed in order to augment the method's diagnostic capabilities. According to Jana et al. [2], visual interpretation is enough for discriminating between benign and malignant formations in cancer patients, while the utility of PET is invaluable for CT indeterminate adrenal lesions. Utilizing quantitative measurements, SUVmax 3.4 was reported to yield 95% sensitivity and 86% specificity [2], tumor-to-liver SUV ratio of 1.68 corresponds to 90, 91.1, and 90.4% sensitivity, specificity, and accuracy, respectively [4], while in a meta-analysis of 21 eligible studies, including 1391 lesions, reported sensitivity, specificity, accuracy, positive and negative likelihood ratio for characterizing adrenal masses as malignant or benign are 0.97, 0.91, 0.98, 11.1, and 0.04, respectively [3]. The method's high negative and

A. V. Nikaki (✉)
Docrates Cancer Center, Helsinki, Finland


J. A. Andreou et al. (eds.), *Artificial Intelligence in PET/CT Oncologic Imaging*,
https://doi.org/10.1007/978-3-031-10090-1_10

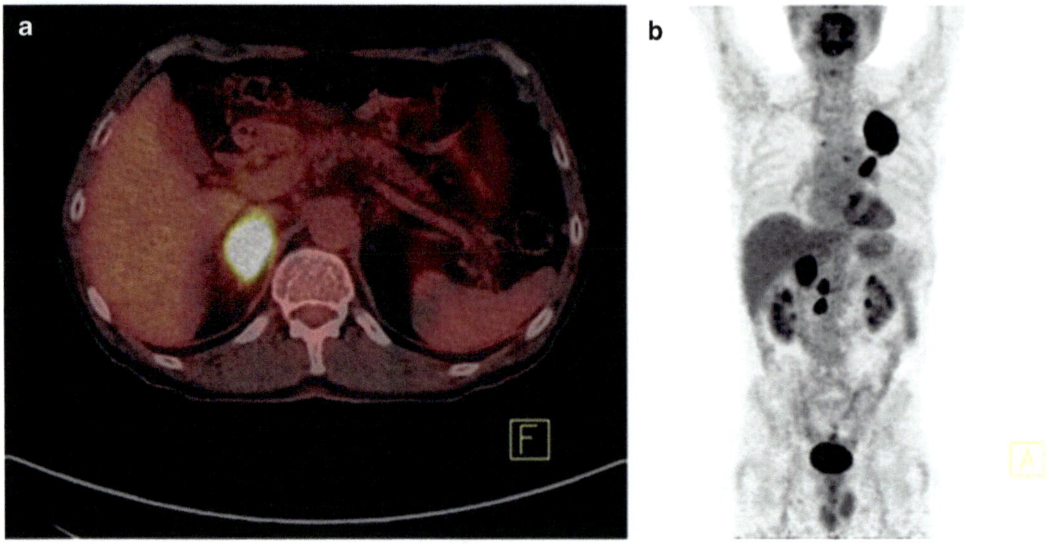


**Fig. 10.1** (**a**), (**b**) Adrenal metastasis in a patient with non-small-cell lung cancer—high FDG uptake

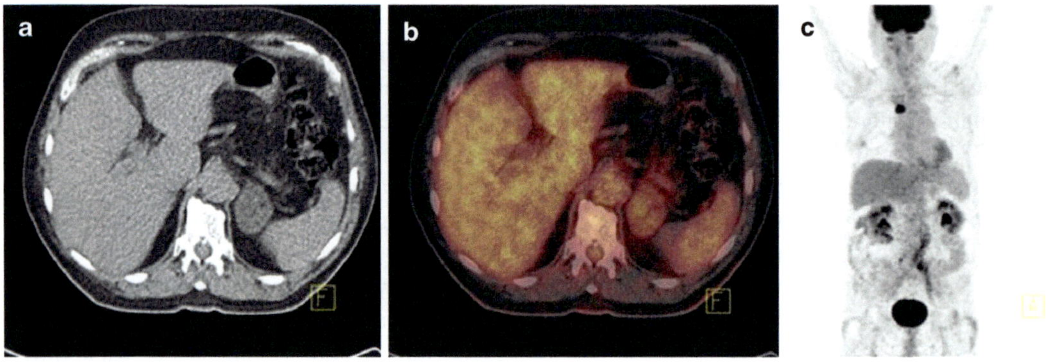


**Fig. 10.2** (**a**), (**b**), (**c**) Adrenal myelolipoma in a patient with non-small-cell lung cancer—FDG uptake lower than liver uptake

positive predictive values of ~93% are also confirmed in a later prospective study [8], and FDG uptake is reported as a significant predictor for malignancy [9]. Further, newer PET/CT device with advanced technology, i.e., time-of-flight PET/CT detectors or addition of CT histogram analysis from PET/CT-derived data, may add to the, anyway high, method's diagnostic potentiality, regardless of qualitative or quantitative measurements [7, 10, 11]. Thus further exploration of adrenal masses with other imaging techniques is considered unnecessary. However, mild uptake, equally increased metabolic activity in both adrenal glands, and size of less than 1 cm should be dealt with caution, as they might provoke false interpreting results [3, 7]. Lipid-poor and generally benign adrenal adenomas, hyperplasia as well as pheochromocytomas (PCCs), and tuberculosis constitute causes of false-positive results [2, 7, 9, 12].

## 10.3 PET/CT in Primary Tumors' Evaluation

Primary tumors of the adrenal glands arise either from the cortex, called adrenocortical carcinomas (ACC), or from the medulla, the most common being pheochromocytoma (PCC).

PCCs are paragangliomas (PGs) that arise from adrenal medulla and are usually diagnosed by their biochemical-functional profile in addition to a CT scan or MRI that reveal an adrenal mass. I-131- or I-123-MIBG complements further diagnostic approach, while somatostatin receptor scintigraphy has also been used [13]. Current approaching strategies if PCC is suspected may include gene profile expression and specific radiopharmaceutical utilization, according to the mutations detected. Although studies are scattered and patient sample is small in most of them, several positron emitting radiopharmaceuticals have been used in PCC investigation, summarized in a review of Havekes et al. [13] with F-18-dihydroxyphenylalanine (FDOPA) to present higher diagnostic accuracy in detection of PCCs as compared to I-123-MIBG. In addition, PET radiopharmaceuticals can be used for multifocal and metastatic disease detection or exclusion and recurrence assessing [13]. In a small sample of 12 patients with suspected or known relapse of PG, FDOPA-PET was reported superior to I-123-MIBG in assessing the burden of disease and changed therapeutic management in one patient [14]. Positive and negative predictive values of FDOPA-PET for the detection of PCCs-PGs are reported 94% and 85%, respectively, yielding an accuracy of 91%, with false results in Von Hippel-Lindau (VHL) and succinate dehydrogenase subunit B (SDHB)-related paraganglioma [15]. FDOPA uptake is not significantly different among the various genotypic tumor mutations [15]. In a direct comparison of FDOPA with MR/CT angiography, the authors highly recommend FDOPA-PET/CT as a diagnostic approach in patients with clinical symptoms of head and neck PG recurrence in the absence of somatostatin Ga-68-labeled agents [16].

Somatostatin analogs, such as DOTATOC, DOTATATE, and DOTANOC, labeled with positron emitting radionuclides—Ga-68—have also been used for evaluation of metastatic disease [13]. In a prospective study, Naswa et al. [17] demonstrated the superiority of Ga-68-DOTANOC over I-131-MIBG in evaluation of PCCs-PGs, concluding in alteration of therapeutic management of six patients. Evaluating the role of Ga-68-DOTATATE in PCCs-PGs at initial staging and follow-up, the authors proposed the utilization of this radiopharmaceutical in high-risk patients and patients with mutations correlated with familial syndromes [18]. However, during the process of dedifferentiation, tumors may lose their primary molecular characteristics, and therefore less specific radiopharmaceuticals, such as F-18-FDG, may be more suitable for imaging. In metastatic SDHB-associated PGs, FDG was reported to yield the highest sensitivity of the modalities used, up to 100% [19]. FDG-PET was also demonstrated to have higher sensitivity, as compared to I-123-MIBG and CT in the evaluation of metastatic disease in biochemically established PCCs and PGs, with a specificity of 90.2% [20].

Adrenocortical carcinoma is a rare tumor, with poor prognosis and high rates of recurrence. Metomidate (MTO), the methyl ester of etomidate, with its high and specific adrenocortical binding, labeled with the positron emitting C-11, has been evaluated in adrenal glands' pathology. Although C-11-MTO-PET could not differentiate between malignant and benign lesions, reported sensitivity and specificity for distinguishing adrenocortical versus non-adrenocortical pathology reach 89% and 96% compared to histopathologic findings [21]. A tumor-to-normal gland uptake cutoff ratio of 1.4 is associated with a risk of 99.5% for adrenocortical tumor [21]. Higher SUV values were reported for aldosterone-secreting tumors, compared to nonfunctional adenomas and to adrenocortical carcinoma [21, 22]. False-negative results were reported for lesions <1 cm and large necrosis [21]. C-11-MTO could potentially serve as complementary to CT and MRI for evaluation of adrenal pathology [22, 23]. Razifar et al. [24] reported improvement of image quality, reduction of image noise, and increase of structure contrast by using principal component analysis—masked volume wise (MVW). Medication, such as adrenal steroid inhibitors and chemotherapeutic agents, may reduce C-11-MTO uptake both in adrenocortical carcinoma lesions and in normal tissues [25]. While C-11-MTO-PET is specific to adrenocortical versus non-adrenocortical pathology evaluation, FDG-PET has been proposed for discriminating benign versus malignant lesions in adrenal glands. FDG-PET, with a sensitivity of ~90%, is proposed to be used complementary to CT for detection of recurrent and metastatic adrenocortical carcinoma. High mitotic rate is found to significantly relate to FDG uptake [26]. Although authors report that FDG avidity and FDG uptake volume are significantly correlated with overall survival [26] in their group of patients, such correlation between FDG uptake in the primary tumor with overall survival (OS) neither in metastatic nor in the non-metastatic patients is verified for initial staging patients in another study [27] and further investigation needs to be carried out. C-11-MTO and F-18-FDG may be utilized supplementarily, since they answer specific and different clinical questions. Further studies are required until both find their exact position in adrenocortical pathology evaluation.

Neuroblastoma consists of the most frequent extracranial tumor in children. Imaging modalities used during the workshop of neuroblastoma include ultrasound, CT, MRI, and bone and MIBG scintigraphy. Although neuroblastoma tumors usually concentrate FDG, FDG-PET could likely be reserved for non-MIBG avid neuroblastoma and perhaps for early response assessment if baseline FDG-PET showed at least moderate FDG uptake, as well as for follow-up [28, 29]. As compared to I-123-MIBG scintigraphy, FDG-PET appears less effective in evaluation of neuroblastoma disease burden; thus it cannot replace I-123-MIBG scintigraphy in everyday practice. However, FDG-PET bears significant prognostic value, since (a) FDG uptake higher than the respective MIBG uptake, (b) high tumoral SUVmax, and (c) identification of bone disease in PET are all correlated with lower survival interval in refractory or recurrent neuroblastoma patients going to receive I-131-MIBG therapy [30]. F-18-FDOPA has also been evaluated in advanced stage neuroblastoma at initial staging and during follow-up in suspicion of recurrence; the authors reported sensitivity and accuracy of 90% in a lesion-based analysis, higher than the respective values of I-123-MIBG, thus proposing FDOPA as potential radiopharmaceutical for neuroblastoma exploration either at initial staging or at restaging of the disease, as well as in inconclusive MIBG results [31].

## 10.4 Towards Artificial Intelligence

Artificial intelligence (AI) is a long-living term which describes the potentiality of computers to perform tasks that otherwise would need human intelligence to be achieved. Imaging acquisition as well as imaging interpretation could benefit from AI algorithms providing higher quality services in oncologic patients. Hybrid systems, PET/CT and PET/MRI are considered data-rich methods, which make them excellent tools for AI models application [32]. A systematic review [33] was attempted for AI implementation in FDG-PET imaging in oncologic patients. Although most of the studies concerned lung cancer, AI models may help in tumor detection, staging and restaging as well as in evaluation of patients' prognosis. Further investigation is required in order to implement Deep Learning (DL) techniques in clinical practice.

## 10.5 Conclusion

F-18-FDG-PET/CT in the evaluation of adrenal glands' tumors is currently widely applied in cancer patients, in search of metastatic adrenal lesions, particularly in non-small cell lung cancer patients; in rare cases in noncancer patients and suspicion of cancer, it may serve as a complementary tool in cases of inconclusive CT and MRI. For the exploration of primary adrenal tumors of the medulla, several radiopharmaceuticals, such as FDOPA and Ga-68-somatostatin receptors' analogs, have been used, while C-11-MTO is specific for distinguishing adrenocortical versus non-adrenocortical pathology. However, further research is required so as the above-described positron emitting radiopharmaceuticals reach their definite applications. Of interest would be the application of AI algorithms in the investigation of adrenal gland mass lesions, either it may concern the cortex or the medulla, primary or metastatic, using several different radiopharmaceuticals.

## References


1. Tessonnier L, Sebag F, Palazzo FF, et al. Does 18F-FDG PET/CT add diagnostic accuracy in incidentally identified non-secreting adrenal tumours? Eur J Nucl Med Mol Imaging. 2008;35(11):2018–25.
2. Jana S, Zhang T, Milstein DM, et al. FDG-PET and CT characterization of adrenal lesions in cancer patients. Eur J Nucl Med Mol Imaging. 2006;33(1):29–35.
3. Boland GW, Dwamena BA, Jagtiani Sangwaiya M, et al. Characterization of adrenal masses by using FDG PET: a systematic review and meta-analysis of diagnostic test performance. Radiology. 2011;259(1):117–26.
4. Ozcan Kara P, Kara T, Kara Gedik G, et al. The role of fluorodeoxyglucose-positron emission tomography/computed tomography in differentiating between benign and malignant adrenal lesions. Nucl Med Commun. 2011;32(2):106–12.
5. Xu B, Gao J, Cui L, et al. Characterization of adrenal metastatic cancer using FDG PET/CT. Neoplasma. 2012;59(1):92–9.
6. Terzolo M, Stigliano A, Chiodini I, et al. AME position statement on adrenal incidentaloma. Eur J Endocrinol. 2011;164:851–70.
7. Perri M, Erba P, Volterrani D, et al. Adrenal masses in patients with cancer: PET/CT characterization with combined CT histogram and standardized uptake value PET analysis. AJR Am J Roentgenol. 2011;197(1):209–16.
8. Ansquer C, Scigliano S, Mirallié E, et al. 18F-FDG PET/CT in the characterization and surgical decision concerning adrenal masses: a prospective multicentre evaluation. Eur J Nucl Med Mol Imaging. 2010;37(9):16691678.
9. Kunikowska J, Matyskiel R, Toutounchi S, et al. What parameters from 18F-FDG PET/CT are useful in evaluation of adrenal lesions? Eur J Nucl Med Mol Imaging. 2014;41(12):2273–80.
10. Boland GW, Blake MA, Holalkere NS, Hahn PF. PET/CT for the characterization of adrenal masses in patients with cancer: qualitative versus quantitative accuracy in 150 consecutive patients. Am J Roentgenol. 2009;192(4):956–62.
11. Koopman D, van Dalen JA, Stigt JA, et al. Current generation time-of-flight (18)F-FDG PET/CT provides higher SUVs for normal adrenal glands, while maintaining an accurate characterization of benign and malignant glands. Ann Nucl Med. 2016;30:145–52.
12. Stone WZ, Wymer DC, Canales BK. Fluorodeoxyglucose-positron-emission tomography/computed tomography imaging for adrenal masses in patients with lung cancer: review and diagnostic algorithm. J Endourol. 2014;28(1):104–11.
13. Havekes B, Kathryn King K, Edwin W, Lai EW, et al. New imaging approaches to pheochromocytomas and paragangliomas. Clin Endocrinol (Oxf). 2010;72(2):137–45.
14. Rufini V, Treglia G, Castaldi P, et al. Comparison of 123I-MIBG SPECT-CT and 18F-DOPA PET-CT in the evaluation of patients with known or suspected recurrent paraganglioma. Nucl Med Commun. 2011;32(7):575–82.
15. Rischke HC, Benz MR, Wild D, et al. Correlation of the genotype of paragangliomas and pheochromocytomas with their metabolic phenotype on 3,4-dihydroxy-6-18F-fluoro-L-phenylalanin PET. J Nucl Med. 2012;53(9):1352–8.
16. Heimburger C, Veillon F, Taïeb D, et al. Head-to-head comparison between 18F-FDOPA PET/CT and MR/CT angiography in clinically recurrent head and neck paragangliomas. Eur J Nucl Med Mol Imaging. 2017;44(6):979–87. https://doi.org/10.1007/s00259-016-3605-0.
17. Naswa N, Sharma P, Nazar AH, et al. Prospective evaluation of 68Ga-DOTA-NOC PET-CT in phaeochromocytoma and paraganglioma: preliminary results from a single centre study. Eur Radiol. 2012;22(3):710–9.
18. Maurice JB, Troke R, Win Z, et al. A comparison of the performance of 68Ga-DOTATATE PET/CT and 123I-MIBG SPECT in the diagnosis and follow-up of phaeochromocytoma and paraganglioma. Eur J Nucl Med Mol Imaging. 2012;39(8):1266–70.
19. Timmers HJ, Kozupa A, Chen CC, et al. Superiority of fluorodeoxyglucose positron emission tomography to other functional imaging techniques in the evaluation of metastatic SDHB-associated pheochromocytoma and paraganglioma. J Clin Oncol. 2007;25(16):2262–9.
20. Timmers HJ, Chen CC, Carrasquillo JA, et al. Staging and functional characterization of pheochromocytoma and paraganglioma by 18F- fluorodeoxyglucose (18F-FDG) positron emission tomography. J Natl Cancer Inst. 2012;104(9):700–8.
21. Hennings J, Lindhe O, Bergström M, et al. [11C] metomidate positron emission tomography of adrenocortical tumors in correlation with histopathological findings. J Clin Endocrinol Metab. 2006;91(4):1410–4.
22. Hennings J, Sundin A, Hägg A, Hellman P. 11C-metomidate positron emission tomography after

dexamethasone suppression for detection of small adrenocortical adenomas in primary aldosteronism. Langenbecks Arch Surg. 2010;395(7):963–7.
23. Hennings J, Hellman P, Ahlström H, Sundin A. Computed tomography, magnetic resonance imaging and 11C-metomidate positron emission tomography for evaluation of adrenal incidentalomas. Eur J Radiol. 2009;69(2):314–23.
24. Razifar P, Hennings J, Monazzam A, et al. Masked volume wise principal component analysis of small adrenocortical tumours in dynamic [11C]-metomidate positron emission tomography. BMC Med Imaging. 2009;22(9):6.
25. Khan TS, Sundin A, Juhlin C, et al. 11C-metomidate PET imaging of adrenocortical cancer. Eur J Nucl Med Mol Imaging. 2003;30(3):403–10.
26. Leboulleux S, Dromain C, Bonniaud G, et al. Diagnostic and prognostic value of 18- fluorodeoxyglucose positron emission tomography in adrenocortical carcinoma: a prospective comparison with computed tomography. J Clin Endocrinol Metab. 2006;91(3):920–5.
27. Tessonnier L, Ansquer C, Bournaud C, et al. 18F-FDG uptake at initial staging of the adrenocortical cancers: a diagnostic tool but not of prognostic value. World J Surg. 2013;37(1):107–12.
28. Boubaker A, Bischof Delaloye A. Nuclear medicine procedures and neuroblastoma in childhood. Their value in the diagnosis, staging and assessment of response to therapy. Q J Nucl Med. 2003;47(1):31–40.
29. Chawla M, Kumar R, Sandeep A, et al. Role of positron emission tomography-computed tomography in staging and early chemotherapy response evaluation in children with neuroblastoma. Indian J Nucl Med. 2010;25(4):147–55.
30. Papathanasiou ND, Gaze MN, Sullivan K, et al. 18F-FDG PET/CT and 123I-metaiodobenzylguanidine imaging in high-risk neuroblastoma: diagnostic comparison and survival analysis. J Nucl Med. 2011;52(4):519–25.
31. Piccardo A, Lopci E, Conte M, et al. Comparison of 18F-dopa PET/CT and 123I-MIBG scintigraphy in stage 3 and 4 neuroblastoma: a pilot study. Eur J Nucl Med Mol Imaging. 2012;39(1):57–71.
32. Zaharchuk G, Davidzon G. Artificial intelligence for optimization and interpretation of PET/CT and PET/MR images. Semin Nucl Med. 2021;51(2):134–42.
33. Sadaghiani MS, Rowe SP, Sheikhbahaei S. Applications of artificial intelligence in oncologic 18F-FDG PET/CT imaging: a systematic review. Ann Transl Med. 2021;9(9):823.

# PET/CT in Renal Cancer

11

Alexandra V. Nikaki

## 11.1 Introduction

The incidence of renal cell carcinoma (RCC) at all stages is rising, with clear cell histologic type being the commonest [1]. However, it has been reported that 15% of small renal masses are benign [2]. Partial or total nephrectomy is the current treatment for RCC. Contrast-enhanced computed tomography (CECT)-renal protocol [3] is the imaging modality of choice in the detection and differentiation of solid renal masses versus cystic ones, even small ones of size <2 cm; however, it faces certain limitations consisting of its lower ability to differentiate between benign and malignant lesions, as well as indolent from aggressive phenotype [2, 3]. The role of magnetic resonance imaging (MRI) is currently mostly restricted to characterization of equivocal computed tomography (CT) findings, evaluation of perirenal fat and venous cava thrombosis. The urge of functional characterization of renal masses has brought the utilization of PET/CT in the foreground [2, 3].

## 11.2 18F-FDG-PET for Renal Cancer Investigation

### 11.2.1 Renal Mass Characterization and Initial Staging

Although FDG-PET has an established or promising role in initial staging and restaging of the majority of malignances, results are less optimal when renal masses are validated. Primarily physiologic renal excretion of the radiopharmaceutical and secondary inflammatory or indolent processes can provoke false positive results. Moreover, the variable degree of FDG uptake by the renal masses as well as the spatial resolution of PET scanners can mislead to false negative diagnosis [2, 4].

Studies concerning the exploration of the value of FDG-PET imaging procedure in initial staging and restaging patients with renal cancer are only scattered, occupying a small sample of patients and the majority of them reveal no or little added information as compared to conventional imaging procedures. Although differences in FDG uptake in the means of SUV values between high- and low-grade clear cell RCC, as well as between high-grade clear RCC and normal kidney tissue are demonstrated [5], the reported sensitivity for RCC diagnosis and staging varies in the range of 32–100% and 47–75%, respectively [2, 4].

A. V. Nikaki (✉)
Docrates Cancer Center, Helsinki, Finland


J. A. Andreou et al. (eds.), *Artificial Intelligence in PET/CT Oncologic Imaging*,
https://doi.org/10.1007/978-3-031-10090-1_11

First promising results for the utilization of FDG-PET in the exploration and characterization of RCC, with a reported sensitivity of 94% [6], equal to that of CT, were not verified in more recent studies, although it should be mentioned that studies are subjected to referral bias, since most patients were only referred to PET examination, if they were to be treated with surgical excision after CT and/or MRI indication [3, 6–8]. Aide et al. [7] demonstrated the high number of false negative PET examinations in evaluating suspicious renal masses, thus reporting a sensitivity of 47%, however a higher specificity (80%); the authors also reported the discordance between high FDG uptake by small low-grade renal malignances and low FDG uptake by large high-grade renal malignances, although the median size of visualized tumors was actually higher than that of nonvisualized ones. The last was also confirmed by Ozulker et al. [8] reporting an average 8.3 ± 4.3 cm for FDG-PET visualized tumors versus 3.5 ± 1.3 for nonvisualized ones; however, the authors also reported statistically significant higher Fuhrman grade in visualized tumors as compared to nonvisualized malignances. Accuracy was ~50%.

FDG-PET is reported to have a good sensitivity in characterizing the extent of disease, especially in detecting distant metastasis, thus showing higher accuracy than CT, concerning, more frequently, bone [7, 9, 10] and adrenal metastasis [7], renal vein and inferior vena cava infiltration, and tumor thrombus [8]. Advanced local disease, lymph node assessment, and predominantly distant metastasis are well identified by FDG-PET with higher sensitivity than CT and bone scintigraphy, thus concluding in alteration of patients' management in 9–13% of cases, or even more according to more optimistic studies [6–10]. FDG avidity in metastatic lesions is demonstrated to be higher as compared to the primary site of the tumor, possibly indicating different biology and GLUT expression [3, 9]. Sensitivities in detecting metastatic disease range between 64% and 100%, more closely to 100% (for a review see Lawrentschuk et al. [4]). False results may occur in oncocytomas [6, 8]. Sensitivity could, likely, be improved by delayed imaging or with the use of diuretics; however, there are conflicting results and further investigation needs to be carried out.

High SUVmax either at the primary or at the metastatic foci as well as increased number of FDG-avid lesions before treatment in metastatic or recurrent RCC patients has been reported to have prognostic significance and to be correlated with reduced overall survival [11, 12]. Further, in a multivariate analysis of 139 RCC patients, Nakajima et al. demonstrated that the total lesion glycolysis (TLG) and the metabolic tumor volume (MTV) along with high pathologic TNM stage were the significant factors for predicting progression-free survival [13].

18F-FDG-PET has been investigated in a small pediatric population sample with Wilms tumor and was reported to correctly identify the primary site of the tumor and lymph node invasion and to accurately rule out distant metastasis; the authors reported that although it could be suitable for imaging Wilms tumor, it does not actually offer added information [14].

### 11.2.2 Relapse and Evaluation of Treatment Response

The role of FDG-PET is perhaps more decisive in the evaluation of possible renal bed recurrence or metastatic disease in restaging patients with renal cell carcinoma, especially considering the post-treatment changes that may influence CT interpretation. Regarding that FDG-PET is not subject to such alterations, it has been found accurate and useful in this portion of patients. Reported sensitivity is 74–100% [6, 15–19]; specificity [15–19] and accuracy [15, 18, 19] are 71–100% and 79–90% respectively (partially varying according to the usage of per-patient or per-lesion evaluation), while prognosis is better for PET negative patients. Lymph node invasion, local relapse, and adrenal metastasis were identified as relapse or metastatic lesions. During surveillance, Park et al. [16] demonstrated positive and negative predictive value of FDG-PET 77.3% and 92.6%, respectively, with an overall accuracy of 85.7% in evaluating possible recurrence and

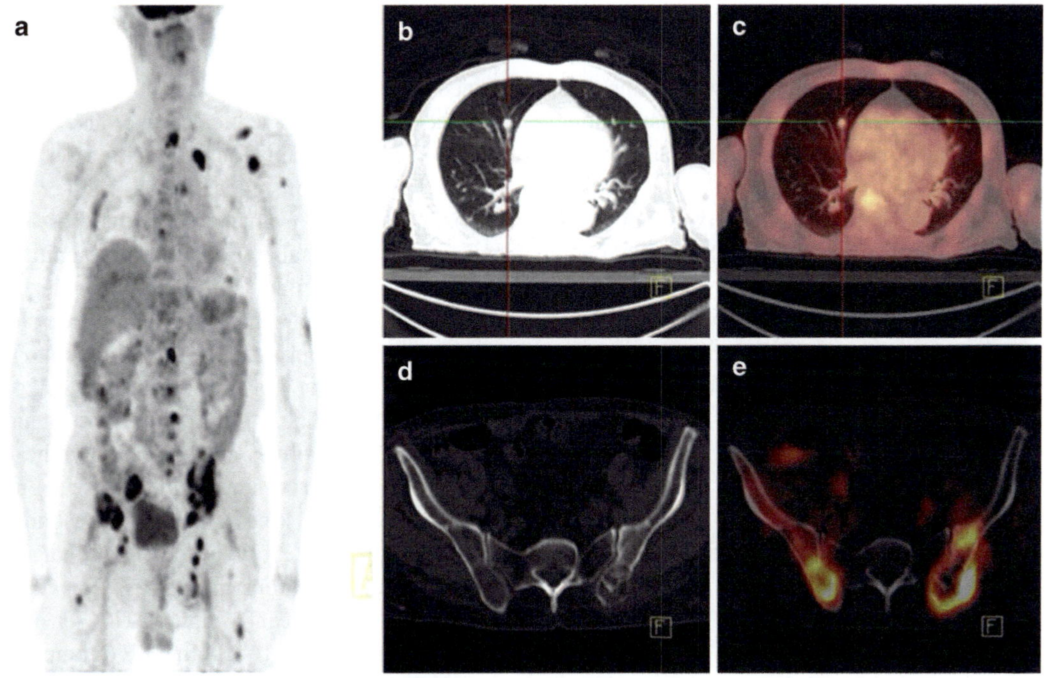


**Fig. 11.1** (**a**) 18F-FDG-PET-MIP imaging reveals multiple metastatic lesions in a patient with renal carcinoma, who underwent surgical resection of the left kidney and had received multiple schemes of chemo and targeted therapy. (**b**), (**c**) Nodule at the right lung (**b**) with 18F-FDG uptake (**c**), indicative of pulmonary metastasis. (**d**), (**e**) Osseous distortion at CT imaging (**d**) with high 18F-FDG uptake at PET (**e**), compatible with osseous secondary invasion

metastatic disease; however, the reported results did not overweight those of other conventional modalities (Fig. 11.1a–e). More recently FDG-PET/CT is demonstrated to influence therapeutic strategy in 43% of patients and to correlate both with overall survival and progression-free survival [19]. SUVmax is considered as an independent factor of survival in advanced RCC cases, recurrent and stage IV [20].

Apart from radical or partial nephrectomy, current therapeutic strategies for renal cancer, especially in advanced or recurrent cases, include tyrosine kinase inhibitors which target VEGF signaling, as well as mTOR inhibitors. However, these approaches do not result, at least initially, in massive tumor shrinkage and size changes, since they act more as cytostatics rather than cytotoxics [3]. On the other hand it would be of great importance to determine which patients mostly benefit from targeted therapies. FDG-PET has been evaluated in the assessment of renal cell cancer response to tyrosine kinase inhibitors—sunitinib and sorafenib. Correlation with overall survival has also been reported. Ueno et al. [21], in their prospective study, demonstrated that SUVmax reduction of >20% early in the course of targeted treatment (~ 30 days after the initiation of treatment) was correlated with longer progression-free interval. Moreover, when patients were categorized in good and intermediate responders according to SUVmax reduction >20 or < 20% in non-increasing masses according to CT criteria, both progression-free and overall survival were statistically significantly different. Therefore, FDG-PET potentially could complement CT in evaluation of response to kinase inhibitors treatment and further discriminate patients with CT findings of stable disease [21]. However, Kayani et al. [11] reported prognostic significance of FDG-PET only 16 weeks after initiation of treatment with sunitinib, and not early in the course of therapy, although FDG-PET may provide information about tumors' biologic nature and sunitinib resistance according to the writers.

As for pediatric population with Wilms tumor, FDG-PET bears a potential role in post-treatment setting and in evaluating pretherapeutic relapse [14].

Conclusively, FDG-PET is likely not used in determining renal malignancy; however, it could play a role in selected cases of suspected distant metastasis during initial staging. Its role is more prominent in providing functional prognostic information and evaluating response to treatment and recurrent disease.

## 11.3 Non-FDG Radiopharmaceutical for RCC Imaging

Considering the limited value of FDG-PET in determining renal cell carcinoma especially in the means of monitoring small renal masses, efforts have been made so as other imaging biomarkers to be manufactured. Carbonic anhydrase IX is a cell surface antigen, highly expressed in >95% of clear cell renal cell carcinoma (ccRCC). Girentuximab (cG250), a chimeric antibody, labeled with I-124 (positron emitting radionuclide) binds with carbonic anhydrase IX and has been proposed for the evaluation of ccRCC [2]. After promising initial results in a small sample of patients [22], a multicenter open-label study was carried out, in which I-124-cG250-PET was performed in patients with renal masses, who were planned for surgical removal. With excellent interobserver agreement, reported average sensitivity and specificity are 86.2 and 85.9 versus 75.5 and 46.8%, respectively, for CECT, while accuracy ranges between 85.6 and 86.9% and higher than the respective reported for CECT and at least comparable to that of biopsy. Positive and negative predictive values are demonstrated 93.9–94.7 and 68.8–70.3%, respectively. Interestingly, I-124-cG250-PET could detect even small lesions of less than 2 cm. I-124-cG250-PET has been characterized as the first molecular imaging procedure which bears specific prognostic information for a specific solid tumor [23]. Despite, however, the first encouraging results, girentuximab-labeled tracers have not gained wide acceptance.

Other radiopharmaceuticals have, also, been proposed for the evaluation of renal masses and RCC. 18F-Fluoromisonidazole, a marker of hypoxia, has been evaluated to define possible oxygen-derivative alterations during sunitinib treatment and baseline 18F-Fluoromisonidazole was found to be linked to progression-free survival in RCC patients treated with sunitinib, however not with overall survival [24]. 18F-Fluorothymidine, a proliferative marker, and 18F-Fluoroethylcholine, a membrane synthesis marker, were also validated in RCC patients receiving tyrosine kinase inhibitor treatment, consisting of a category of potential imaging agents in renal cell carcinoma [25–27]. Nakanishi et al. reported significantly higher AUC, sensitivity, and accuracy for 11C-choline PET compared to 18F-FDG-PET, concluding that RCC patients may benefit more from choline-PET imaging than FDG-PET for staging and restaging [28]. Imaging RCC patients with PSMA-PET is considered less optimal; however metastatic patients may benefit [29]. For bone metastasis evaluation in RCC patients 18F-NaF-PET is reported to be significantly more sensitive than bone scan and CT, a fact which could further have an impact in treatment decisions [30]. However, all these radiopharmaceuticals are under investigation and further validation is required until they gain a role in daily imaging of renal cell carcinoma.

## 11.4 Towards Artificial Intelligence

Artificial Intelligence (AI) is currently invading in PET/CT imaging instrumentation, data acquisition, data processing, and final reporting. Huge efforts have already been made towards algorithms development for machine learning (ML) and imaging interpreting concerning a variety of tumors or nontumor lesions imaged with PET. A systematic approach [31] was attempted for AI FDG-PET imaging in oncologic patients. The majority of the studies concerned lung cancer, followed by head and neck tumors. ML models may serve as useful assistance to physicians for tumor detection, segmentation, staging, prognosis, and evaluation of response. Despite, however, the promising results, AI in PET imaging is still in its early stages and more effort is required in order to implement Deep Learning (DL) techniques in everyday practice. Considering RCC imaging, AI may be even more useful, as current approaches are in some cases of limited value and new radiopharmaceuticals are being explored.

## References


1. Paul C. Renal cell carcinoma. Cancer Biomark. 2011;9(1–6):461–73.
2. Smaldone MC, Chen DY, Yu JQ, Plimack ER. Potential role of (124)I-girentuximab in the presurgical diagnosis of clear-cell renal cell cancer. Biologics. 2012;6:395–407.
3. Khandani AH, Rathmell WK. Positron emission tomography in renal cell carcinoma: an imaging biomarker in development. Semin Nucl Med. 2012;42(4):221–30.
4. Lawrentschuk N, Davis ID, Bolton DM, Scott AM. Functional imaging of renal cell carcinoma. Nat Rev Urol. 2010;7(5):258–66.
5. Takahashi M, Kume H, Koyama K, et al. Preoperative evaluation of renal cell carcinoma by using 18F-FDG PET/CT. Clin Nucl Med. 2015;40(12):936–40.
6. Ramdave S, Thomas GW, Berlangieri SU, et al. Clinical role of F-18 fluorodeoxyglucose positron emission tomography for detection and management of renal cell carcinoma. J Urol. 2001;166(3):825–30.
7. Aide N, Cappele O, Bottet P, et al. Efficiency of [(18) F]FDG PET in characterising renal cancer and detecting distant metastases: a comparison with CT. Eur J Nucl Med Mol Imaging. 2003;30(9):1236–45.
8. Ozülker T, Ozülker F, Ozbek E, Ozpaçaci T. A prospective diagnostic accuracy study of F-18 fluorodeoxyglucose-positron emission tomography/computed tomography in the evaluation of indeterminate renal masses. Nucl Med Commun. 2011;32(4):265–72.
9. Kang DE, White RL Jr, Zuger JH, et al. Clinical use of fluorodeoxyglucose F 18 positron emission tomography for detection of renal cell carcinoma. J Urol. 2004;171(5):1806–9.
10. Wu HC, Yen RF, Shen YY, et al. Comparing whole body 18F–2-deoxyglucose positron emission tomography and technetium-99 m methylene diphosphate bone scan to detect bone metastases in patients with renal cell carcinomas: a preliminary report. J Cancer Res Clin Oncol. 2002;128(9):503–6.
11. Kayani I, Avril N, Bomanji J, et al. Sequential FDG-PET/CT as a biomarker of response to sunitinib in metastatic clear cell renal cancer. Clin Cancer Res. 2011;17(18):6021–8.
12. Namura K, Minamimoto R, Yao M, et al. Impact of maximum standardized uptake value (SUVmax) evaluated by 18-Fluoro-2-deoxy-D- glucose positron emission tomography/computed tomography (18F-FDG-PET/CT) on survival for patients with advanced renal cell carcinoma: a preliminary report. BMC Cancer. 2010;10:667.
13. Nakajima R, Matsuo Y, Kondo T, et al. Prognostic value of metabolic tumor volume and Total lesion glycolysis on preoperative 18F-FDG PET/CT in patients with renal cell carcinoma. Clin Nucl Med. 2017;42:e177–82.
14. Misch D, Steffen IG, Schönberger S, et al. Use of positron emission tomography for staging, preoperative response assessment and posttherapeutic evaluation in children with Wilms tumour. Eur J Nucl Med Mol Imaging. 2008;35(9):1642–50.
15. Nakatani K, Nakamoto Y, Saga T, et al. The potential clinical value of FDG-PET for recurrent renal cell carcinoma. Eur J Radiol. 2011;79(1):29–35.
16. Park JW, Jo MK, Lee HM. Significance of 18F-fluorodeoxyglucose positron-emission tomography/computed tomography for the postoperative surveillance of advanced renal cell carcinoma. BJU Int. 2009;103(5):615–9.
17. Safaei A, Figlin R, Hoh CK, et al. The usefulness of F-18 deoxyglucose whole-body positron emission tomography (PET) for re-staging of renal cell cancer. Clin Nephrol. 2002;57(1):56–62.
18. Kumar R, Shandal V, Shamim SA, et al. Role of FDG PET-CT in recurrent renal cell carcinoma. Nucl Med Commun. 2010;31(10):844–850 507.
19. Alongi P, Picchio M, Zattoni F, et al. Recurrent renal cell carcinoma: clinical and prognostic value of FDG PET/CT. Eur J Nucl Med Mol Imaging. 2016;43(3):464–73.
20. Nakaigawa N, Kondo K, Tateishi U, et al. FDG PET/CT as a prognostic biomarker in the era of molecular-targeting therapies: max SUVmax predicts survival of patients with advanced renal cell carcinoma. BMC Cancer. 2016;16:67.
21. Ueno D, Yao M, Tateishi U, et al. Early assessment by FDG-PET/CT of patients with advanced renal cell carcinoma treated with tyrosine kinase inhibitors is predictive of disease course. BMC Cancer. 2012;12:162.
22. Divgi CR, Pandit-Taskar N, Jungbluth AA, et al. Preoperative characterisation of clear- cell renal carcinoma using iodine-124-labelled antibody chimeric G250 (124I-cG250) and PET in patients with renal masses: a phase I trial. Lancet Oncol. 2007;8(4):304–10.
23. Divgi CR, Uzzo RG, Gatsonis C, et al. Positron emission tomography/computed tomography identification of clear cell renal cell carcinoma: results from the REDECT trial. J Clin Oncol. 2013;31(2):187–94.

24. Hugonnet F, Fournier L, Medioni J, et al. Metastatic renal cell carcinoma: relationship between initial metastasis hypoxia, change after 1 month's sunitinib, and therapeutic response: an 18F-Fluoromisonidazole PET/CT study. J Nucl Med. 2011;52:1048–55.
25. Liu G, Jeraj R, Vanderhoek M, et al. Pharmacodynamic study using FLT PET/CT in patients with renal cell cancer and other solid malignancies treated with sunitinib malate. Clin Cancer Res. 2011;17(24):7634–44.
26. Middendorp M, Maute L, Sauter B, et al. Initial experience with 18F-fluoroethylcholine PET/CT in staging and monitoring therapy response of advanced renal cell carcinoma. Ann Nucl Med. 2010;24(6):441–6.
27. Horn KP, Yap JT, Agarwal N, et al. FDG and FLT-PET for early measurement of response to 37.5 mg daily sunitinib therapy in metastatic renal cell carcinoma. Cancer Imaging. 2015;15:15.
28. Nakanishi Y, Kitajima K, Yamada Y, et al. Diagnostic performance of (11)C-choline PET/CT and FDG PET/CT for staging and restaging of renal cell cancer. Ann Nucl Med. 2018;32:658–68.
29. Rhee H, Blazak J, Tham CM, et al. Pilot study: use of gallium-68 PSMA PET for detection of metastatic lesions in patients with renal tumour. EJNMMI Res. 2016;6:76.
30. Gerety EL, Lawrence EM, Wason J, et al. Prospective study evaluating the relative sensitivity of 18F-NaF PET/CT for detecting skeletal metastases from renal cell carcinoma in comparison to multidetector CT and 99mTc-MDP bone scintigraphy, using an adaptive trial design. Ann Oncol. 2015;26(10):2113–8.
31. Sadaghiani MS, Rowe SP, Sheikhbahaei S. Applications of artificial intelligence in oncologic 18F-FDG PET/CT imaging: a systematic review. Ann Transl Med. 2021;9(9):823.

# 12 PET/CT Findings in Testicular Cancer

Chariklia D. Giannopoulou

A glucose analog, 18F-fluoro-2-deoxy-D-glucose (FDG), is the most used PET tracer in testicular cancer. In general, increased FDG tumor uptake is due to the increased number of glucose transport molecules and the increased activity of hexokinase isoenzymes, making FDG a probe for imaging tumor metabolism, aggressiveness, and viability. FDG-PET/CT provides functional information about the metabolical activity of disease sites, and especially about viability in residual masses that cannot be correctly predicted by anatomical, conventional imaging.

Non-FDG-PET tracers have also been used in testicular germ cell tumors (CGTs) such as 39-deoxy-39-18F-fluorothymidine (18F-FLT)—a probe for imaging cellular proliferation—[1] and radio-labeled integrins [2].

Seminomatous germ cell tumors (SGCT), including their metastases, show high FDG uptake and express significantly greater FDG avidity than nonseminomatous germ cell tumors (NSGCT), whereas mature teratomas have low FDG uptake [3].

False-positive findings are due to the fact that FDG is not a tumor-specific tracer; normal and benign cells may also accumulate it. Apart from the normal distribution (brain, kidneys, and bladder) sites of inflammation, granulomata, and tissues in certain other non-malignant conditions may concentrate FDG. Post-radiotherapy inflammatory reactions, as well as post-chemotherapy metabolic flare may also be responsible for non-specific FDG uptake resulting in false-positive studies.

On the other hand, false-negative findings may be due to lesion's size (foci smaller than 1 cm are at the limits of systems' resolution), to tissue histology: a mature differentiated teratoma has low FDG uptake, or to short time elapsed after chemotherapy.

It is evident that special care should be taken about the timing of PET/CT that should be performed not earlier than 6 weeks post-chemotherapy, in order to obtain maximum accuracy.

## 12.1 Initial Staging: Early Detection of Micrometastases

There is not enough evidence supporting the value of FDG-PET in the staging at presentation of patients with either SGCTs or NSGCTs.

The predictive value of FDG-PET at the initial staging of patients with clinical stage I/II GCTs has been a question of dispute, as it affects patients' management, i.e., the selection of surveillance against primary retroperitoneal

C. D. Giannopoulou (✉)
Nuclear Medicine Department, "Evangelismos" Hospital, Athens, Greece
e-mail: harisg@otenet.gr


J. A. Andreou et al. (eds.), *Artificial Intelligence in PET/CT Oncologic Imaging*,
https://doi.org/10.1007/978-3-031-10090-1_12

lymphadenectomy for NSGCTs, or surveillance versus radiation therapy for SGCTs.

CT is the established method of staging patients with SGCTs. However, the great percentage of false-negative CT results—due to its inability to detect microscopic metastases in approximately 30% of patients—hampers the accurate diagnosis of early-stage disease, and the correct differentiation of stage I from stage IIA NSGCT patients [4].

Anatomical imaging (CT) findings are solely based on lymph node (LN) size and morphology, whereas FDG uptake reflects the metabolical LN status: relatively small LNs may harbor active disease and enlarged LNs may be reactive. Another PET advantage over CT, improving PET sensitivity, is standard whole-body scanning covering areas that are not routinely scanned by CT. On the other hand, PET resolution of about 10 mm may limit sensitivity for the detection of small volume disease; however, newer PET/CT systems may achieve a resolution of 5 mm or less.

FDG-PET/CT could be useful for small-volume metastatic disease diagnosis in patients with early-stage II NSGCT and inconclusive conventional imaging studies.

In a paper from a German multicenter trial, studying the predicting value of FDG-PET in primary staging of retroperitoneal LN metastases in patients with newly diagnosed early-stage NSGC, the PPV and NPV of FDG-PET were 95% and 78%, while for CT, PPV and NPV were 87% and 67%, respectively. The authors concluded that FDG-PET as a primary staging tool for NSGCT yielded slightly better results than CT and that false-negative findings were more frequent with CT, rendering FDG-PET mostly useful as a diagnostic tool in case of inconclusive CT scan [5]. These results are in keeping with those of previous studies [6].

However, an earlier UK study of patients with clinical stage I NSGCT examining the ability of FDG-PET to identify patients without occult metastatic disease was stopped prematurely, because of the high number of FDG-PET false negatives: Of 88 patients with negative PET scans, 33 patients relapsed with an estimated one-year relapse-free rate of 63.3% [7]. In a recently published paper FDG-PET was helpful in the initial staging of 16 patients with equivocal CT studies; however it was not able to predict relapse in the group of high-risk patients [8]

In conclusion, although FDG-PET/CT does not have a distinctive role in staging of patients with SGCTs or NSGCTs, it could be useful for small-volume metastatic disease diagnosis in patients with early-stage II NSGCT and inconclusive conventional imaging studies.

## 12.2 Response to Treatment Assessment: Residual Mass Characterization

Assessing residual disease after treatment in both seminoma and nonseminomatous germ cell tumors of the testis is of great importance in patients' management, as it contributes to patient selection for surgical resection, especially those with masses greater than 1 cm.

## 12.3 Seminomatous GCTs

After seminoma resection, patients with seminomatous testicular GCTs are generally followed up with CT. Surveillance using serum tumor markers is unreliable, because of its limited sensitivity—only 30% of seminoma relapses are marker positive [9].

In patients with post-chemotherapy residual masses, FDG-PET due to its ability to differentiate between necrosis/fibrosis and residual or recurrent viable tumor has been proved sensitive as well as specific for detecting recurrent disease and selecting those patients who could thereafter be treated surgically (Figs. 12.1 and 12.2).

In a large, prospective, multicenter trial [10], FDG-PET was performed in 51 patients with metastatic seminoma and post-chemotherapy residual masses greater than 1 cm, detected by CT. FDG-PET findings were correlated with the histological findings as to tumor viability, or to clinical or radiological (CT) evidence of progressive disease. In that study it was shown that

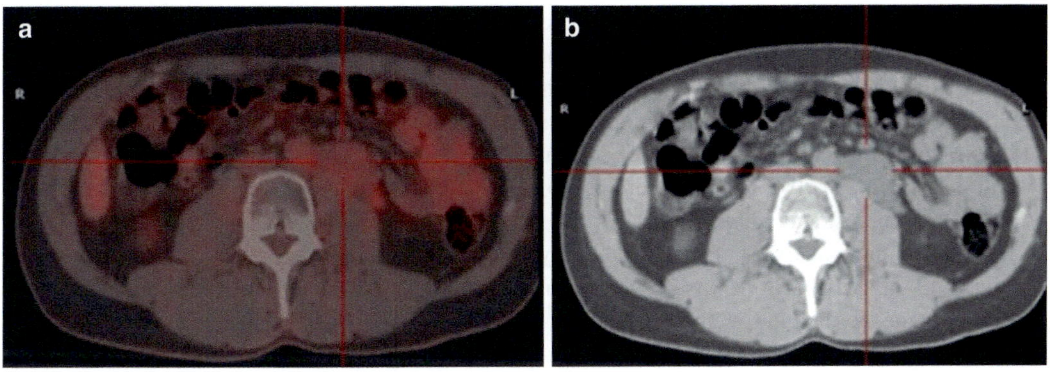


**Fig. 12.1** (**a**) FDG-PET/CT, axial fused image showing residual retroperitoneal mass without increased FDG uptake, in a patient with seminoma, 2 months after the completion of chemotherapy. This is a true negative study, as there was no evidence of active disease after 3 years of follow-up. (**b**) Corresponding CT axial image

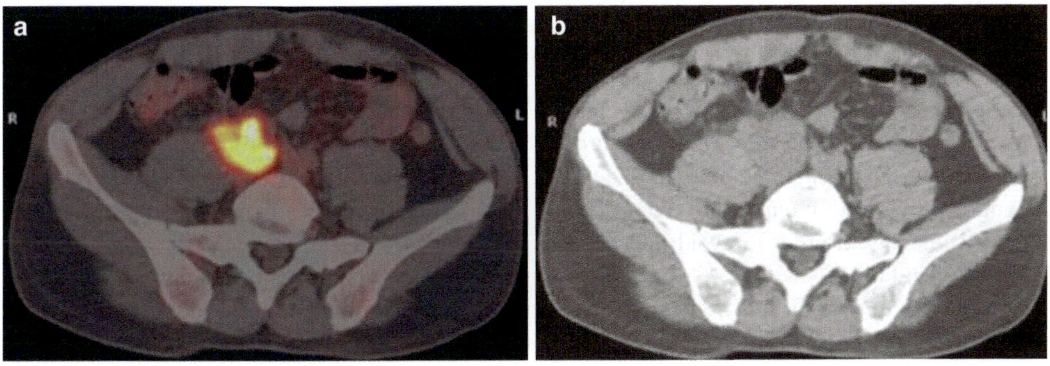


**Fig. 12.2** (**a**) FDG-PET/CT, axial fused image of a 56-year-old patient with stage IIb seminoma, 7 weeks after first-line chemotherapy completion, showing intense FDG uptake in the residual retroperitoneal mass. After surgery, histology revealed viable tumor in the resected mass. (**b**) Corresponding CT axial image

FDG-PET can identify viable tumor with a specificity of 100%, a sensitivity of 80%, a positive predictive value of 100%, and a negative predictive value of 96%, versus CT's respective values of 74% specificity, 70% sensitivity, 37% positive predictive value, and 92% negative predictive value. The authors conclude that FDG-PET performed within 4–12 weeks after chemotherapy can accurately predict viable residual tumor. In patients with residual lesions greater than 3 cm and negative FDG-PET, surgery can be omitted, whereas if PET is positive, residual lesions, even smaller than 3 cm, can be considered as harboring viable tumor; hence surgery can be of benefit [10].

These results are in keeping with a prospective study in 48 patients with metastatic seminoma and CT-documented residual mass after chemotherapy, investigating whether FDG-PET predicts viable tumor. FDG-PET had a sensitivity and specificity of 80% and 100%, respectively, compared with CT sensitivity and specificity being both 73%. In conclusion, in patients with post-chemotherapy seminoma residuals, a positive PET is highly predictive for the presence of viable tumor. A negative PET scan can accurately exclude disease in lesions >3 cm, with a slightly higher sensitivity than CT, thus contributing to avoid unnecessary additional treatment for these patients [11].

In a study by Hintz, the ability of FDG-PET for predicting residual tumor viability was evaluated in 20 patients with seminoma following chemotherapy for advanced disease.

Histopathological findings were correlated with PET results. All patients with viable tumor were identified correctly by FDG-PET. No false-negative results were observed, but nine patients had false-positive PET results. FDG-PET had an overall sensitivity of 100% and specificity of 47% in detecting residual viable tumor [12].

In a recent meta-analysis of nine studies by Treglia at al. [13], FDG-PET was proved as an accurate diagnostic imaging method in the post-chemotherapy management of patients with seminoma—in particular in patients with recurrent/residual lesions >3 cm.

However, the PPV of FDG-PET has been challenged by a retrospective study done in 2018: in a cohort of 90 patients with metastatic seminoma and FDG/PET positive residual retroperitoneal tumor mass, the PPV was only 23%. False-positive FDG has been associated mainly with necrosis, or with sarcoidosis, fibrosis, inflammation, and benign tumors. The authors recommend closely monitoring patients with repeated imaging in order to avoid unnecessary overtreatment [14].

An interim FDG-PET study, after two cycles of cisplatin, etoposide, and bleomycin (PEB) treatment, has been proposed in patients with metastatic seminoma and was compared with a CT study after three or four cycles of therapy. There has been found a significant association between metabolic PET response and tumor shrinkage in patients, resulting in predicting those who do not need additional treatment, in order to reduce toxicity, and in timely identifying cases hard to treat [15]. Similarly, a recent prospective observational study by Raggi et al. in 75 patients with advanced stage seminoma, an interim FDG/PET study after 2 cycles of PEB or EP, showed that those patients with no residual FDG uptake had better relapse-free survival. The authors also concluded that an early interim FDG/PET study may also contribute to optimizing the prognostic risk groups definition [16].

In conclusion, in patients with post-chemotherapy seminoma residuals, a positive PET is an indicator of residual active—viable tumor regardless of lesion size. A negative PET scan can accurately exclude disease in lesions >3 cm. In order to enhance specificity, reducing the incidence of false-positive results, the PET scan should be performed at least 6 weeks after the completion of chemotherapy [17].

In keeping with international guidelines [18–21] PET-CT study is recommended in the post-chemotherapy management of pure seminoma patients, in order to assess whether residual viable tumor is present. In patients with a residual mass > 3 cm, normal levels of serum markers, and negative PET, no further treatment is needed and close surveillance is recommended. If PET scan is positive, surgical resection could be considered, along with biopsy or surveillance.

## 12.4 Nonseminomatous Germ Cell Tumors

Most patients (70%) with advanced metastatic NSGCT will show complete response to first-line chemotherapy, with subsequent normal serum markers and mass disappearance. In the rest 30%, who show partial response to treatment with negative marker levels and persistent residual masses, the major imaging diagnostic challenge is to differentiate, in a noninvasive way, between fibrosis and necrosis, that occurs in approximately half of those patients, from either mature or immature teratomas—that have to be operated upon as they are chemotherapy resistant, tend to grow, and undergo malignant transformation—or viable/active disease.

FDG-PET cannot reliably distinguish mature teratoma from benign residual mass, because mature teratoma has low FDG uptake and cannot be differentiated from fibrotic or necrotic tissue (Fig. 12.3). In a prospective multicenter study of 121 patients with stage IIC or III NSGCT, with histological confirmation [22] FDG-PET predicted correctly tumor viability with a 56% accuracy, comparable to CT accuracy (55%). Sensitivity and specificity of FDG-PET were 70% and 48%. With viable carcinoma as the unique malignant finding, the negative predictive value was 83% for FDG-PET. Authors conclude that this trial demonstrated that FDG-PET cannot add a clear clinical benefit to the standard diag-

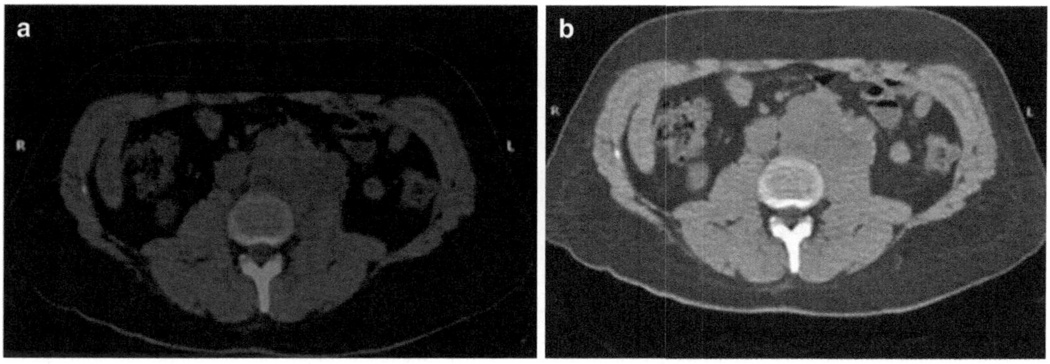

**Fig. 12.3** (**a**) sFDG-PET/CT, axial fused image of a 34-year-old patient with mixed nonseminomatous germ cell tumor 40 days after the completion of cisplatin-based combination chemotherapy. There is no increased FDG uptake noted in the residual retroperitoneal masses shown on corresponding CT axial image (**b**). This is a false-negative study: after surgery, histology revealed mature cystic teratoma in the resected masses

nostic procedures—CT and serum tumor markers—in the prediction of tumor viability in residual masses.

However, in a previous prospective study, Kollmannsberger et al. [23] demonstrated that FDG-PET could correctly characterize residual masses with a specificity of 92% and a sensitivity of 59% in a high-risk population of 45 patients with nonseminomatous germ cell tumors, concluding that positive PET is highly predictive for the presence of viable carcinoma.

Possibly, FDG-PET could contribute to defining the lesions worth operating, i.e., those with high FDG uptake most likely to harbor viable tumor, in patients with multiple residual masses.

In conclusion, current evidence does not support the use of FDG-PET/CT in the management of patients with nonseminomatous germ cell tumors [24] as FDG-PET has no clear additional role in predicting residual mass histology in patients with advanced metastatic NSGCT after the completion of chemotherapy.

## References


1. Pfannenberg C, Aschoff P, Dittmann H, et al. PET/CT with 18F-FLT: does it improve the therapeutic management of metastatic germ cell tumors? J Nucl Med. 2010;51:845–53.
2. Aide N, Briand M, Bohn P, et al. avb3 imaging can accurately distinguish between mature teratoma and necrosis in 18F-FDG-negative residual masses after treatment of non-seminomatous testicular cancer: a preclinical study. Eur J Nucl Med Mol Imaging. 2011;38:323–33.
3. Vela A, Deslandes E, Vera P, et al. The management of residual masses after chemotherapy in metastatic seminoma. BJU Int. 1999;83:649–53.
4. Hilton S, Herr HW, Teitcher JB. CT detection of retroperitoneal lymph node metastases in patients with clinical stage I testicular nonseminomatous germ cell cancer: assessment of size and distribution criteria. Am J Roentgenol. 1997;169:521–5.
5. De Wit M, Brenner W, Hartmann M, et al. 18F-FDG–PET in clinical stage I/II non-seminomatous germ cell tumours: results of the German multicentre trial. Ann Oncol. 2008;19:1619–23.
6. Lassen U, Daugaard G, Eigtved A, et al. Whole-body FDG-PET in patients with stage I non-seminomatous germ cell tumours. Eur J Nucl Med. 2003;30:396–402.
7. Huddart RA, O'Doherty MJ, Padhani A, et al. 18 fluorodeoxyglucose positron emission tomography in the prediction of relapse in patients with high-risk, clinical stage I nonseminomatous germ cell tumors: preliminary report of MRC trial TE22–the NCRI testis tumour clinical study group. J Clin Oncol. 2007;25:3090–5.
8. Cook GJ, Sohaib A, Huddard RA, Dearnaley DP, et al. The role of 18F-FDG PET/CT in the management of testicular cancers. Nucl Med Commun. 2015;36:702–8.
9. Sohaib SA, Koh D, Husband JE, et al. The role of imaging in the diagnosis, staging and management of testicular cancer. Am J Roentgenol. 2008;191:387–95.
10. De Santis M, Becherer A, Bokemeyer C, et al. 2–$^{18}$fluoro-deoxy-D-glucose positron emission tomography is a reliable predictor for viable tumor in postchemotherapy seminoma: an update of the prospective multicentric SEMPET trial. J Clin Oncol. 2004;22:1034–9.
11. Becherer A, De Santis M, Karanikas G, et al. FDG PET is superior to CT in the prediction of viable

tumour in post-chemotherapy seminoma residuals. Eur J Radiol. 2005;54:284–8.
12. Hinz S, Schrader M, Kempkensteffen C, et al. The role of positron emission tomography in the evaluation of residual masses after chemotherapy for advanced stage seminoma. J Urol. 2008;179:936–40.
13. Treglia G, Sageghi R, Annunziata S, et al. Diagnostic performance of fluorine-18-fluorodeoxyglucose positron emission tomography in the postchemotherapy management of patients with seminoma: systematic review and meta-analysis. Biomed Res Int. 2014;2014:852681.
14. Cathomas R, Klingbiel D, Bernard B, et al. Questioning the value of Fluorodeoxyglucose positron emission tomography for residual lesions after chemotherapy for metastatic seminoma: results of an international global germ cell cancer group registry. J Clin Oncol. 2018;36(34):3381–7.
15. Necchi A, Nicolai N, Alessi A. Interim (18) F-fluorodeoxyglucose positron emission tomography for early metabolic assessment of response to cisplatin, etoposide, and bleomycin chemotherapy for metastatic seminoma: clinical value and future directions. Clin Genitourin Cancer. 2016;14:249–54.
16. Raggi D, Bandini M, Giannatempo P, et al. Prognostic role of early interim fluorodeoxyglucose positron emission tomography in patients with advanced seminoma undergoing standard treatment. Clin Genitourin Cancer. 2021;19:237–45.
17. Decoene J, Winter C, Albers P, et al. False-positive fluorodeoxyglucose positron emission tomography results after chemotherapy in patients with metastatic seminoma. Urol Oncol. 2015;33:23.e15–21.
18. Motzer RJ, Agarwal N, Beard C, et al. Testicular cancer clinical practice guidelines in oncology. J Natl Compr Canc Netw. 2012;10:502–35.
19. Schmoll HJ, Jordan K, Huddart R, et al. Testicular seminoma: ESMO clinical practice guidelines for diagnosis, treatment and follow-up. Ann Oncol. 2010;21(S5):140–6.
20. Warde P, Huddart R, Bolton D, et al. Management of localized seminoma, stage I-II: SIU/ICUD consensus meeting on germ cell tumors GCT shanghai 2009. Urology. 2011;78:S435–43.
21. Honecker F, Aparicio J, Berney D, et al. ESMO consensus conference on testicular germ cell cancer: diagnosis, treatment and follow-up. Ann Oncol. 2018;29:1658–86.
22. Oechsle K, Hartmann M, Brenner W, et al. Positron emission tomography in nonseminomatous germ cell tumors after chemotherapy: the German multicenter positron emission tomography study group. J Clin Oncol. 2008;26:5930–5.
23. Kollmannsberger C, Oechsle K, Dohmen B, et al. Prospective comparison of [18F] fluorodeoxyglucose positron emission tomography with conventional assessment by computed tomography scans and serum tumour markers for the evaluation of residual masses in patients with nonseminomatous germ cell carcinoma. Cancer. 2002;94:2353–62.
24. Schmoll H-J, Jordan K, Huddart R, et al. Testicular non-seminoma: ESMO clinical practice guidelines for diagnosis, treatment and follow-up. Ann Oncol. 2010;21(suppl_5):v147–v54.

# PET/CT in Prostate Cancer

# 13

Alexandra V. Nikaki and Vassilios Prassopoulos

## 13.1 Introduction

The evolving role of nuclear medicine and particularly of PET/CT over time in prostate cancer is represented by the expansion of applications of already used radiopharmaceuticals in everyday clinical practice, by newly utilized radiopharmaceuticals, as well as by the introduction of new imaging modalities such as PET/MRI. Radiopharmaceuticals used for prostate cancer imaging include $^{11}$C- and $^{18}$F-Choline, $^{18}$F-Fluciclovine, $^{18}$F- and $^{68}$Ga-Bombesin, $^{18}$F-Dihydrotestosterone, $^{89}$Zr-STEAP monoclonal antibody, $^{18}$F-Sodium Fluoride, $^{18}$F-Fluorodeoxyglucose, and finally $^{68}$Ga- and $^{18}$F-Prostate-Specific Membrane Antigen (PSMA).

## 13.2 Imaging of Prostate Cancer with PET/CT

The role of $^{11}$C-**Choline**, an FDA and NCCN guideline-approved radiopharmaceutical, is quite established in the era of prostate imaging, particularly with regard to Choline-PET/CT utilization in the investigation of biochemical relapse where high detection rates are demonstrated. Pooled sensitivity and specificity of $^{11}$C-Choline-PET for recurrent prostate cancer including 1270 participants is demonstrated 89% in a recent meta-analysis [1]. However, for preoperative lymph node evaluating, as with diffusion-weighted imaging, moderate sensitivity ~70% is reported [2]. PET-guided treatment, oligometastatic therapeutic planning, radiation delineation, and dose escalation are some of the newer applications that Choline-PET is investigated. Castellucci et al., evaluating a large series of patients, propose the performance of $^{11}$C-Choline-PET in biochemical recurrence patients aimed for salvage therapy, particularly in cases of increased PSA-doubling time, in order to exclude extrapelvic malignant lesions [3]. Besides, confirmation of oligometastatic disease is of great importance as it largely affects the therapeutic strategy. Choline-PET may lead to a treatment change in ~40% of prostate cancer patients [4]. Furthermore, $^{11}$C-choline-PET has been suggested for neoadjuvant treatment evaluation in high-risk or locally advanced prostate cancer cases [5]. $^{11}$C- and $^{18}$F-Choline-PET has been used for radiation treatment contouring in prostate cancer patients, providing added value to MRI scheduling alone in the era of escalated radiation therapy to specific recognized targets (Dominant Intraprostatic Lesions, DILs). Several thresholds and manners for identification of DILs using PET have been described. Automatic delineation using a cutoff

A. V. Nikaki (✉)
Docrates Cancer Center, Helsinki, Finland

V. Prassopoulos
Hygeia Hospital, Marousi, Attiki, Greece
e-mail: vprasso@otenet.gr


J. A. Andreou et al. (eds.), *Artificial Intelligence in PET/CT Oncologic Imaging*,
https://doi.org/10.1007/978-3-031-10090-1_13

of 60% of SUVmax has been demonstrated as the preferable approach [6, 7]. Although, for visual analysis, PET is suggested to be performed before the initiation of anti-androgen treatment [6], further investigation is still required. Performance of Choline-PET is associated with PSA and PSA-doubling time values as well as Gleason scores [8].

A new FDA-approved radiopharmaceutical, a leucine amino acid derivative **$^{18}$F-fluciclovine** (anti-$^{18}$F-FACBC), has been developed for prostate cancer imaging with, also, promising results. Uptake is clearly observed in cancer sites in newly diagnosed prostate cancer patients. Moreover correlation with 3 T MRI is demonstrated, as well as good tolerance of the radiopharmaceutical, good image quality and correlation of SUV and radiopharmaceuticals' kinetics over time [9], although overlap between malignant and benign lesions was recorded in primary prostate cancer [10]. Positive findings are reported to correlate with PSA and PSA-doubling values [11]. For prostate/prostatic bed investigation, sensitivity, specificity, accuracy, positive and negative predictive value for anti-3-[(18)F]FACBC are, respectively, 90.2%, 40.0%, 73.6%, 75.3%, and 66.7%, while the respective values for extra-prostatic lesions are 55.0%, 96.7%, 72.9%, 95.7%, and 61.7% [12]. FACBC-PET is demonstrated superior to CT in prostate cancer relapse patients [13]. In a direct comparison with $^{11}$C-Choline-PET imaging in recurrent prostate cancer patients $^{18}$F-FACBC seems to have slightly higher specificity, sensitivity, and positive predictive values with a statistically significant difference as far as TP, TN, FP, and FN results are concerned, while $^{18}$F-FACBC seems to perform better in cases of low PSA ($p = 0.0001$ for PSA <1 ng/mL). Among others the authors also favorably comment the physical properties, production feasibility, and tracer distribution within the body and tumor uptake [14]. Furthermore fluciclovine-PET is investigated in radiotherapy treatment contouring with so far positive results [15].

**PSMA**, a transmembrane protein, was identified as a potential target for prostate cancer imaging, as it is overexpressed in prostate cancer cells, as well as may serve as a target for therapy in the thera(g)nostics era ([16] for a review see Hofman and Iravani). Ga-68 and F-18 labeled PSMA compounds are the most utilized in Europe. Advantages of Ga-68 are its physical characteristics and its in-site production through $^{68}$Ge/$^{68}$Ga generators. But, although some differences have been described between different PSMA tracers for PET imaging, there is no clear proof to date that one of those radiopharmaceuticals has actually improved diagnostic characteristics compared with another and therefore when we refer to PSMA-PET we in fact refer to any of the PSMA-PET tracers [17]. Schwenck et al. [18] directly compared the PSMA-PET with $^{11}$C-choline-PET in a group of 123 initial and biochemically relapsed prostate cancer patients. In the relapse group abnormal lesions in prostatic bed/prostate, lymph nodes, and bones showed significantly higher uptake of PSMA than of choline; the detection rate of pathologic lymph nodes ($p < 0.001$)—particularly smaller ones—and bone metastasis (98% vs. 64%) was significantly higher for $^{68}$Ga-PSMA. In a per-patient and in per-regional-lymph-node basis detection rate differences were also observed. Notable was the fact that the discrepancy in the detection rate of lymph nodes concerned more low-PSA (<1 ng/mL) prostate cancer cases in favor of PSMA-PET. Altogether $^{68}$Ga-PSMA-11 PET presented with 83% detection rate of at least one metastatic lesion vs 79% for $^{11}$C-choline-PET. Concentrating on TNM staging and oligometastatic disease, PSMA-PET imaging was found to have a higher impact in N and M staging compared to that of Choline-PET. As far as the initial staging group is concerned, higher uptake of $^{68}$Ga-PSMA was observed, as well as more lymph nodes and bone lesions detected, although no difference in per-patient basis.

PSMA-PET tracers are, thus, gaining acceptance in prostate cancer patients imaging during staging and restaging. Specificity, negative and positive predictive values of $^{68}$Ga-labeled PSMA ligand HBED-CC in a retrospective study of 319 recurrent prostate cancer patients in a lesion-based analysis are 100%, 91.4%, and 100%, while the detection rate in per patient analysis is 82.8%

[19]. Pooled estimated positivity for $^{68}$Ga-PSMA-PET, in a recent meta-analysis, is 42% for PSA levels <0.2 ng/mL reaching 76% for PSA 1.0–1.99 ng/mL and 95% for PSA >2 ng/mL, while similar findings are reported for PSA-doubling time [20]. In ProPSMA trial, a multicenter randomized trial, for staging high-risk prostate cancer patients, PSMA-PET had 27% greater accuracy than that of conventional imaging [21]. PSMA-PET is the most sensitive modality for depicting metastatic disease; however prognosis based only on metastases found in PSMA-PET is missing [22]. It is reported that the detection rate of 50% of lymph nodes requires >2.3 mm lymph node diameter and of 90% $\geq$ 4.5 mm [23]. Discussion exists about the necessity of baseline PSMA-PET when evaluating treatment response. Figure 13.1 shows PSMA-PET/CT before and after hormone therapy in a prostate cancer patient with favorable outcome.

Biochemical recurrence, oligometastatic disease, and imaging after androgen deprivation therapy are only a few questions regarding the performance of PSMA-PET, and numerous studies are currently evaluating its value in prostate cancer patients. New guide recommendations have been proposed for PSMA-PET imaging. For initial staging high score (appropriate) indication includes unfavorable intermediate-, high-risk, or very-high-risk prostate cancer ± negative or equivocal or oligometastatic disease conventional imaging. For biochemical recurrence indication includes the increase or persistence of PSA after radical prostatectomy or after definitive radiotherapy. Last, for Castration-resistant cancer high score indication includes negative conventional imaging [17]. Figures 13.2 and 13.3 show the incremental contribution of PSMA-PET/CT in biochemical recurrence.

Consensus criteria were recently established proposing the use of PSMA-PET/CT for investigation of metastatic disease at any stage of the screening process, as well as for biochemical recurrence investigation, while it should be omitted in low-risk cases. PSMA-PET/CT can lead to stage alteration, directing to further consideration and perhaps to alternative clinical treatment decisions [22]. Concern is expressed about how deprivation therapy has an effect on the interpretation of PSMA-PET imaging results. Hormone therapies may have an impact on PSMA uptake including flare phenomenon, and Fanti et al. being particularly careful propose at least 3-month initiation of therapy before performing a PSMA-PET [22, 24]. A molecular imaging TNM (miTNM) has been proposed [25] for standardization of reporting local disease, pelvic and extrapelvic involvement, as well as for improving diagnostic confidence when reporting using a five-point scale. Blood pool, liver or spleen, and parotid uptake function as thresholds for reporting PSMA expression [25].

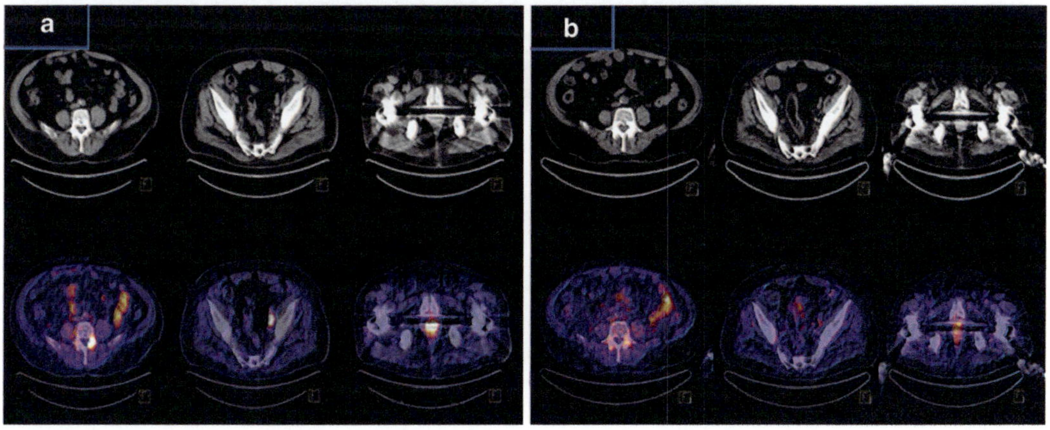


**Fig. 13.1** CT (upper row) and $^{68}$Ga-PSMA-PET/CT fused images (lower row) before (**a**) and after (**b**) hormone therapy in a prostate cancer patient—favorable outcome

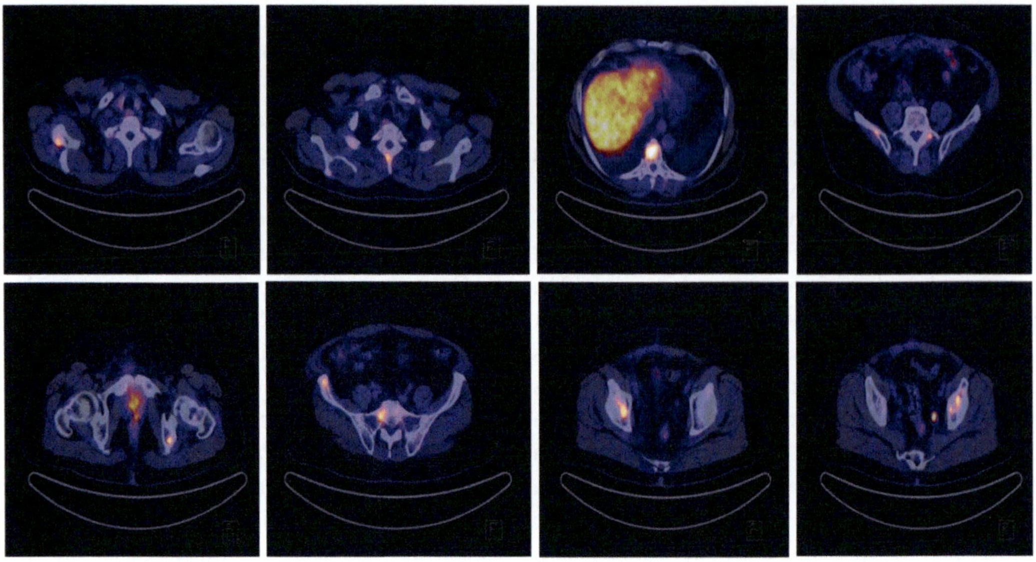

**Fig. 13.2** $^{68}$Ga-PSMA-PET/CT fused images. Biochemical recurrence after prostatectomy, Gleason Score 9, PSA 20.35. Multiple skeletal lesions and a left pelvic lymph node

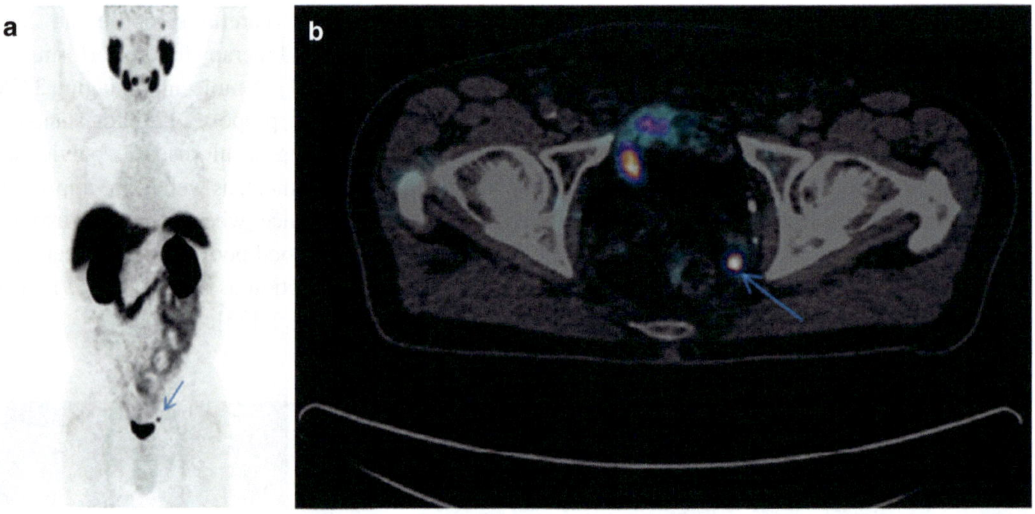


**Fig. 13.3** Ga-68-PSMA-PET/CT. (**a**): MIP image, (**b**): transverse PET/CT. A 68 years old patient with history of surgery because of prostate adenocarcinoma [Gleason score 6 (3 + 3)]. PSA levels were elevated to 0.3 ng/dL. A small (4 mm) left pelvic lymph node uptake is noted (arrows) (SUVmax 9.2). Radiotherapy and 3 months later no detectable PSA levels (<0.001 ng/dL). Ga-68-PSMA-PET/CT can detect site of recurrence even in cases with low PSA levels

## 13.3 Artificial Intelligence in the Service of Prostate Cancer Patients

The term Artificial intelligence (AI) has been in use for long time to describe the ability of computers to do tasks that would require human intelligence to be performed. In practice, artificial intelligence in imaging device and processing, meaning the application of computer algorithms for image interpretation, is currently widely applied and investigated both in the acquisition processing and in the reconstruction face, gaining growing acceptance in the imaging field. For PET instrumentation modern AI refers essentially to the time-of-flight and the localization of photon interaction [26]; for radiopharmaceuticals it stands for the development of new tracers/radiopharmaceuticals using computing AI technology [27], while radiomics directs to the transformation of the image to measurable data, through which information about the tumor/lesion biology or further about the patient's prognosis can be derived [28]. The advantage of hybrid PET/CT or PET/MR systems is that either one or both the anatomic and the functional compartment can be used for machine training and validation. Using textural analyses and radiomic features derived from the CT component of the hybrid PET/CT systems, as well as MR parameters derived from PET/MR systems several investigators developed and/or used AI CT or MRI-derived methods to detect tumor lesions concerning the primary tumor, the lymph nodes, and distant metastases in prostate cancer patients [29–31], concluding that AI tools may serve at least comparable to expert physicians [30]. Furthermore, radiomic features, derived from any imaging method, can be used for machine learning or in neural network systems in order to create predictive models (deep radiomics) [28].

Several challenges are confronted every day in the effort to implement AI in everyday practice. These are even more in prostate cancer imaging, correlated to the organ's proximity to the bladder—which yields high activity measurements, or derived from the small or the multiple or the non-avid cancerous foci in the prostate, as well as the physiologic distribution of tracer uptake [32]. Still being at its outset, a few studies have been published using AI and Deep Learning (DL) for the primary tumor segmentation and quantification, lymph node and metastasis evaluation, as well as outcome and survival prediction.

Mortensen et al. developed and trained a convolutional neural network (CNN) algorithm for prostate segmentation using data from both the PET and CT compartments of the PET/CT device with the utilization of F-18 choline (FCH). Researchers compared PET values such as SUVmean, SUVmax, TLU, and $Vol_{abn}$ derived from manually drawn prostate areas to CNN automatic derived prostate areas and found a good match between them [33]. Polymeri et al. [34] evaluated DL CNN-based algorithm obtaining training data from one PET system and apply it to a validation group scanned by a different PET device, thus showing that algorithms, when trained properly, may be used in a larger scale. This was even evaluated in a larger cohort for lymph node detection using different PET systems in different hospitals [35]. Using choline-PET, differences were reported between observers and automated systems, yet correlation between quantification values and survival was mentioned; lastly, concerning prostate volume evaluation, the automated method tended to overestimate the small prostates while overestimate the large ones [34]. Yi et al. developed and validated radiomics methods in order to predict the probability of an invisible Ga-PSMA-PET prostate area to be cancerous, thus avoiding further biopsies or pointing to biopsy necessitation [36]. The investigators used the 10 more profound predictive radiomic features derived from standard and delayed PET images for machine training and external testing. Reported AUCs in the validation group of trained model was 0.903 for the standard images, 0.856 for the delayed ones, and 0.925 for both, all of which significantly higher than that of PSA Density, while accuracies ranged between 79.4% and 87.0%. Taking into account that the measurements may be applied for the right and left prostate lobe separately, further application of this prediction model could be the evaluation of the "negative" prostate site in known one-sided prostate cancer. Zamboglou et al. using different approach applied AI radiomic features from PSMA-PET in the investigation of primary tumor to discriminate cancerous from noncancerous prostate tissue [37].

Detecting lymph nodes using AI methods is considered even more challenging, as lymph nodes do not concern a specific organ easily segmented in CT and secondly the higher percentage of nonspecific uptake of the radiopharmaceutical leads to more false-positive findings. These obstacles need to be surpassed before AI algorithms become a routine in daily practice. However lymph node status depicted by AI CNN-based tools is demonstrated to be related to survival in prostate cancer patients. Furthermore AI can perform as good as a physician, although overestimating lymph node involvement, and AI tools can be trained for better performance. These initial tools can serve as the basis for more advanced ones and/or for other tracers' utilization [35]. Capobianco et al. reported that it is possible to train a convolutional neural network to find Ga-68-PSMA uptake lesions in the entire axial body and further classify them according to the PROMISE miTNM system, showing agreement with the expert's estimation and opinion. In addition, the authors showed that it is possible to use information from other PET tracers such as FDG for training the system, which actually may lead to improvement of the performance of the system [38]. Evaluating the pelvic area including bone and lymph node lesions using a developed deep neural network a precision and recall of 99% was reached for skeletal detection and 94% and 89% respectively for lymph node involvement estimation on Ga-68-PSMA-PET/CT [39].

Using a developed automated software ("aPROMISE—automated Prostate Molecular Imaging Standardized Evaluation") bearing deep learning methods so as to segment the organs in low-dose CT and further to measure the uptake of the radiopharmaceutical in these organs, high accuracy of the method for organ segmentation is reported. Also high sensitivity is demonstrated of 91.5%, 90.6%, and 86.7%, respectively, for regional lymph node detection in high-risk localized disease patients, for all lymph nodes, and skeletal metastasis [40]. Finally, AI and CNN models can be applied in prostate cancer patients with biochemical recurrence undergoing $^{18}$F-fluciclovine-PET imaging. Analyzing pelvic images, AUC for the slice-based approach 2D-CNN is 0.971. AUC for the case-based approaches using the 2D-CNN and the 3D-CNN was respectively 0.750 and 0.699 [41].

Alongi et al. developed ML radiomics algorithm to discover features for high-risk prostate cancer progression estimation derived from FCH-PET imaging. From the 106 features initially extracted out of 4876 features analyzed, the combination of 13 was found to express the highest sensitivity, specificity, and accuracy in DA classification [42]. Further, in another study, using ML feature selection, from manual tumor delineation, a prognostic model was trained using features that mostly related to patients risks. The investigators used discriminant analysis (DA) for classification of features according to TNM as well as in the whole cohort to predict the presence of progressive disease during follow-up and although different features were depicted for better tumor, nodal, and metastatic prognostication, the fact is that such ML models are feasible and may be useful for PD prediction in this group of patients with a similar level of risk [43]. In a prospective study evaluating risk stratification in prostate cancer patients undergoing $^{18}$F-DCFPyL PET-CT using radiomics extraction and machine learning-based algorithms the authors concluded that the PSMA expression metrics derived from the primary tumor was a good marker for predicting tumor's histopathology and metastatic propensity. Different features were identified for a variable of predictions, i.e., Gleason score or lymph node disease with a variable association to SUV metrics, with intensity-based features to be more important for lymph node invasion prediction and textural ones for Gleason score. Reported AUCs were 0.86–0.76 for predicting Gleason score, extracapsular extension, lymph node, and distant metastasis. The authors demonstrated the role of partial volume correction to the radiomics estimations as well as the threshold set for the metrics [44].

**Theranostics,** in Nuclear Medicine, is a term which arises from the combination of the words therapy and diagnosis, to describe the utilization of the same target for radiopharmaceutical manufacturing for both imaging and therapeutic purposes. For prostate cancer the use of F-18 or Ga-68 PSMA for PET/CT imaging and Lu-177 PSMA for treatment is the epitome of a "theranostics" example. The introduction of Lu-177 PSMA in the treatment strategies for prostate cancer patients is supported by several trials, as well as by the increasing number of ongoing ones. The VISION trial, which randomized metastatic castration-resistant prostate cancer patients receiving either 177Lu-PSMA-617 plus standard care or standard care alone, showed that radiographic progression-free survival (PFS) was improved to 8.7 months in the first group of patients versus 3.4 months for the second one (hazard ratio 0.40), while overall survival respectively was 15.3 versus 11.3 months (hazard ratio 0.62). Patients in the 177Lu-PSMA-617 plus best standard of care group were reported to have a diminished death risk of 38% [45]. The TheraP trial (PSMA radionuclide therapy vs. cabazitaxel) demonstrated that radiolabeled PSMA treatment was associated with higher PSA response, longer PFS, and fewer high-grade adverse events [46].

Personalized treatment takes into account patient's special characteristics such as age, body mass, or comorbidity, as well as tumor's characteristics such as Gleason score, PSMA expression, or PSA values in prostate cancer cases. For radionuclide therapy dosimetric calculations constitute the basis for individualized treatments. AI models may serve as an immense assistance in every step during radionuclide diagnostic- based personalized radionuclide therapy [for a review see 47]. Specifically such models may be implicated in quantitative imaging acquisition, during registration of the images, and segmentation of the organs as well as of the abnormal and normal tissues and the assessment of time-activity curves; Radiomics and Deep Learning models may be used for dosimetric calculations and prediction of the absorbed dose so in the tumoral tissues, as in the organs that need to be spared. Finally algorithms may be used for the prediction of the treatments' outcome and patients' prognosis [47].

As newer radiopharmaceuticals and technologies appear in oncologic patients' service, further assessment is required until each is applied in the most useful manner. AI can become an undisputed tool in PET/CT imaging and radionuclide therapy providing objective quantitative assessment within seconds, assisting both experienced physicians and beginners.

## References


1. Fanti S, Minozzi S, Castellucci P, et al. PET/CT with (11)C-choline for evaluation of prostate cancer patients with biochemical recurrence: meta-analysis and critical review of available data. Eur J Nucl Med Mol Imaging. 2016;43(1):55–69.
2. Vag T, Heck MM, Beer AJ, et al. Preoperative lymph node staging in patients with primary prostate cancer: comparison and correlation of quantitative imaging parameters in diffusion-weighted imaging and 11C-choline PET/CT. Eur Radiol. 2014;24(8):1821–6.
3. Castellucci P, Ceci F, Graziani T, et al. Early biochemical relapse after radical prostatectomy: which prostate cancer patients may benefit from a restaging 11C-choline PET/CT scan before salvage radiation therapy. J Nucl Med. 2014;55(9):1424–9.
4. Von Eyben FE, Kairemo K. Acquisition with (11) C-choline and (18)F-fluorocholine PET/CT for patients with biochemical recurrence of prostate cancer: a systematic review and meta-analysis. Ann Nucl Med. 2016;30(6):385–92.
5. Schwarzenböck SM, Knieling A, Souvatzoglou M, et al. [11C]choline PET/CT in therapy response assessment of a neoadjuvant therapy in locally advanced and high risk prostate cancer before radical prostatectomy. Oncotarget. 2016;7(39):63747–57.
6. Chan J, Carver A, Brunt JN, et al. Effect of androgen deprivation therapy on intraprostatic tumour volume identified on 18F choline PET/CT for prostate dose painting radiotherapy. Br J Radiol. 2017;90(1071):20160818.
7. Chang JH, Joon DL, Lee ST, et al. Histopathological correlation of (11)C-choline PET scans for target volume definition in radical prostate radiotherapy. Radiother Oncol. 2011;99(2):187–92.
8. Umbehr MH, Muntener M, Hany T, et al. The role of 11C-choline and 18F-fluorocholine positron emission tomography (PET) and PET/CT in prostate cancer: a systematic review and meta-analysis. Eur Urol. 2013;64:106–17.
9. Sörensen J, Owenius R, Lax M, Johansson S. Regional distribution and kinetics of [18F]fluciclovine (anti-

[18F]FACBC), a tracer of amino acid transport, in subjects with primary prostate cancer. Eur J Nucl Med Mol Imaging. 2013;40(3):394–402.
10. Turkbey B, Mena E, Shih J, et al. Localized prostate cancer detection with 18F FACBC PET/CT: comparison with MR imaging and histopathologic analysis. Radiology. 2014;270(3):849–56.
11. Kairemo K, Rasulova N, Partanen K, Joensuu T. Preliminary clinical experience of trans-1-Amino-3-(18)F-fluorocyclobutanecarboxylic acid (anti-(18)F-FACBC) PET/CT imaging in prostate cancer patients. Biomed Res Int. 2014;2014:305182.
12. Schuster DM, Nieh PT, Jani AB, et al. Anti-3-[(18)F] FACBC positron emission tomography-computerized tomography and (111)in-capromab pendetide single photon emission computerized tomography-computerized tomography for recurrent prostate carcinoma: results of a prospective clinical trial. J Urol. 2014;191(5):1446–53.
13. Odewole OA, Tade FI, Nieh PT, et al. Recurrent prostate cancer detection with anti-3-[18F]FACBC PET/CT: comparison with CT. Eur J Nucl Med Mol Imaging. 2016;43(10):1773–83.
14. Nanni C, Zanoni L, Pultrone C, et al. 18F-FACBC (anti1-amino-3-18F-fluorocyclobutane-1-carboxylic acid) versus 11C-choline PET/CT in prostate cancer relapse: results of a prospective trial. Eur J Nucl Med Mol Imaging. 2016;43(9):1601–10.
15. Akin-Akintayo OO, Jani AB, Odewole O, et al. Change in salvage radiotherapy management based on guidance with FACBC (Fluciclovine) PET/CT in postprostatectomy recurrent prostate cancer. Clin Nucl Med. 2017;42(1):e22–8.
16. Hofman MS, Iravani A. Gallium-68 prostate-specific membrane antigen PET imaging. PET Clin. 2017;12(2):219–34.
17. Jadvar H, Calais J, Fanti S, et al. Appropriate use criteria for prostate-specific membrane antigen PET imaging. J Nucl Med. 2022;63(1):59–68.
18. Schwenck J, Rempp H, Reischl G, et al. Comparison of 68Ga-labelled PSMA-11 and 11C-choline in the detection of prostate cancer metastases by PET/CT. Eur J Nucl Med Mol Imaging. 2017;44:92. https://doi.org/10.1007/s00259-016-3490-6.
19. Afshar-Oromieh A, Avtzi E, Giesel FL, et al. The diagnostic value of PET/CT imaging with the 68Ga-labelled PSMA ligand HBED-CC in the diagnosis of recurrent prostate cancer. Eur J Nucl Med Mol Imaging. 2015;42(2):197–209.
20. Perera M, Papa N, Christidis D, et al. Sensitivity, specificity, and predictors of positive 68Ga–prostate-specific membrane antigen positron emission tomography in advanced prostate cancer: a systematic review and meta-analysis. Eur Urol. 2016;70(6):926–37.
21. Hofman MS, Lawrentschuk N, Francis RJ, et al. Prostate-specific membrane antigen PET-CT in patients with high-risk prostate cancer before curative-intent surgery or radiotherapy (proPSMA): a prospective, randomised, multicentre study. Lancet. 2020;395:1208–16.
22. Fanti S, Goffin K, Hadaschik BA, et al. Consensus statements on PSMA PET/CT response assessment criteria in prostate cancer. Eur J Nucl Med Mol Imaging. 2021;48:469–76.
23. Jilg CA, Drendel V, Rischke HC, et al. Diagnostic accuracy of Ga-68-HBED-CC-PSMA-ligand-PET/CT before salvage lymph node dissection for recurrent prostate cancer. Theranostics. 2017;7(6):1770–80.
24. Emmett L, Yin C, Crumbaker M. Rapid modulation of PSMA expression by androgen deprivation: serial 68 Ga-PSMA-11 PET in men with hormone-sensitive and castrate-resistant prostate cancer commencing androgen blockade. J Nucl Med. 2019;60(7):950–4.
25. Eiber M, Herrmann K, Calais J, et al. Prostate cancer molecular imaging standardized evaluation (PROMISE): proposed miTNM classification for the interpretation of PSMA-ligand PET/CT. J Nucl Med. 2018;59(3):469–78.
26. Ullah MN, Levin CS. Application of artificial intelligence in PET instrumentation. PET Clin. 2022;17(1):175–82.
27. Ataeinia B, Heidari P. Artificial intelligence and the future of diagnostic and therapeutic radiopharmaceutical development: in silico smart molecular design. PET Clin. 2021;16(4):513–23.
28. Orlhac F, Nioche C, Klyuzhin I, et al. Radiomics in PET imaging: a practical guide for newcomers. PET Clin. 2021;16(4):597–612.
29. Peeken JC, Shouman MA, Kroenke M, et al. A CT-based radiomics model to detect prostate cancer lymph node metastases in PSMA radioguided surgery patients. Eur J Nucl Med Mol Imaging. 2020;47(13):2968–77.
30. Hartenstein A, Lübbe F, Baur ADJ, et al. Prostate cancer nodal staging: using deep learning to predict 68 Ga-PSMA-positivity from CT imaging alone. Sci Rep. 2020;10(1):3398.
31. Papp L, Spielvogel CP, Grubmüller B. Supervised machine learning enables non-invasive lesion characterization in primary prostate cancer with [68Ga]Ga-PSMA-11 PET/MRI. Eur J Nucl Med Mol Imaging. 2021;48(6):1795–805.
32. Ma K, Harmon SA, Klyuzhin IS, et al. Clinical application of artificial intelligence in positron emission tomography: imaging of prostate cancer. PET Clin. 2022;17(1):137–43.
33. Mortensen MA, Borrelli P, Poulsen MH, et al. Artificial intelligence-based versus manual assessment of prostate cancer in the prostate gland: a method comparison study. Clin Physiol Funct Imaging. 2019;39(6):399–406.
34. Polymeri E, Sadik M, Kaboteh R, et al. Deep learning-based quantification of PET/CT prostate gland uptake: association with overall survival. Clin Physiol Funct Imaging. 2020;40:106–13.
35. Borrelli P, Larsson M, Ulén J, et al. Artificial intelligence-based detection of lymph node metastases by PET/CT predicts prostate cancer-specific survival. Clin Physiol Funct Imaging. 2021;41(1):62–7.

36. Yi Z, Hu S, Lin X, et al. Machine learning-based prediction of invisible intraprostatic prostate cancer lesions on 68 Ga-PSMA-11 PET/CT in patients with primary prostate cancer. Eur J Nucl Med Mol Imaging. 2021;49(5):1523–34. https://doi.org/10.1007/s00259-021-05631-6. PMID: 34845536
37. Zamboglou C, Carles M, Fechter T, et al. Radiomic features from PSMA PET for non-invasive intraprostatic tumor discrimination and characterization in patients with intermediate- and high-risk prostate cancer—a comparison study with histology reference. Theranostics. 2019;9:2595–605.
38. Capobianco N, Sibille L, Chantadisai M, et al. Whole body uptake classification and prostate cancer staging in 68Ga PSMA 11 PET/CT using dual tracer learning. Eur J Nucl Med Mol Imaging. 2021;49(2):517–26. https://doi.org/10.1007/s00259-021-05473-2.
39. Zhao Y, Gafita A, Vollnberg B, et al. Deep neural network for automatic characterization of lesions on 68Ga-PSMA-11 PET/CT. Eur J Nucl Med Mol Imaging. 2020;47:603–13.
40. Johnsson K, Brynolfsson J, Sahlstedt H, et al. Analytical performance of aPROMISE: automated anatomic contextualization, detection, and quantification of [18F] DCFPyL (PSMA) imaging for standardized reporting. Eur J Nucl Med Mol Imaging. 2021;49(3):1041–51. https://doi.org/10.1007/s00259-021-05497-8.
41. Lee JJ, Yang H, Franc BL, et al. Deep learning detection of prostate cancer recurrence with 18F-FACBC (fluciclovine, Axumin®) positron emission tomography. Eur J Nucl Med Mol Imaging. 2020;47:2992–7.
42. Alongi P, Laudicella R, Stefano A, et al. Choline PET/CT features to predict survival outcome in high risk prostate cancer restaging: a preliminary machine-learning radiomics study. Q J Nucl Med Mol Imaging. 2020; https://doi.org/10.23736/S1824-4785.20.03227-6.
43. Alongi P, Stefano A, Albert Comelli A, et al. Radiomics analysis of 18F-choline PET/CT in the prediction of disease outcome in high-risk prostate cancer: an explorative study on machine learning feature classification in 94 patients. Eur Radiol. 2021;31:4595–605.
44. Cysouw MCF, Jansen BHE, van de Brug T, et al. Machine learning-based analysis of [18F]DCFPyL PET radiomics for risk stratification in primary prostate cancer. Eur J Nucl Med Mol Imaging. 2021;48:340–9.
45. Rohith G. VISION trial: $^{177}$Lu-PSMA-617 for progressive metastatic castration-resistant prostate cancer. Indian J Urol. 2021;37(4):372–3.
46. Hofman MS, Emmett L, Sandhu S, et al. [$^{177}$ Lu] Lu-PSMA-617 versus cabazitaxel in patients with metastatic castration-resistant prostate cancer (TheraP): a randomised, open-label, phase 2 trial. Lancet. 2021;397(10276):797–804.
47. Brosch-Lenz J, Yousefirizi F, Zukotynski K, et al. Role of artificial intelligence in theranostics: toward routine personalized radiopharmaceutical therapies. PET Clin. 2021;16:627–41.

# The Role of $^{18}$FDG-PET/CT in Malignant Lymphomas Clinical Implications

14

Theodoros P. Vassilakopoulos, Athanassios Liaskas, Alexia Piperidou, Maria Ioakim, and Vassilios Prassopoulos

## 14.1 Introduction

PET/CT has a key role in final response assessment after treatment in most types of malignant lymphomas, as well as in baseline staging and interim (mid-treatment) evaluation [1, 2]. Its application is widely established in Hodgkin lymphoma (HL) and aggressive B cell lymphomas, including diffuse large B cell lymphoma (DLBCL), primary mediastinal large B cell lymphoma (PMLBCL), and other related subtypes. Although recent recommendations suggest the use of PET/CT for baseline staging and response assessment in follicular lymphomas, mantle cell lymphoma (MCL), Burkitt lymphoma, and "nodal" T cell lymphomas [anaplastic large cell (ALCL), peripheral T cell (PTCL), and angioimmunoblastic T cell lymphoma (AITL)], the accumulated clinical experience with these subtypes is considerably less [1–7]. The role of PET/CT is much more controversial in non-follicular low-grade lymphomas and primary extranodal lymphomas other than DLBCL [6, 8].

T. P. Vassilakopoulos (✉) · A. Liaskas · A. Piperidou · M. Ioakim
Department of Haematology, National and Kapodistrian University of Athens, Laikon General Hospital, Athens, Greece

V. Prassopoulos
Departments of Nuclear Medicine and PET/CT, Hygeia Hospital, Athens, Greece

The various lymphoma subtypes are not equally FDG-avid and this mainly depends on their histologic features, aggressiveness, and biologic characteristics. "Routinely FDG-avid lymphomas" include HL, DLBCL, and other aggressive B cell lymphomas, lymphoblastic and Burkitt lymphoma, follicular and MCL, nodal marginal zone lymphoma, and systemic ALCL, since they are almost invariably 18-FDG-avid (>90% and usually >95–100% of the cases) [1, 2, 9, 10]. Other aggressive T cell lymphomas, mainly the non-ALCL "nodal" types, such as PTCL and AITL as well as extranodal NK/T cell lymphomas, are typically but not invariably 18-FDG-avid (>80–100% of the cases in various studies) [1, 2, 9, 10]. In contrast, other indolent lymphomas are even more "variably 18-FDG-avid." Thus, several forms of extranodal lymphomas, including MALT and cutaneous B and T cell lymphomas, small lymphocytic, splenic marginal zone lymphoma as well as some rare lymphoma subtypes, may not be satisfactorily evaluated by PET/CT, displaying frequencies of FDG avidity between 50% and 80% [1].

## 14.2 PET/CT in Initial Staging

The rationale of using FDG-PET in the initial staging of lymphomas is based on its improved accuracy in determining disease extent, as compared to conventional imaging [1, 2]. PET/CT is



J. A. Andreou et al. (eds.), *Artificial Intelligence in PET/CT Oncologic Imaging*,
https://doi.org/10.1007/978-3-031-10090-1_14

more sensitive than CT, mainly because it can detect disease in normal-sized lymph nodes or facilitate the evaluation of extranodal disease [1, 2]. The extent of disease upstaging or—less frequently—downstaging varies according to histology and will be discussed later. Further to more accurate staging, baseline PET/CT can facilitate the interpretation of the end-of-treatment (EOT) PET/CT response assessment serving as a basis for comparison. Finally, baseline PET/CT may provide new prognostic factors related to tumor burden and metabolic activity, which are increasingly evaluated in detail, although they have not yet become standard prognostication tools.

### 14.2.1 Role of PET in the Initial Staging of Lymphomas

Baseline PET/CT is strongly recommended for initial staging of the routinely FDG-avid lymphomas [1, 2] (Figs. 14.1a, 14.2a, 14.3a, 14.4a, 14.5a, 14.7a). In HL, the number and density of Hodgkin-Reed-Sternberg cells in the tumor vary and FDG uptake occurs mainly by the inflammatory tumor microenvironment. PET/CT identifies 25–30% more lesions and leads to upstaging an average of 18% of patients in various studies compared to conventional staging [2]. Conversely, up to 10% of the patients (average 4% in various studies) [2] can be downstaged [1, 2, 11, 12]. Such changes might lead to major treatment modification in up to 1/4 of the patients (average 11% in the studies reviewed by Barrington et al.) [2]. In a more common scenario, the identification of more disease sites may affect radiotherapy (RT) fields, even in the absence of stage shift [12]. However, most of the knowledge on treatment approaches is based on conventional staging [11, 12]. Thus, it is not yet clearly proven that stage shift according to PET/CT should guide treatment decisions in HL. In addition, the clinical benefit to be gained from the widening of the RT fields to include anatomically subclinical disease sites may be of concern with respect to potential long-term sequelae. This is becoming

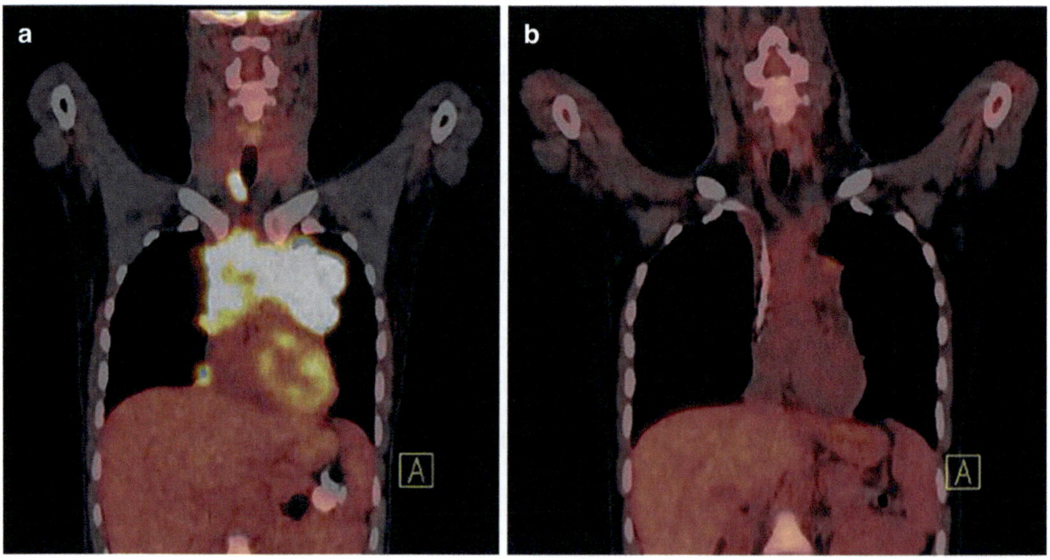


**Fig. 14.1** (**a**) Baseline staging in a patient with Hodgkin lymphoma. Intense FDG uptake is shown in a bulky mediastinal mass. Right cervical and right epiphrenic nodal involvement is also shown. (**b**) Post chemotherapy evaluation revealed a residual mediastinal abnormality with FDG uptake higher than the mediastinal blood pool but not exceeding that of the liver. This would have been interpreted as positive, i.e., suggestive of residual active disease based on the 2007 IHP criteria. However, interpreted as Deauville 5-point scale score 3 (Table 14.1), it is now considered compatible with complete metabolic response based on the 2014 Lugano criteria (Table 14.2)

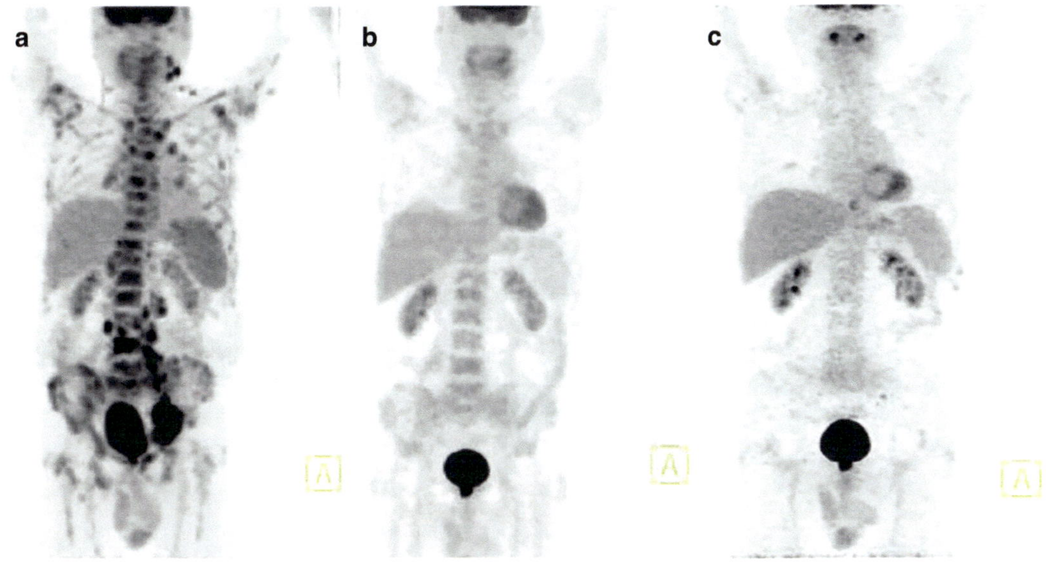

**Fig. 14.2** (**a**) Baseline staging in a patient with diffuse large B-cell lymphoma. Disseminated lymphadenopathy including a left pelvic mass and multiple focal osseous/bone marrow lesions suggestive of bone marrow involvement are consistent with stage IV disease. (**b**) Interim PET after two cycles of R-CHOP is completely negative. (**c**) Post R-CHOP evaluation is also negative, as correctly predicted by the negative interim examination

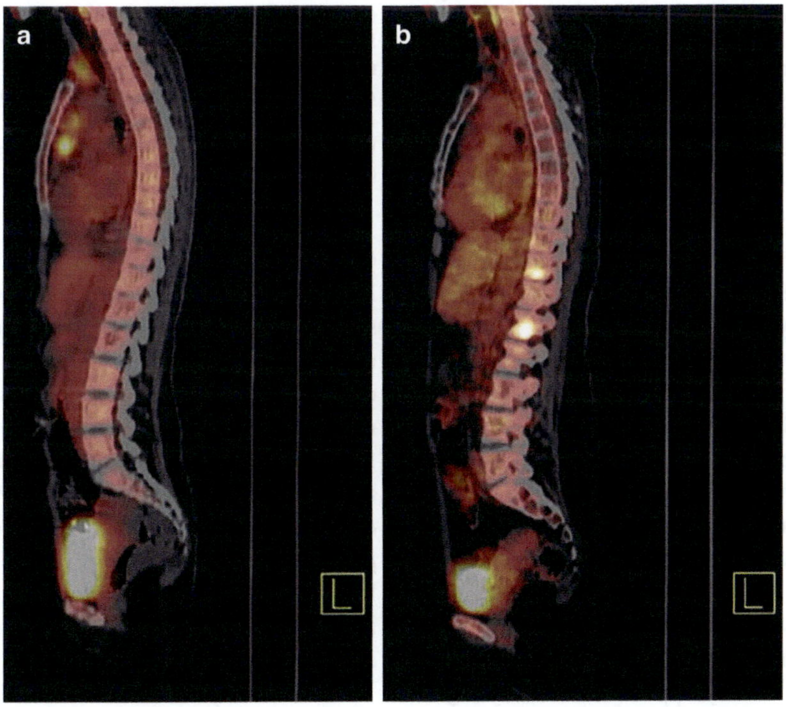

**Fig. 14.3** (**a**) Baseline staging in a patient with Hodgkin lymphoma, indicating cervical and mediastinal involvement. Conventional staging had revealed mildly enlarged paraortic nodes, which were not demonstrable by PET/CT. Thus, the patient was downstaged from clinical stage IIIA to PET-stage IIA. (**b**) PET/CT at the time of relapse in the same patient. PET/CT had been normalized following ABVD × 6. Three months after the completion of involved field radiotherapy the patient presented with lumbar pain and elevated ESR and C-Reactive Protein levels. MRI revealed osseous abnormalities, which were confirmed by PET/CT. PET/CT normalized again after IGEV salvage chemotherapy and BEAM with autologous stem cell support

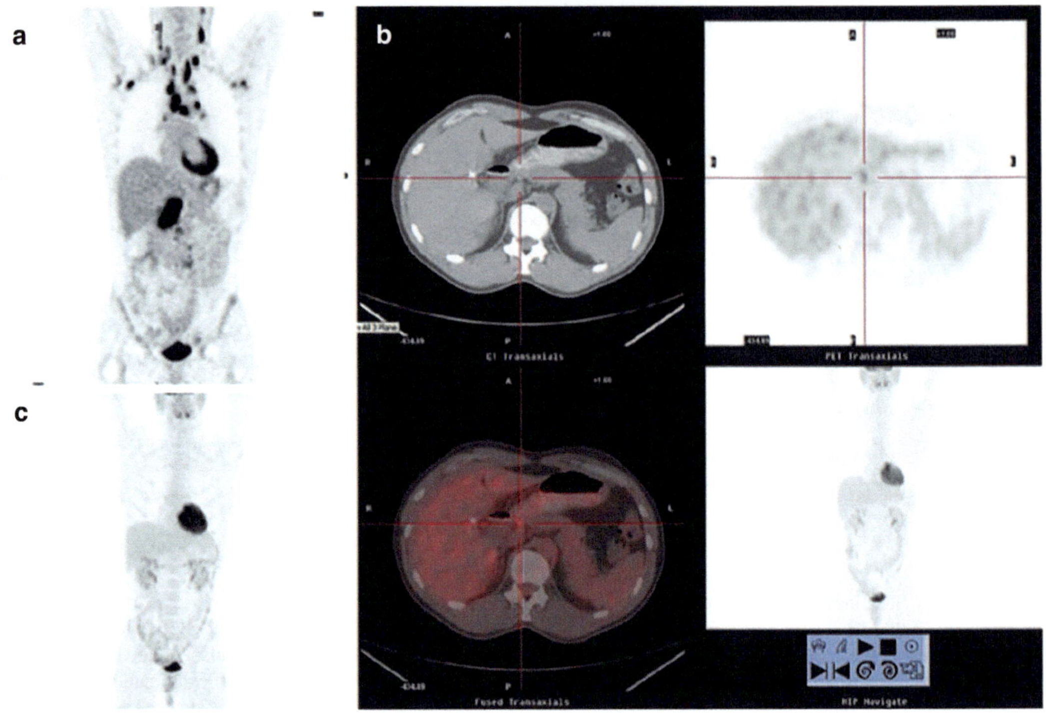

**Fig. 14.4** (**a**) Baseline staging in a patient with Hodgkin lymphoma. The patient had disseminated nodal disease, including a mass at the hepatogastric junction, and a positive bone marrow biopsy (stage IVB). (**b**) Interim PET after two cycles of ABVD revealed complete resolution of FDG uptake except of the hepatogastric mass, which was reduced in size and had residual FDG uptake just above that of the liver. Interim PET was interpreted as positive, Deauville score 4. The patient received intensified chemotherapy with six cycles of BEACOPP-escalated. (**c**) Negative end-of-treatment PET in the same patient. He remains in complete remission 8.5 years after the positive interim PET/CT (Courtesy of Drs Datseris I and Rondogianni Ph, Department of Nuclear Medicine and PET/CT, Evangelismos General Hospital, Athens, Greece)

particularly relevant, given the trend to adopt smaller RT fields and doses or even omit RT in appropriately selected patients.

The situation is similar in DLBCL, the commonest form of aggressive B cell lymphomas, and PMLBCL, in which PET/CT is also strongly recommended for initial staging [1, 2]. However, the effect on treatment decisions with standard rituximab-based chemoimmunotherapy may be less important, with the potential exception of abbreviated immunochemotherapy regimens in localized DLBCL. The effect on potential RT fields may not be so relevant in DLBCL, since RT is not routinely applied in the majority of patients in many centers.

In other routinely FDG-avid lymphomas, especially follicular lymphomas and MCL, PET/CT is also recommended for initial staging [1, 2]. However, a meaningful impact on treatment strategy is not expected, since the disease is already disseminated in the vast majority of cases. In the unusual cases of early stage disease, mainly seen in a minority of patients with follicular lymphoma (less frequently in NMZL and even more rarely in MCL), PET/CT may confirm that the disease is indeed localized and potentially curable with involved field or regional RT. Baseline PET evaluation is generally not recommended in lymphoma subtypes which are not routinely FDG-avid (Fig. 14.6) [1, 2].

PET/CT may also contribute to the identification and histologic confirmation of transformed disease in patients with known indolent lymphomas. The degree of FDG uptake has been pro-

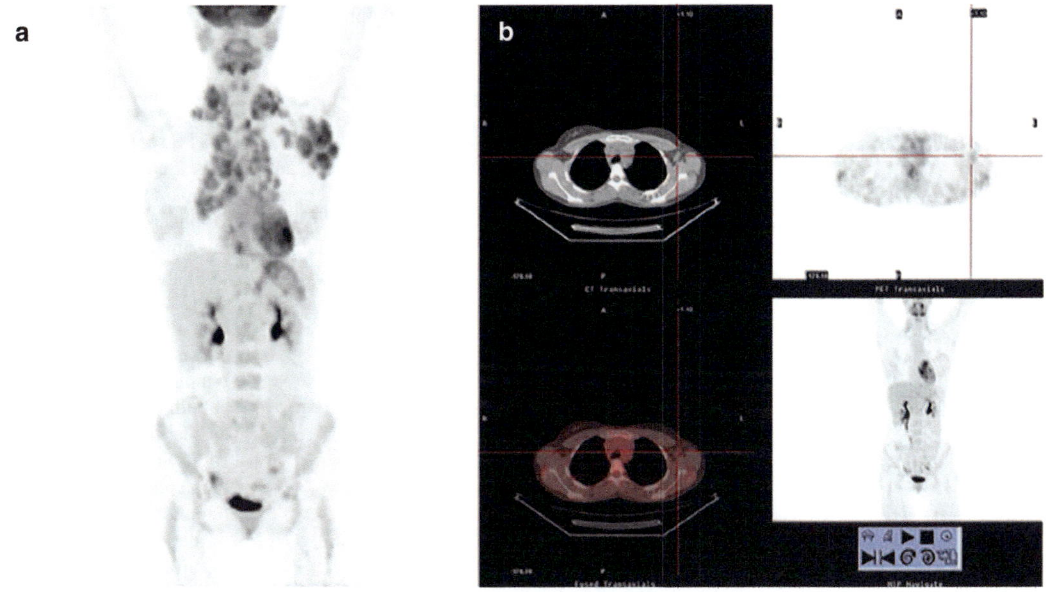


**Fig. 14.5** (**a**) Baseline staging in a patient with Hodgkin lymphoma demonstrating stage IIB disease with extensive supradiaphragmatic nodal involvement. (**b**) Interim PET revealed a residual left axillary abnormality with FDG uptake above the surrounding background but below the mediastinal blood pool. Interim PET was interpreted as negative, Deauville score 2. The patient continued on ABVD. Posttreatment PET/CT was negative. Following involved field radiotherapy, the patient remains in complete remission 8 years after the negative interim PET/CT (Courtesy of Drs Datseris I and Rondogianni Ph, Department of Nuclear Medicine and PET/CT, Evangelismos General Hospital, Athens, Greece)

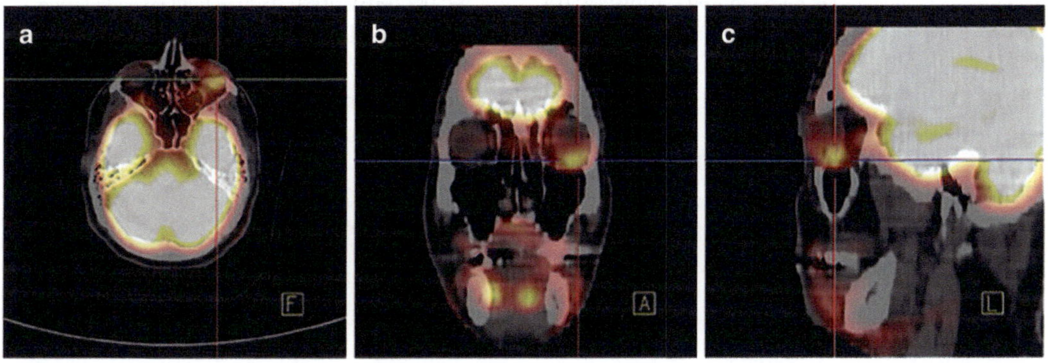


**Fig. 14.6** Extranodal marginal zone lymphoma of the left eye. A mass with increased FDG uptake is shown. Marginal zone lymphomas are not routinely FDG-avid. PET/CT is not routinely recommended either for baseline staging or for posttreatment evaluation in this entity

posed to be correlated with tumor grade, proliferative activity, and aggressiveness and to be of prognostic value [9]. Studies using semi-quantitative measurements based on SUVmax suggest that SUVmax >10 is usually seen in aggressive or transformed indolent lymphomas [9]. The optimal threshold to detect Richter transformation in chronic lymphocytic leukemia (CLL) may range between 5 and 10 with varying effects on sensitivity, specificity, positive and negative prognostic value and may differ in the era of novel agents [13, 14].

**Table 14.1** 2014 Revised criteria for response assessment in malignant lymphomas

| | Complete response (CR) | Partial response (PR) | No response/stable disease (SD) | Progressive disease (PD) |
|---|---|---|---|---|
| *Pet-Based Criteria*[a] | | | | |
| Lymph nodes | D5-PS score 1, 2, or 3 (±residual masses) | D5-PS score 4 or 5—but reduced compared to baseline—and residual mass(es) of any size<br>•At interim evaluation: responding disease<br>•At final evaluation: residual disease (treatment failure) | D5-PS score 4 or 5—but no significant change in FDG uptake compared to baseline (applicable at both interim and final evaluation) | D5-PS score 4 or 5 and increase in FDG uptake compared to baseline (applicable at both interim and final evaluation)<br>AND/OR<br>New FDG-avid lesions consistent with lymphoma (applicable at both interim and final evaluation)<br>Biopsy or follow-up PET encouraged if lymphomatous nature of the lesion(s) is uncertain |
| Extralymphatic sites | D5-PS score 1, 2, or 3 (±residual masses)[b] | | | |
| Non-measured lesions | Not applicable | Not applicable | Not applicable | |
| Organ enlargement | Not applicable[b] | Not applicable | Not applicable | |
| Bone marrow | No FDG-avid disease[b] | Residual uptake higher than normal marrow but less than baseline (diffuse uptake permitted)[c] | No change from baseline | New or recurrent FDG-avid foci |
| *Conventional (CT) Criteria*[a] | | | | |
| Target lymph nodes/masses and/or extralymphatic sites | Nodal regression to LDx ≤1.5 cm AND No extralymphatic sites | Up to 6 sites in total: ≥50% decrease in SPD[d] | Up to 6 sites in total: <50% decrease in SPD and no progressive disease criteria met | PPD progression of ≥1 individual node/lesion, which should be abnormal (all the following):<br>• LDx >1.5 cm and.<br>• Increase by ≥50% from PPD nadir and.<br>• Increase of LDx or SDx (compared to nadir) by 0.5 cm or 1.0 cm for lesions ≤2 and > 2 cm respectively.<br>AND/OR new sites, defined as:<br>• Regrowth of previously resolved lesions.<br>• New node >1.5 cm in any axis.<br>• New extranodal site >1.0 cm in any axis; if <1.0 cm, it should be unequivocal and attributable to lymphoma |

**Table 14.1** (continued)

| | Complete response (CR) | Partial response (PR) | No response/stable disease (SD) | Progressive disease (PD) |
|---|---|---|---|---|
| Non-measured lesions | Absent | No increase (regressed or absent/normal) | No increase falling into the definition of progression (see below) | Clear progression or new lesions |
| Organ enlargement | Regression to normal | Spleen regression by >50% (in its length beyond normal) | No increase falling into the definition of progression (see below) | •Prior splenomegaly: Increase of splenic length by >50% of the extent of its prior increase beyond baseline<br>•No prior splenomegaly: Increase ≥2 cm from baseline |
| Bone marrow | Morphologically normal; negative IHC, if indeterminate | Not applicable | Not applicable | New or recurrent involvement |

*PET* positron emission tomography, *D5-PS* Deauville 5-point scale, *CT* computed tomography, *FDG* fluorodeoxyglucose, *IHC* immunohistochemistry, *LDx* longest transverse diameter of a lesion, *MRI* magnetic resonance imaging, *PET* positron emission tomography, *PPD* cross product of the *LDx* and perpendicular diameter, *SDx* shortest axis perpendicular to the *LDx*, *SPD* sum of the product of the perpendicular diameters for multiple lesions

Terms used throughout this table: (1) Target lesions (target lymph nodes/masses and/or extralymphatic sites) or Measured Dominant Lesions: They include the dominant lesions, i.e., those which are the major determinants of response. They should include up to 6 of the largest nodes/nodal masses or extranodal lesions, being representative of the total tumor burden. Further selection criteria include: a. to be clearly measurable bidimensionally; b. to be located at as much as disparate anatomic regions as possible, including both mediastinal and retroperitoneal areas, if involved. Measurable nodes and extranodal lesions should have an LDx of >1.5 cm and >1.0 cm respectively. (2) Non-Measured Lesions: They include: a. any nodal or extranodal disease, which has not been selected as "Measured Dominant Disease" according to the above definition; b. lesions considered abnormal, but failing to fulfill the requirements for measurability; c. any site of suspected disease, which is assessable but is difficult to be followed by quantitative measurements (serous effusions, bone lesions, leptomeningeal disease, etc.)

[a]PET-based criteria are recommended for FDG-avid lymphoma subtypes (defined in Chap. 4). Conventional (CT) criteria are recommended for non-FDG-avid lymphoma subtypes (defined in Chap. 4)

[b]An uptake higher than mediastinum or liver can be compatible with complete metabolic response, if observed at sites that might have high physiologic uptake or high uptake due to "activation" (i.e., chemotherapy or growth factor-induced), such as the Waldeyer's ring, GI tract, spleen, or marrow. In such cases, FDG uptake at sites of initial involvement should not exceed the surrounding normal tissue, even if this is "physiologically" high

[c]Caution: Persistent focal lesions might be further evaluated by MRI, biopsy, or a new PET

[d]Further instructions to assess partial response, when small residuals are present, are provided in the corresponding article (see below). Adapted and modified from Cheson BD, Fisher RI, Barrington SF, et al. Recommendations for initial evaluation, staging and response assessment of Hodgkin and non-Hodgkin lymphoma: The Lugano classification. J Clin Oncol 2014; 32:3059–3067; (Table 3). Reproduced from "PET/CT in lymphomas: A case-based Atlas", Springer 2016, by the same Editors

Finally, baseline PET/CT may be used to determine the metabolic tumor volume (MTV) and total lesion glycolysis (TLG), which is a combined evaluation of both tumor burden and metabolic activity. These parameters—and other radiomic markers—can be of prognostic significance, as described later.

**Table 14.2** Summary of selected studies evaluating the outcome of EOT-PET-negative patients with Hodgkin lymphoma after the completion of chemotherapy and prior to any radiotherapy

| Author, year, ref | Pts | Stages | Chemotherapy | Definition of negative EOT-PET | Radiotherapy | Relapse (progression) free survival |
|---|---|---|---|---|---|---|
| *Localized stages* | | | | | | |
| Fuchs [84]<br>HD16, RT arm | 328 | I/II, few EORTC unfavorable[a] | ABVD × 2 | D5PS score 1–2 | 100% | 93% at 5 years (PFS) |
| Radford [83]<br>RAPID, RT arm, per protocol | 183 | I/IIA, no bulky mediastinum | ABVD × 3 | D5PS score 1–2 | 100% | 97% at 3 years (PFS) |
| Borchmann [85]<br>HD17, RT arm | 274 | I/II with ≥1 r.f. but not IIB E or bulky | BEACOPP-esc ×2 plus ABVD ×2 | D5PS score 1–2 | 100% | 98% at 5 years (PFS) |
| Vassilakopoulos [79] | 157 | I/II A/B | ABVD × 4–6 | IHP criteria | 96% | 96% at 4 years (RFS) |
| Barrington [88]<br>RAPID, RT arm, ITT | 209 | I/IIA, no bulky mediastinum | ABVD ×3 | D5PS score 1–2 | 88% | 96% at 5 years (EFS) |
| Barnes [81] | 83 | I/II A/B, non-bulky | ABVD ×4–6 | "neg or likely neg for neoplastic disease" | ≤56%[b] | 94% at 4 years (PFS) |
| Barrington [88]<br>RAPID, no RT arm, ITT | 211 | I/IIA, no bulky mediastinum | ABVD ×3 | D5PS score 1–2 | 1% | 90% at 5 years (EFS) |
| Radford [83], 2015<br>RAPID, no RT arm, per protocol | 209 | I/IIA, no bulky mediastinum | ABVD ×3 | D5PS score 1–2 | 0% | 91% at 3 years (PFS) |
| Fuchs [84]<br>HD16, RT arm | 300 | I/II, few EORTC unfavorable[a] | ABVD ×2 | D5PS score 1–2 | 0% | 86% at 5 years (PFS) |
| Borchmann [85]<br>HD17, RT arm | 323 | I/II with ≥1 r.f. but not IIB E or bulky | BEACOPP-esc ×2 plus ABVD ×2 | D5PS score 1–2 | 0% | 96% at 5 years (PFS) |
| *Advanced stages* | | | | | | |
| Vassilakopoulos [79] | 56 | III/IV | ABVD ×6–8 | IHP criteria | 12% | 80% at 4 years (RFS) (88% versus 69% for stages III vs. IV) |
| Engert [80, 87]<br>HD15, CR/CRu (no or < 2.5 cm residual); no PET evaluation | 884 | IIB X/E, III/IV | BEACOPP-esc ×6 or 8 or BEACOPP-14 | IHP criteria | not planned | 92% at 4 years (PFS) AND 85% at 10 years (PFS) |
| Engert [80, 87]<br>HD15, PET-negative residual ≥2.5 cm | 548 | IIB X/E, III/IV | BEACOPP-esc ×6 or 8 or BEACOPP-14 | IHP criteria | 1% | 93% at 4 years (PFS) AND 88% at 10 years (PFS) |

[a]Early stages according to GHSG definition, but few early unfavorable according to the EORTC definition because of bulk definition and age

[b]Among 96 patients, 56% received radiotherapy but 13/96 had a positive PET and presumably received RT more frequently (decision based on physician's choice)

### 14.2.2 PET in the Assessment of Bone Marrow Involvement

Numerous studies have investigated the role of PET in the assessment of bone marrow (BM) involvement. The comparative accuracy of PET/CT and bone marrow biopsy (BMb) highly depends on the specific lymphoma subtype under evaluation.

#### 14.2.2.1 Hodgkin Lymphoma

According to current recommendations, bone marrow biopsy (BMb) can be omitted in HL, if baseline PET/CT is performed [1, 2]. The omission of BMb in this setting is also proposed by the latest version of the ESMO guidelines at a level of evidence III (from prospective cohort studies) and grade B strength of recommendation (generally recommended) [15]. However, a BMb still remains necessary in cases with no baseline PET/CT available. Indeed, PET/CT uncovers more cases of BM involvement [11, 16–19] while treatment decisions are not typically affected in the rare cases with a positive BMb but a negative PET/CT, as analyzed below. Patients with BM involvement by PET/CT may have similarly poor outcomes irrespective of BMb status, but this information is still based on rather limited data [16, 18]. Notably, PET/CT is suggestive of BM involvement only if focal lesions are present. In contrast, diffuse increased uptake, even with intensity >liver, is due to reactive BM changes caused by the cytokine milieu present in HL and should not be confused with BM involvement [1, 2, 16–18, 20].

In a large study of 454 HL patients, who were staged by both PET/CT and bone marrow biopsy [16] (Fig. 14.4a), 6% (27 patients) had BM involvement. However, more than twice (13% or 59 patients) had multi- ($n$ = 31), bi- ($n$ = 9), or unifocal ($n$ = 19) PET/CT bone lesions and a negative BMb. No cases of BM involvement were detected among patients with diffusely increased 18-FDG uptake. Only 4/454 patients (<1%) had a positive BMb in the absence of PET/CT evidence of BM disease, and BMb did not lead to treatment modification, since all of them had already advanced disease (stage shift from III to IV). The experience of the German Hodgkin Study Group (GHSG) in the HD16–18 trials was similar [19]. Only 20/832 (2.4%) patients had a positive BMb but five fold more patients ($n$ = 110) had a PET/CT evidence of BM disease. The negative predictive value was 99.9% as only 1/703 patients without BM disease on PET/CT had a positive BMb. In both studies, patients with both positive PET/CT and BM biopsy had much more frequently multifocal lesions, suggesting that among patients with PET/CT-based evidence of BM involvement, those who also have positive BMb have more extensive BM disease. Similarly, only 1.1% of patients with HL and a negative BM PET/CT had a positive BMb in a meta-analysis of 955 patients, including the first previously mentioned study [21] while the overall frequency of a positive BMb in the presence of a negative PET/CT was 1.9% in a study of 1085 patients [22]. Our experience, based on 172 patients, is very similar, further demonstrating that there is not even a small high-risk subgroup [17, 23], in which BMb could offer additional information. Furthermore, it appears that the outcomes of patients with positive BMb and those with PET/CT evidence of BM involvement but negative BMb are equally poor, but this should be further confirmed [16–18]. Thus, the biologic and prognostic significance of BM involvement detected by means of PET/CT only appears to be similar to that of histologically proven BM disease in HL [16–18]. Finally, PET/CT might facilitate the identification of foci of increased uptake in order to guide bone marrow biopsy, since bone marrow involvement can be patchy and incremental information could be lost.

#### 14.2.2.2 Diffuse Large B Cell and Primary Mediastinal Large B Cell Lymphoma [24–33]

In DLBCL the frequency of BM involvement is 10–15% and PET/CT is again suggestive of BM involvement only if focal lesions with increased uptake are present (Fig. 14.2a). BM involvement may be either concordant (large cell) or discordant (small cell) compared to lymph node histology with an almost equal frequency [24].

This phenomenon, which is of prognostic significance, cannot be effectively demonstrated by PET/CT [25].

According to the 2014 Lugano recommendations, BMb could be safely omitted in DLBCL staged by PET/CT, because the probability of a positive BMb is low in the absence of focal BM lesions on PET/CT and, even in such cases, treatment strategy is not typically affected [1, 2]. However, a BMb was still indicated for the detection of discordant histology in DLBCL, if this was relevant for patient management or required by a clinical trial [1, 2]. Extending these thoughts, current ESMO and NCCN guidelines propose to omit BMb if PET/CT is suggestive of BM involvement but keep BMb in staging procedure in case of a negative PET/CT in order to detect discordant or low-volume (<10–20%) BM involvement [34, 35]. The scientific basis for these recommendations is analyzed below.

Although BMb might be omitted in the majority of DLBCL patients, it is more informative compared to HL, because more patients may have positive biopsies with negative PET/CT. PET/CT reveals on average twice more cases of BM involvement than BMb in DLBCL [26–32].

However, in contrast to HL, approximately 1/3 of patients with positive BMb (range, 14–50%) have a negative PET/CT, accounting for 1.5–8% of the total DLBCL population in various studies [26–31, 33, 36]. If BMb is omitted, several cases of BM involvement may be overlooked, but most of them have already features of advanced disease and management is not affected (see Lugano recommendations [1, 2]). This was recently shown clearly in a combined analysis of the PETAL and OPTIMAL trials [33]. However, PET+/BMb- cases may have a better prognosis than BMb + cases, so that BM involvement could be an adverse prognostic factor only if demonstrated at the histologic level [27, 29–32]. Thus, although of limited value, the exact role of BMB in DLBCL remains to be further investigated [31, 32, 37]. Special caution should be taken in patients with no evidence of BM disease on PET/CT and apparently limited stage, who are scheduled for abbreviated immunochemotherapy regimens, in whom a BMb would be most useful [15, 35].

In PMLBCL, the baseline probability of BM involvement is extremely low and it would be reasonable to omit BMb in the absence of relevant findings in PET/CT, especially because a positive result would not alter treatment strategy [32, 38, 39]. However, there is no formal recommendation on this for the time being.

#### 14.2.2.3 Other Lymphoma Subtypes

In indolent lymphomas, including follicular lymphomas and MCL, BM biopsy remains the gold standard for the evaluation of BM disease, which is much more prevalent than in HL and DLBCL. PET/CT may not reveal bone marrow involvement by low-grade lymphoma [9] and BMb cannot be omitted [1, 2].

### 14.2.3 Potential Prognostic Impact of Baseline PET Parameters

The calculation of total metabolic tumor volume (TMTV) by baseline PET/CT may provide a better estimation of the true tumor burden compared to conventional imaging. Furthermore, total lesion glycolysis (TLG) provides a combined evaluation of both TMTV and intensity of metabolic activity (SUV mean of each lesion) [40]. These parameters, which are derived from baseline PET/CT, may provide important prognostic information in individual lymphoma subtypes.

Further to rather small studies in which TMTV was demonstrated as an independent prognostic factor for PFS [41] and OS [41, 42] in HL, the impact of TMTV and TLG has been significant in the context of randomized trials or larger patient series as well, both for early stage disease [43, 44] and for advanced disease, where TMTV may stratify patients with a negative interim PET into distinct prognostic subgroups [45–48].

Similarly, small or medium-sized studies (<200 patients) have shown the prognostic impact of TMTV [49–53] and TLG [54, 55] in DLBCL, which appears to be independent from conventional prognostic systems and molecular profiling. In addition, a very recent large study of >1000 patients clearly demonstrated the additive impact of TMTV to the IPI in DLBCL in the form of International Metabolic Prognostic Index [56]. TMTV and TLG were also independent prognostic factors after adjustment for IPI and cell-of-origin within the large population (>1000 patients with DLBCL) enrolled in the GOYA trial comparing CHOP plus rituximab or obinutuzumab [57]. Furthermore, within the REMARC randomized clinical trial which included only patients with a response to R-CHOP (and consequently more favorable prognosis), baseline TMTV still remained a strong independent prognostic factor and this was independent from the administration of lenalidomide maintenance or not [58].

In PMLBCL, for which established and reproducible prognostic factors are generally lacking, baseline PET parameters may also be valuable: Within the IELSG26 study, 103 patients were treated predominantly with R-MACOP-B (84%) or R-CHOP (16%), both followed by RT [59]. Baseline SUVmax, MTV, and TLG of the mediastinal disease were associated with outcome, but only high TLG, observed in 1/3 of patients, was an independent prognostic factor, overcoming the significance of the other PET parameters, bulky disease, and other conventional prognostic factors. The 5-year PFS and OS for patients with low vs. high TLG were 99% vs. 64% ($p < 0.0001$) and 100% vs. 80% respectively ($p = 0.0001$) [59]. The prognostic significance of TMTV was confirmed by a LySA study as well as by MD Anderson and Dana Farber data under R-da-EPOCH chemotherapy [60, 61].

Other baseline PET-derived metabolic parameters may also provide important prognostic information in HL and aggressive B cell lymphomas. The distance between the 2 lesions that are farthest apart (Dmax or lesion dissemination), a measure of tumor dissemination, may add to the prognostic significance of MTV or even overcome it in DLBCL and cHL [62–64]. Metabolic heterogeneity refers to the intratumoral distribution of $^{18}$FDG uptake, which reflects the glucose metabolism of both the tumor cells and their microenvironment as well as other processes, such as necrosis, apoptosis, proliferation, and angiogenesis. High metabolic heterogeneity confers adverse prognosis in PMLBCL in addition to TLG [65]. In DLBCL, high metabolic heterogeneity does not correlate with TMTV and may also confer an adverse impact on prognosis [66, 67].

Baseline PET parameters have also been evaluated in other lymphoma subtypes. A high MTV predicted the outcome of high-tumor burden follicular lymphomas independently from the well-established FLIPI2 prognosticator in a pooled analysis of 3 multicenter studies [68], while it predicted outcomes independently from cell-free DNA in another study [69]. In contrast, neither baseline MTV nor TLG or SUVmax predicted the outcome of follicular lymphoma patients treated within the GALLIUM study with Obinutuzumab or rituximab plus chemotherapy (predominantly bendamustine) followed by antibody maintenance [70]. In MCL, baseline MTV and TLG—but not SUVmax—were independent predictors of PFS in a series of 87 patients [71]. Baseline MTV also predicted PFS and OS in "nodal" T cell lymphomas independently from other clinical factors and had a synergistic prognostic impact with the T cell prognostic index (PIT) [72], while it was subsequently shown to offer prognostic information independent from interim PET as well [73]. Similar data were recently published for TLG in peripheral T cell lymphomas [74]. Finally, a similar prognostic effect for TLG (and SUVmax) was shown in patients with extranodal NK/T cell lymphomas [75].

Although interesting, all this information deserves further prospective evaluation in large-scale studies along with many established clinical and biological prognostic factors before implemented in clinical practice. Standardization of the procedures is also essential for reliable clinical application.

## 14.3 PET/CT in Response Assessment After Completion of Therapy

### 14.3.1 Criteria for Response Assessment and Definitions of PET Positivity

The most important information provided by PET, as far as response evaluation is concerned, is the differentiation between viable lymphomatous tissue and necrotic or fibrotic tissue within residual masses, which are apparent on CT. Furthermore,

EOT-PET/CT may uncover occult disease in normal-sized lymph nodes or bone marrow disease, which may not be demonstrable by trephine biopsy. In 2005, Juweid et al. published a retrospective study in patients with aggressive NHL, predominantly DLBCL, who underwent PET and CT after 4–8 cycles of chemotherapy [76]. They noticed that patients otherwise categorized as CRu (Complete Remission unconfirmed) based on Cheson's 1999 criteria were usually PET-negative, and, overall, had a favorable outcome with PFS similar to that of the CR group. Patients in partial remission (PR) had strikingly different outcomes when PET was negative or positive. In the "early" PET era, response assessment had been traditionally based on the International Harmonization Project (IHP) criteria described in 2007 [77, 78]. According to that set of criteria, a positive PET at the EOT was defined in relation to the size of the residual lesion: For residuals <2 cm, any focal or diffuse FDG uptake above the background in a location not compatible with normal anatomy/physiology was considered positive. However, for residuals ≥2 cm a mild uptake above background was still compatible with CR, i.e., PET positivity was defined as FDG uptake exceeding that of the mediastinal blood pool structures (Figs. 14.1b, 14.2c, 14.4c, 14.7c).

More recently, the EOT response criteria were revised, adopting the Deauville 5-point scale (D5PS), which had been initially used for interim response assessment (Table 14.1). The D5PS was incorporated in the currently used Lugano criteria [1, 2]. According to current recommendations any FDG uptake up to that of the mediastinal blood pool (corresponding to D5PS 1–2) is considered compatible with CR irrespective of the size of the residual mass. Furthermore, a low-grade positivity, higher than the mediastinal blood pool and up to the uptake of the liver (D5PS 3; Table 14.1), is also considered as a favorable response. Thus, clear PET positivity at the EOT is defined as any uptake above that of the liver, corresponding to D5PS 4 or 5 (Figs. 14.1b, 14.2c, 14.4c, 14.7c). It should be noted that the D5PS score should be determined visually; the classification should not be relied on simple SUVmax comparisons between the uptake of the lesion and that of the liver or the mediastinal blood pool.

The currently used set of criteria for the evaluation of response in malignant lymphomas incorporating both PET/CT and anatomic findings are summarized in Table 14.1 [1, 2, 32] (Figs. 14.1b, 14.2c, 14.4c, 14.5c, 14.7c).

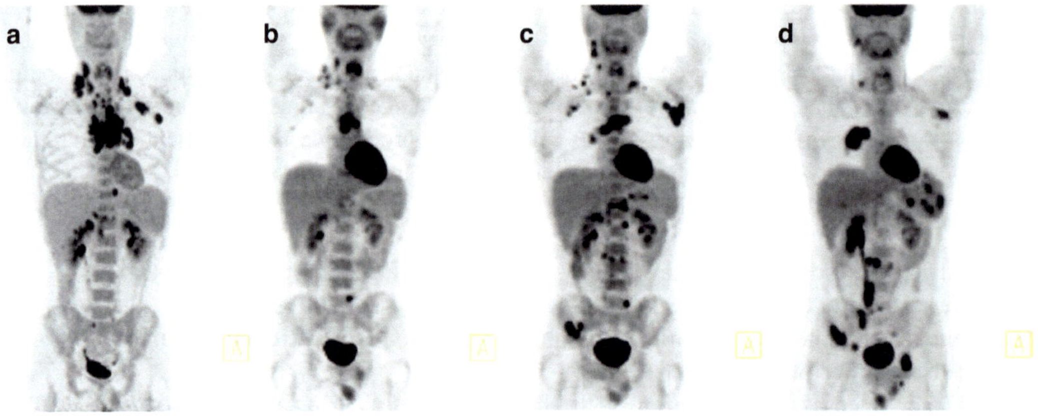


**Fig. 14.7** (**a**) Baseline staging in a patient with Hodgkin lymphoma: Extensive supradiaphragmatic as well as infradiaphragmatic involvement consistent with stage IIIB disease. (**b**) Interim PET after two cycles of ABVD revealed persistence of multiple nodal sites on both sides of the diaphragm with FDG uptake markedly greater than that of the liver. A new focal osseous lesion is also seen. Interim PET was interpreted as positive, Deauville score 5. The patient continued on ABVD. (**c**) End-of-treatment PET after a total of six ABVD cycles demonstrated further progression. The patient had progressive disease by conventional restaging as well. (**d**) Further progression later on, during disease course in the same patient. Multiple focal splenic lesions are noted

### 14.3.2 Who Should Have an EOT-PET-Based Response Assessment and When?

PET/CT is routinely used for final response assessment in patients with HL and aggressive B cell lymphomas. It is also currently recommended as the optimal tool for final response assessment in all other FDG-avid subtypes, especially in follicular lymphomas. However, the accuracy parameters related to EOT-PET depends on the precise histologic subtype, being highest for HL but lower for aggressive non-Hodgkin lymphomas. Although clearly recommended for final response assessment, PET/CT may not be so informative in low-grade follicular lymphomas and MCL, since these diseases are incurable and a negative PET/CT is merely reflecting an improved PFS and prolonged survival but not "true" disease eradication. When used in variably 18-FDG-avid histologic subtypes, which is not recommended as a general rule, it is essential to have a baseline PET/CT available in order to confirm that the tumor is 18-FDG-avid (Fig. 14.6).

EOT-PET/CT evaluation should preferably be performed 4–6 weeks (and at least 3 weeks) after chemotherapy and immunotherapy and 8–12 weeks after RT, in order to avoid false positive findings due to inflammatory processes and false negative due to stunning from cytostatic drugs [1, 2, 77, 78]. As far as interim PET is concerned it should better be performed as close to the next chemotherapeutic cycle as possible (see next topic).

### 14.3.3 Clinical Data in Individual Lymphoma Subtypes

As already stated, accuracy parameters, i.e., positive and negative predictive value (PPV, NPV) of EOT-PET/CT, depends on the histologic subtype (Hodgkin lymphoma vs. individual subtypes of non-Hodgkin lymphomas), but also on the chemotherapy regimen applied (standard or intensive) and the a priori probability of relapse, as reflected by clinical stage or other prognostic factors.

#### 14.3.3.1 Hodgkin Lymphoma

The long-term outcome of patients with HL who achieve a PET-negative status at the end of first-line chemotherapy, depends on stage, chemotherapy regimen, and use of RT, as summarized in Table 14.2 [79–88]. A negative PET/CT after standard ABVD chemotherapy predicts a 5-year relapse-free survival (RFS) of ~95% in stages I/II, where ABVD is typically followed by RT (Fig. 14.5c), and ~ 80% in stages III/IV, in which only few patients are irradiated (Fig. 14.4c) [79].

Within the RAPID trial, patients with non-bulky clinical stage I/IIA and a strictly negative PET (D5PS 1 or 2) after ABVD×3 were randomized to receive 30 Gy involved field (IF)-RT or no further treatment, achieving a 3-year PFS of 97% versus 91% respectively ($p = 0.026$) [83]. In the German Hodgkin Study Group (GHSG) HD16 trial of patients with localized, favorable HL (early stages) treated with ABVD×2, the 5-year PFS was 93% versus 86% who received consolidative IF-RT or not, if EOT-PET was strictly negative (D5PS 1 or 2) [84]. Within the GHSG HD17 trial of patients with localized, unfavorable HL (intermediate stages) treated with intensified therapy (BEACOPP-escalated ×2 plus ABVD×2) consolidative RT could be omitted without clinically meaningful loss of efficacy, if EOT-PET was strictly negative (D5PS 1 or 2). Even among patients with bulky disease, the 5-year PFS was 97% regardless of the administration of consolidative RT. [86] These data may have important implications for the design of follow-up strategies [89].

Regarding advanced HL treated with ABVD, the HD607 trial demonstrated that RT can be omitted in patients who achieve a negative PET status, defined as D5PS score 1–3, both at the interim and EOT evaluation despite the presence of bulky disease ≥5 cm [90]. The 6-year PFS was 92% versus 90% for irradiated and non-irradiated patients and the difference was not significant whatever the definition of bulk (5, 7, or 10 cm) [91]. If advanced stage patients are treated with more aggressive chemotherapy such as BEACOPP-escalated or variants, the 5-year RFS for patients with a residual mass of >2.5 cm and a negative post-chemotherapy PET/CT is approximately 90% without RT [80], falling to 88% at 10 years [87]. Within the HD15 study of the GHSG, this was comparable to the 85% observed as 10-year PFS in patients with conventional CR or residual masses <2.5 cm, who did not undergo EOT-PET/CT evaluation [87].

Despite additional RT, early stage patients who remain PET/CT-positive after ABVD chemotherapy have a 5-year RFS of 40–65% (Fig. 14.1b) [81, 82, 88, 92]. Higher 18-FDG uptake is predictive of treatment failure in this setting and could have an impact on therapeutic strategies, but this needs further clarification [88, 92]. In the above-mentioned RAPID trial, patients with favorable (defined as non-bulky) stage I/IIA HL who remained PET-positive (D5PS 3, 4 or 5) after ABVDx3 received one more ABVD cycle and IF-RT. The outcome was favorable for those with D5PS 3–4, but it was dismal for those with D5PS 5: The 5-year PFS was 95%, 88%, and 62% for patients with D5PS score 3, 4, and 5 respectively [88]. This difference was translated to overall survival difference as well. In the GHSG HD16 trials of early (favorable) stages, among patients receiving ABVD×2 plus IF-RT, the 5-year PFS was 93%, 88%, and 81% for patients with D5PS score 1–2, 3–4, or 4, respectively, while the corresponding figures were 98%, 94%, and 82% within the HD17 trial after BEACOPP-escalated ×2 plus ABVD×2 plus consolidative RT. [84, 86] This suggests that D5PS score ≥ 4 is an unfavorable prognostic factor despite additional RT (caution to be exercised to the definition of score 4; cases with conventional D5PS score 5 may have been included in the absence of new lesions).

In advanced stages, the figures are similar to early stages after ABVD, but it appears that, after more intensive chemotherapy such as BEACOPP-escalated, RT to >2.5 cm PET-positive residuals may be much more efficient for disease control with long-term RFS just below 85% [87]. The degree of conventional radiographic response appears to correlate with disease control after BEACOPP-based therapy and RT: Patients whose residual masses had been reduced by >40% in their largest diameter compared to baseline had similar outcomes with PET-negative patients with 4-year PFS of 92%. The prognosis was worse for patients with reductions ≤40%, who had a 4-year PFS of 73% [93].

#### 14.3.3.2 Primary Mediastinal Large B Cell Lymphoma

A negative PET/CT after R-CHOP, R-MACOP-B, or R-da-EPOCH is associated with 90–95% cure rates in PMLBCL, even when RT is omitted in many patients [38, 39, 94–98]. According to the Vancouver experience, even patients with D5PS score 3 after R-CHOP may enjoy a > 90% long-term disease control rate without consolidative RT [97], which is similar to the outcomes achieved with RT in all these patients [98].

If irradiated, PET/CT-positive residual masses are effectively controlled in 65–70% of cases provided that the disease is responsive by conventional imaging [39, 95, 96, 98, 99]. In particular the rate of long-term disease control in patients with D5PS score 4 following R-CHOP (or R-MACOP-B) is exceptionally high in the range of 80–87% [39, 97, 98]. Among the latter patients, those with D5PS score 4 and "lower" FDG uptake may have equally favorable outcomes compared to PET-negative patients with long-term PFS >90%, while those with higher SUVmax (for example ≥5) probably have significantly inferior outcomes [99, 100]. Although patients with D5PS score 5 have inferior outcomes [39, 98–101] >40% of them can achieve long-term disease control with consolidative RT if they have achieved PR by conventional imaging [98]. However, salvage chemotherapy intending to autologous transplant is preferrable for patients with D5PS score 5 and conventionally defined stable or progressive disease [98].

If patients are treated with the more intensive combination R-dose adjusted-EPOCH (R-da-EPOCH), EOT-PET/CT can be interpreted more conservatively. Patients with D5PS scores 1–2 are not candidates for consolidative RT, but RT is also omitted in patients with D5PS 3 and 4. Serial PET/CT evaluation typically shows regression or stability even in D5PS score 4 during follow-up with no further intervention [102–104]. The few patients with D5PS score 5 after R-da-EPOCH can be effectively salvaged with RT if they have achieved PR by conventional methods but should be again forwarded to salvage chemotherapy intending to autologous transplant if they have conventionally defined stable or progressive disease [105].

Because of the considerable curative potential of RT, patients with PMLBCL should not be referred for high-dose therapy and autologous transplantation solely based on a positive PET/CT after immunochemotherapy and this is especially true if the uptake is not marked [94]. It should be also noted that certain patients who have low-grade positivity after immunochemotherapy remain PET/CT positive at a similar degree after RT as well without experiencing disease progression, suggesting that mild positivity (at the lower range of D5PS score 4) may be compatible with cure in this entity [99, 101, 102]. Finally, the question whether RT could be safely omitted in PET-negative patients after immunochemotherapy (other than R-da-EPOCH) is currently evaluated by the IELSG-37 randomized trial.

#### 14.3.3.3 Diffuse Large B Cell Lymphoma

A negative PET/CT after R-CHOP carries a lower NPV in DLBCL compared with HL and PMLBCL [106–113]. The long-term event-free survival (EFS) in these patients after a negative PET/CT post R-chemotherapy is roughly 70–85% (Table 14.3) and the probability of relapse may depend on their baseline relapse risk, as reflected by the International Prognostic Index (IPI) and its components [106, 109, 110], the cell of origin [106] as well as on the depth of conventional radiographic response (CR versus PR) (Fig. 14.2c), the size of the residual mass, and the number of residual lesions [108].

Recently, two large studies including patients with predominantly advanced DLBCL evaluated EOT-PET after R-CHOP (or obinutuzumab-CHOP) using the D5PS [112, 113]. Both demonstrated a 3-year disease control rate of 82–83% without consolidative RT. Within the GOYA trial including >1000 patients, a positive EOT-PET (D5PS score 4–5) was an independent prognostic factor after adjustment for IPI or the cell-of-origin. Unexpectedly, among patients with complete metabolic response (D5PS score 1–3), those with IPI 0–2 had inferior 2.5-year PFS to those with IPI 3–5 (77% versus 88%, $p < 0.0001$), while ABC DLBCL expectedly fared worse than their GCB counterparts (2.5-year PFS 80% versus 89%, $p < 0.05$) [112]. According to the British Columbia experience on 723 patients, the 3-year disease control was 83% and inferior outcomes were predicted independently by baseline B-symptoms and BM involvement. The individual IPI factors were not independently associated with the outcome but the IPI per se and the cell-of-origin were not assessed. Interestingly, the outcome of patients with a negative EOT-PET was the same in the presence of bulky disease or not and independently of the presence of skeletal or craniofacial involvement, which were traditionally irradiated in some institutions [113]. The feasibility to omit RT in patients with bulky disease who achieve a PET-negative status following R-CHOP-based therapy was also confirmed in the setting of the OPTIMAL randomized trial, which was limited to elderly DLBCL patients [114].

Patients with DLBCL who remain PET/CT-positive after R-CHOP have a < 40–50% probability to remain disease-free [107–110], but even this figure suggests that false positive findings are not infrequent (Table 14.3). Within the GOYA trial only 12% of the 1092 patients had a positive EOT-PET defined as D5PS score 4–5 and still enjoyed a 3-year PFS of 49% [112]. IPI was not predictive in this subgroup, but ABC DLBCL remained worse than GCB (44% versus 63% disease control). Unfortunately, there was no mention of the potential impact of the exact D5PS score (4 versus 5), which may be critical for the outcome.

The British Columbia group also focused on the EOT-PET-positive subgroup and the role of RT. Among 723 patients with advanced DLBCL (stage III/IV or I/IIB or bulky) treated with R-CHOP, the rate of EOT-PET positivity was much higher reaching 25% (178/723) [113]. The

**Table 14.3** Summary of selected studies evaluating the role of EOT-PET after the completion of full-course rituximab-based chemoimmunotherapy

| Author, year, ref | Pts | IPI ≥3 | Chemotherapy | Radiotherapy | End-of-treatment PET positivity | | Progression Free Survival | | | | Prognostic factors for the outcome of PET-neg patients/ other comments |
|---|---|---|---|---|---|---|---|---|---|---|---|
| | | | | | Definition | Frequency # (%) | iPET-neg | iPET-pos | At *n*-years | *p*-value | |
| Thomas 2010 [107] | 125[a] | 40% | R-CHOP or similar: 84%<br>R-EPOCH: 9%;<br>Other: 7% | 20% | NR | 31 (25%) | ~75% (neg)<br>71% (indet) | 30–40% (overall sv) | 5 years | NR | Higher IPI |
| Dabaja 2013 [108] | 300[b] | 27% | R-CHOP-21: 81%<br>R-HyperCVAD: 14%<br>Other: 5% | No | NR | 52 (17%) | 84%, if CR by CT<br>64%, if PR by CT | 42% | 5 years | <0.0001 | Stage III/IV, composite score (bulk, Ki67, SUVmax), >1 residual site on CT or ≥ 2 cm residual (DSS, OS) or conventional PR (OS) |
| Freeman 2021[113] | 723[c] | 52% | R-CHOP | ~15%[c] | IHP/ D5PS | 206 (28%)[c] | 83%[c] | 76% (+RT)<br>34% (−RT) | 3 years | <0.001 | B-symptoms and bone marrow involvement |
| Vassilakopoulos 2014 [109] | 151[d] | 38% | R-CHOP-21 or similar | NR[c] | IHP | 34 (23%) | 86%[d] | 40% | 4 years | <0.0001 | Performance status ≥2 |
| Mamot 2015 [111] | 138 | 28% | R-CHOP-14 + R ×2 | No | D5PS ≥4 | 25 (21%)[e] | 72% | 24% | 3 years | <0.001 | NR |
| Witzig 2018 [110] | 742[e] | 99% | R-CHOP: 98%,<br>R-EPOCH: 2% | No | PET-neg only[e] | 0 (0%) | 77% | NA | 2 years | NA | 5-year PFS much lower (~60%, but death of any cause included, median age 64 years) |
| Kostakoglu 2021 [112] | 1092[f] | 44% | R-CHOP versus G-CHOP | No | D5PS ≥4 | 131 (12%) | 82% | 49% | 3 years | <0.0001 | IPI 0–2 inferior to 3–5; ABC inferior to GCB |

[a]Among 215 consecutive DLBCL patients, 125 were included based on EOT-PET availability; 20% had indeterminate results and were analyzed together with PET-neg patients (similar outcomes)
[b]169 further patients were excluded, because they had received radiotherapy after chemotherapy (possible positive selection)
[c]Selected on the basis of advanced stage [III/IV (74%) or II either B or bulky (26%)] AND the presence of >2 cm residual mass but no primary progression (possible negative selection). PET interpreted according to IHP criteria between 2005 and 2014 and the D5PS thereafter. RT was given almost exclusively to PET-positive patients. In the subgroup of patients evaluated by the D5PS the 3-year TTP was 83%, 69%, and 33% for PET-neg, PET-pos irradiated, and PET-pos not irradiated
[d]Selected on the basis of conventional radiographic response (CR/CRu/PR) and PET/CT availability. RT was given mainly in selected PET-positive patients (percentage not provided). Deaths of any cause in remission were not considered as events
[e]According to investigator's assessment, patients were randomized to receive everolimus maintenance or placebo
[f]Patients had to be PET-negative after R-chemotherapy, before randomization to everolimus versus placebo (no difference detected)

study was focused on patients who had not experienced disease progression until the time of EOT-PET, so that they were considered as responders with residual disease. Among the 178 patients with a positive EOT-PET defined as D5PS score 4–5, 86 received RT and achieved a 3-year time-to-progression (TTP) of 69%, which was only slightly inferior to EOT-PET-negative patients (83%). This impressive success rate should be further confirmed, since it depends on optimal patient selection. In contrast, the 3-year TTP for the 92 patients that had disease not amenable to RT was only 33%. However, even in this unfavorable setting, 1/3 of the patients remain without disease progression. Notably, despite some overlap, the median SUVmax of progressors was substantially higher to that of the minority of patients who remain in remission [16.3 (up to 36.0) versus 4.5 (up to 18.1)] [113].

#### 14.3.3.4 Follicular Lymphoma

EOT-PET carries prognostic significance for patients with FL. Dupuis et al. reported that a positive EOT-PET after 6 cycles of R-CHOP significantly affected PFS regardless of iPET status and FLIPI score [115]. A pooled analysis using EOT-PET/CT scans from 439 patients enrolled in three landmark studies (PRIMA, PET-FL, and FOLL05) showed that D5PS >4 was associated with significantly lower PFS (16.9 vs. 74 months for EOT-PET-positive and -negative patients respectively) [116]. Also, the secondary analysis of PET results from GALLIUM study reported that patients who achieved complete metabolic response had better PFS and OS irrespective of whether they received rituximab- or obinutuzumab-based treatment, or whether they achieved CR in conventional imaging [117]. Currently, restaging with EOT-PET is recommended for prognostication, but not for treatment modification decisions or patient surveillance.

#### 14.3.3.5 Mantle Cell Lymphoma

EOT-PET is considered optional in patients with MCL and its role remains unsettled, as treatment strategies in patients with MCL are heterogenous. A study of 32 cases treated with Rituximab-Bendamustine demonstrated that patients who achieved complete metabolic response by D5PS had significantly higher PFS [118]. Similarly, in a study of 72 patients treated with alternating R-CHOP/R-high-dose cytarabine, a positive EOT-PET (D5PS score 4–5) was associated with worse PFS [119]. The LyMA-PET project demonstrated that SUVmax and D5PSS in iPET and EOT-PET had not prognostic significance; however SUVmax in iPET and ΔSUVmax (reduction of SUVmax between iPET and EOT-PET) in EOT-PET were associated with OS and PFS, respectively [120].

#### 14.3.3.6 T Cell Lymphomas

The utility of EOT-PET in T cell lymphomas remains rather poorly defined, as T cell lymphomas consist of various histological subtypes with diverse clinical and biological characteristics and heterogenous treatment approaches. In a study of 114 patients with PTCL, iPET had not prognostic significance but a positive EOT-PET (D5PS score 4–5) was significantly associated with worse PFS and OS [121]. In another study of 140 patients with PTCL treated mainly with CHOP or CHOP-like regimens, the authors aimed to explore the role of interim (after 2 or 3–4 cycles of chemotherapy) and EOT-PET/CT. PET positivity was again defined as D5PS score 4–5. Patients with positive interim PET had significantly compromised 2-year PFS and OS. EOT-PET was also predictive as the 2-year PFS and OS were 83% and 94% vs. 6% and 27% for EOT-PET-negative and -positive patients, respectively.

## 14.4 Interim Response Assessment

Early prediction of response to therapy is of major importance, not only as a powerful prognostic factor but also as a potential basis for early treatment modification. Functional changes that precede the anatomic ones could potentially be more accurate in predicting treatment response early in the course of therapy.

### 14.4.1 Who Might Benefit from Interim PET-Based Early Response Assessment?

Early response assessment has provided a major prognostic clue for patients with advanced HL or localized HL with adverse prognostic factors [122, 123] and provides a useful tool for early treatment intensification. The prognostic effect of interim PET (iPET) is less marked, although still significant, for patients with DLBCL, but it cannot be used for early treatment modification in the absence of effective alternative chemotherapy. In the specific setting of PMLBCL, the outcomes according to iPET appear to be conflicting [124]. Data on other lymphoma subtypes, including T cell lymphomas, are sparse. Relevant studies regarding iPET are discussed below.

The D5PS was initially described for the evaluation of iPET and remains the standard tool for this purpose in HL [1, 2]. In DLBCL, the D5PS is less reproducible and is associated with inferior prognostic discrimination. An approach based on the reduction of SUVmax between baseline and iPET (ΔSUVmax at a cutoff of 66%) is prognostically superior and sufficiently reproducible. Thus, the calculation of ΔSUVmax is the recommended approach for iPET interpretation in the specific setting of DLBCL (see below) [1, 2].

### 14.4.2 Clinical Data in Individual Lymphoma Subtypes

#### 14.4.2.1 Hodgkin Lymphoma

According to the D5PS (Table 14.1), a negative iPET may not be nominally negative: Any positivity in previously involved sites with 18-FDG uptake up to that of the liver is acceptable as a favorable interim response (D5PS scores 1,2,3) and this assessment should be made visually (Fig. 14.5b). Any uptake higher than the liver is considered positive (scores 4,5) (Figs. 14.4b, 14.7b). Using the D5PS, the International Validation Study demonstrated that, under ABVD chemotherapy, the 3-year PFS for patients with negative and positive iPET was 95% vs. 28% [125]. Such figures may apply not only to advanced HL, but also to intermediate stage HL (localized stages with ≥1 unfavorable features). However, the outcome of iPET-positive patients with localized disease and no adverse factors, especially no bulky disease, may be much better than the ~30% reported above [82, 122, 126]. Furthermore, the excellent outcome for iPET-negative patients with intermediate, and particularly advanced, stages has not been reproduced in subsequent studies using ABVD, as discussed below.

Under BEACOPP-escalated, the NPV of iPET is also very high, with >90% of iPET-negative patients achieving continuous CR. Nevertheless, the PPV is much lower compared with ABVD-treated patients: Large datasets within the context of randomized trials have recently revealed PFS rates between 70% and > 90% with continued BEACOPP-escalated for a total of 6 cycles in case of iPET positivity after the second cycle [127–130]. In the HD18 trial of the GHSG, 46% of advanced stage patients remained iPET-positive after BEACOPP-escalated ×2 (defined loosely as D5PS ≥3) and ~ 54% of them were still positive by the current definition of D5PS ≥4 [131]. The 3-year PFS for all these patients was ~93–94%; it was 91% for patients with D5PS ≥4.

### 14.4.3 Is It Reasonable to Modify Treatment of HL in Response to Interim PET Results?

In order to justify treatment modification in response to iPET result, two conditions must be met: Firstly, the outcome of iPET-positive patients could be possible to improve by an alternative therapy, and, secondly, the NPV should be sufficiently high to avoid relapses in the vast majority of iPET-negative patients.

Regarding the first condition, there are overwhelming data indicating that treatment intensification may produce long-term PFS rates of ~65% (vs. ~30% expected based on historical data with continued ABVD) in patients with advanced or even intermediate (early unfavorable) stage HL, who remain PET/CT-positive after 2 ABVD cycles (Fig. 14.4b) [90, 91, 132–137]. This is typically achieved by switching chemotherapy from ABVD to BEACOPP-escalated for at least 4 cycles [90, 91, 132–136, 138] but early salvage therapy and autologous stem cell transplantation may also produce similar results [139]. These data are summarized in reference #138.

Although clinical trials are mainly investigating PET-adapted therapy for advanced disease, the only randomized evidence for the superiority of treatment intensification with BEACOPP-escalated in HL comes from the H10 trial for localized stages [140]. In H10, 361/1925 (19%) of patients had persistent PET/CT positivity after ABVD×2, loosely defined according to the IHP criteria and roughly corresponding to D5PS score ≥ 3. Only 97/361 (27%) had no adverse factors, while 264 (73%) had ≥1 risk factor. These 361 patients were randomized to receive: (1) 1 or 2 further ABVD cycles (according to the absence or presence of risk factors) plus 30 Gy involved node RT (standard arm) or (2) 2 cycles of BEACOPP-escalated plus 30 Gy involved node RT (experimental arm) irrespective of risk factor classification. PFS was improved by only 2 cycles of BEACOPP-escalated with 5-year rates of 91% versus 77% in the experimental and the standard arm respectively ($p = 0.002$). Importantly, a marginally significant but clinically meaningful improvement was noted for 5-year OS as well (96% versus 89%, $p = 0.062$) [140]. However, in a subsequent analysis presented in abstract form, it became evident that the benefit of switching to BEACOPP-escalated was limited only to patients with D5PS score 4–5, while those with D5PS score 3 were effectively treated by ABVD×2 plus RT. [141]

In the specific setting that first-line therapy is based on BEACOPP-escalated instead of ABVD, the long-term PFS of iPET-positive patients may be in the range of 70 to >90%, as stated above [128, 131]. In this setting, improvement of the outcome of iPET-positive patients appears difficult. For example, the addition of rituximab was not successful in improving the outcome of iPET+ patients after BEACOPP-escalated ×2, in the GHSG HD18 trial [131].

While the first of the required conditions is partially fulfilled, the second one is becoming particularly important for the final success of iPET-directed therapy: Although major early studies had shown that the NPV of iPET could be >90% under ABVD, more recent studies and maturing data suggest that it may not be so perfect as initially thought in patients with truly advanced HL: In the US S0816 trial, the 2-year PFS of 271 patients with stage III/IV HL treated with ABVD×6 was 82% (and was projected to be reduced to ~–70–75% at 4–5 years!) and did not differ according to the D5PS score (80%, 84%, and 81% for scores 1, 2, or 3) [134, 137]. In the RATHL trial, the 3-year PFS for iPET-negative patients with continued ABVD or AVD was 84–86%, but it was only 82% for younger (<60 years old) stage III/IV patients [133]. Within the HD0801 trial (81% stage III/IV), the 2-year PFS was 81% [139], while the 3-year PFS was 87% in the HD607 trial, which included only 67% stage III/IV patients [90]. Smaller studies also provided similar results with long-term PFS for iPET-negative patients clearly <90% and as low as 71–77% [135, 136, 142]. These data have been extensively reviewed in reference #138. It is not currently known if there is a reproducible subgroup of iPET-negative patients after ABVD who remain at a high risk of failure.

The a priori risk of failure as reflected by stage IV (or extranodal involvement) or other prognostic factors may affect the NPV of iPET and should be further investigated [133, 136, 143]. A large mediastinal mass ≥ 7 cm was predictive of relapse in iPET-negative patients in another retrospective study [144]. The significance of any bulk ≥5 cm was also demonstrated in strictly iPET-negative, non-bulky stage I/IIA patients in the RAPID trial [145]. Serum lactate dehydrogenase elevation was the only predictor of conversion from iPET-negative to EOT-PET-positive and anemia was modestly associated with PFS in the HD0801 study [146, 147], while only the IPS predicted—albeit loosely—treatment failure in iPET-negative patients of the HD0607 trial [148]. Within the latter trial, baseline TMTV and IPS could define 3 groups of iPET-negative patients with highly diverse outcomes: TMTV<471 mL and IPS 0–1 (7% of patients), either elevated (80% of patients) and both elevated (TMTV≥471 mL and IPS >1; 13% of patients) with 3-year PFS of 98%, 85%, and 56% [46]. Similarly, within the H10 trial for localized HL, TMTV >147 mL (observed in only 16% of iPET-negative patients) was associated with significantly, but numerically slightly inferior outcome with 5-year PFS of 82% versus 95% for those with lower TMTV [43]. Biological prognostic factors may also be relevant, such as high content of CD68+ tumor-associated macrophages plus diffuse or rosetting PD1+ cells in the microenvironment or STAT1 negativity of tumor cells [149]. Persistence of residual TARC levels >800 pg/mL after ABVD×2 may also discriminate a rather small subgroup (19% of iPET-negative patients) with inferior outcome (4-year PFS 74% versus 89%) [150]. Despite all these data there is no evidence that any prognostic factor or combination can define a sizeable subgroup of iPET-negative patients with sufficiently poor outcome to justify a different approach from the beginning.

Apart from starting with ABVD and escalating to BEACOPP, an alternative iPET-driven strategy can be starting with BEACOPP-escalated and de-escalating chemotherapy in case of a negative iPET.

Very promising results have been reported by the LySA 2011 trial, in which this reverse iPET-driven strategy was applied to 823 patients with advanced stage HL according to the GHSG definition, i.e., stage III/IV or IIB with mediastinal bulk and/or extranodal involvement [127, 128]. The standard arm consisted of fixed treatment with BEACOPP-escalated ×6 and the experimental arm consisted of BEACOPP-escalated ×6 in case of a positive iPET after 2 cycles or BEACOPP-escalated ×2 plus ABVD ×4 if iPET was negative. The study had a non-inferiority design with a margin of 10%. The experimental arm was not inferior to the standard one with 5-year PFS rates of 86.7% versus 87.5% [128]. The 5-year PFS for iPET-negative patients was similar for the two arms reaching ~90%. For iPET-positive patients it was ~71%. It should be noted that iPET positivity was defined as metabolic activity exceeding 140% of the liver activity and only 12–13% of the patients remained iPET-positive after BEACOPP-escalated ×2 [127].

In the GHSG HD18 trial (again advanced stages according to the GHSG definition) the standard arm consisted of fixed treatment with BEACOPP-escalated (×8 or ×6 in a subsequent amendment) and the experimental arm consisted of BEACOPP-escalated (×8 or ×6 in a subsequent amendment) in case of a positive iPET after 2 cycles or BEACOPP-escalated ×4 (total cycles) if iPET was negative [130]. The definition of iPET positivity was D5PS score ≥ 3 and 48% of the patients remained iPET-positive. The 5-year PFS after BEACOPP-escalated ×4 or ×6 in patients with D5PS score 1–2 (iPET-negative) was ~91% in both arms and overall survival was numerically better with the abbreviated 4-cycle regimen [129]. The 5-year PFS for the iPET-positive population was ~88% (numerically higher in case of D5PS score 3 compared to ≥4) in sharp contrast with the 71% observed in the AHL 2011 trial with the same treatment. However, the rate of iPET positivity was 48% versus 12–13% in the two trials due to the different thresholds used and this is the possible explanation for this large discrepancy.

#### 14.4.3.1 Diffuse Large B Cell Lymphoma

In DLBCL, iPET is also predictive of the outcome after R-CHOP or similar immunochemotherapy, but differences are not so marked compared with HL. The use of iPET to guide treatment decisions is not currently recommended [1, 2] because there is still no proven salvage therapy capable of improving the outcome of patients with a positive iPET, while the NPV of iPET is rather low.

As stated above, the D5PS is not so widely accepted in this setting, because of their moderate reproducibility and prognostic capacity [151] (Fig. 14.2b). Alternatively, a satisfactory iPET response can be defined by a > 66% reduction in SUVmax between baseline and interim assessment [1, 2, 151]. In the NHL International Validation Study, based on 114 DLBCL patients treated with standard R-CHOP-21 or intensified R-CHOP-14 or R-ACVBP-14, where no PET-driven treatment modification was made, the 3-year PFS was 79% vs. 44% in patients with >66% and ≤ 66% SUVmax reductions after 2 cycles of immunochemotherapy [151]. The 66% SUVmax reduction criterion was superior to the D5PS in a subanalysis of the CALGB 50303 trial (R-CHOP-21 or R-da-EPOCH), as well as in the UKCRN-ID 1760 and the SAKK 38/07 trials (both adopting R-CHOP-21 or R-CHOP-14), in which no treatment modification was made according to iPET results [152–154].

In the LNH-2007-3B trial, higher risk, young DLBCL patients randomly received either R-CHOP-14 or R-ACVBP-14 and underwent iPET assessments after 2 and 4 cycles, which modified subsequent treatment strategy. The study confirmed that visual analysis was not accurate enough. The cutoff for SUVmax reduction was set at 66% for PET-2 and 70% for PET-4 [155]. The 4-year PFS according to PET-2 was 80% vs. 56%, while it was 84% vs. 35% according to PET-4 [156]. The prognostic significance of iPET using the 66% SUVmax reduction criterion was also confirmed in the PETAL randomized trial and a GELTAMO phase 2 trial, both of which included treatment intensification for iPET-positive patients [157]. In the PETAL trial, 2-year PFS was 79% for iPET-negative versus 46% for iPET-positive patients despite treatment intensification in the latter ($p < 0.0001$). Using the D5PS the difference was much less marked and the corresponding figures were 79% versus 71% ($p = 0.0068$). Neither the addition of 2 rituximab infusions in iPET-negative patients nor treatment intensification in the form of a Burkitt protocol resulted in any improvement in the outcome of patients with aggressive lymphomas [158]. The corresponding 2-year OS rates were 88% versus 59% ($p < 0.0001$). The prognostic significance of iPET was independent from that of IPI [158, 159].

Overall, the use of the SUVmax reduction criterion over the D5PS score in DLBCL is supported by the results of studies of fixed or PET-driven modified treatment as well as by expert opinions [151–161].

The prognostic significance of iPET in DLBCL in various studies using either or both of the above criteria, either under the same continued treatment or after treatment escalation, is summarized in Table 14.4 [111, 124, 151, 153–159, 162–167].

#### 14.4.3.2 Primary Mediastinal Large B Cell Lymphoma

At present, existing data are too limited to support the recommendation of interim response assessment and iPET-based treatment modification in PMLBCL [168–170]. However, data on

**Table 14.4** Summary of selected studies evaluating the role of interim PET during rituximab-based chemoimmunotherapy

| Author, year, ref | Pts | Initial treatment | iPET positivity | | | Escalation regimen | Progression (or event) free survival | | | |
|---|---|---|---|---|---|---|---|---|---|---|
| | | | Time-point | Definition | Frequency # (%) | | iPET-neg | iPET-pos | At *n*-years | *p*-value |
| Safar 2012 [164] | 112 | R-CHOP-14/21 or R-ACVBP | 2 cycles | Any uptake >MRU | 42 (38%) | Treatment unchanged, according to the initial regimen | 84% | 47% | 3 years | <0.0001 |
| Safar 2012 [164] | 85 | R-CHOP-14/21 or R-ACVBP | 2 cycles | ΔSUVmax≤66% | 30 (35%) | | 77% | 38% | 3 years | 0.002 |
| Itti 2013 [151] | 114 | R-CHOP-14/21 or R-ACVBP | 2 cycles | D5PS ≥4 | 51 (45%) | Treatment unchanged, according to the initial regimen | 81% | 59% | 3 years | 0.003 |
| Itti 2013 [151] | 114 | R-CHOP-14/21 or R-ACVBP | 2 cycles | ΔSUVmax≤66% | 25 (22%) | | 79% | 44% | 3 years | 0.0002 |
| Mamot 2015 [111] | 125 | R-CHOP-14 | 2 cycles | D5PS ≥4 | 58 (46%) | Treatment unchanged (plus R-CHOP×4 + R ×2) | 76% | 41% | 2 years | <0.001 |
| Mamot 2015 [111] | 138 | R-CHOP-14 | 2 cycles | ΔSUVmax≤66% | 19 (14%) | | 61% | 42% | 2 years | 0.10[a] |
| Casasnovas 2011 [155] | 200 | R-CHOP-14 ×4 vs. R-ACVBP ×4 | 2 cycles<br>4 cycles | ΔSUVmax≤66%<br>ΔSUVmax≤70% | 29/183 (16%)<br>24/183 (13%) | PET2−/4-: Continued regimen<br>PET2+/4-: MTXi.v. + (Z)-BEAM/ASCT<br>PET2±/4+: Salvage therapy<br>*Decisions according to IHP criteria* | 80%<br>83% | 56%<br>40% | 4 years<br>2 years | 0.0005<br><0.0001 |
| Duehrsen 2016 [168] | 606 | R-CHOP-21 ×2 (plus ×4 ± R×2, if iPET-neg) | 2 cycles | ΔSUVmax≤66% | 63 (10%) | Randomized to Burkitt protocol vs. R-CHOP-21 ×6 | 76%[b] | 41%[b] | 2 years | <0.0001 |
| Sehn 2014 [167] | 150 | R-CHOP-21 × 4 (plus ×2, if iPET-neg) | 4 cycles | IHP | 50 (33%) | R-ICE ×4 ± RT | 91%[c] | 59% | 4 years | 0.0001 |
| Swinnen ECOG, 2015 [167] | 76 | R-CHOP-21 × 3 (plus ×3, if iPET-neg) | 3 cycles | D5PS ≥4 (ECOG modified) | 13 (17%) | R-CHOP ×1 + R-ICE ×3 | 71% | 33% | 3 years | |
| Hertzberg 2017 [165] | 143 | R-CHOP-14 × 4 (plus ×2 + R×2, if iPET-neg) | 4 cycles | IHP criteria (but all had D5PS ≥4) | 42 (29%) | R-ICE ×3 + Z-BEAM/ASCT | 74% | 67%[b] | 2 years | 0.32 |

| | | | | | | | | | | |
|---|---|---|---|---|---|---|---|---|---|---|
| Pardal E 2014 [157] | 66 | R-MegaCHOP ×3 (plus ×3, if iPET-neg) | 3 cycles | IHP | 30 (45%) | R-IFE ×2 + BEAM/ASCT (decisions according to IHP) | 81% | 57% | 4 years | 0.02 |
| Pardal E 2014 [157] | 51 | R-MegaCHOP ×3 (plus ×3, if iPET-neg) | 3 cycles | D5PS ≥4 | 21 (42%) | | 83% | 57% | 4 years | 0.02 |
| Pardal E 2014 [157] | 51 | R-MegaCHOP ×3 (plus ×3, if iPET-neg) | 3 cycles | ΔSUVmax≤66% | 9 (18%) | | 81% | 33% | 4 years | <0.001 |
| Yim SK 2019 [162] | 220 | R-CHOP ×6–8 | 3 cycles | D5PS ≥4 | 49 (22.3%) | Treatment unchanged | 72.6% | 39.3% | 5 years | <0.001 |
| Wight 2021 [163] | 188 | R-CHOP in 96% of pts | 2 cycles (3 in 48 pts) | D5PS ≥4 | 60 (33%) (33, 18% D5PSS5) | Treatment unchanged | 80% (Incl. 4) | 30% (only 5) | 2 years | <0.001 |
| Mikhaeel G 2021 [153] | 189 | R-CHOP-21 ×8 (84%) OR R-CHOP-14 ×6 + R ×2 (16%) | 2 cycles | D5PS ≥4 | 70 (37%)[d] | Treatment unchanged | 82% | 76%[d] | 2 years | 0.25 |
| Mikhaeel G 2021 [153] | 189 | | 2 cycles | ΔSUVmax≤66% | 21 (11%) | | ~87% | ~67% | 2 years | 0.03 |
| Zucca E 2020 [154] | 138 | R-CHOP-14 ×6 + R ×2 | 2 cycles | D5PS ≥4 | 72 (52%)[e] | Treatment unchanged | 83% | 68%[e] | 5 years | 0.06 |
| Zucca E 2020 [154] | 137 | | 2 cycles | ΔSUVmax≤66% | 18 (13%) | | 81% | 49% | 5 years | 0.003 |
| Schoder 2020 [152] | 111 | R-CHOP-21 ×6–8 (4 if stI/II) | 2 cycles | D5PS ≥4 ΔSUVmax≤66% | 51 (46%) | Treatment unchanged | 88% | 81% | 4 years | 0.44 |
| Costa 2016 [219] | 147 | R-CHOP×2 | 2 cycles | D5PS ≥4 | 51 (45.9%) | Treatment unchanged | 87.7% | 81.2% | 2 years | 0.44 |
| Jiang 2018 [220] | 106 | R-CHOP-like ×4 | 4 cycles | D5PS ≥4 | 43 (41%) | Treatment unchanged | 78% | 33% | 2 years | <0.001 |
| Kim 2016 [221] | 118 | R-CHOP×2/3 | 2 or 3 cycles | D5PS ≥4 | 35 (30%) | Treatment unchanged | 79% | 51% | 2 years | 0.0004 |
| Li 2019 [222] | 129 | CHOP×4 or R-CHOP×4 | 4 cycles | D5PS ≥4 | 31 (40%) | Treatment unchanged | 85% | 49% | 2 years | 0.009 |

(continued)

**Table 14.4** (continued)

| Author, year, ref | Pts | Initial treatment | iPET positivity | | | Escalation regimen | Progression (or event) free survival | | | |
|---|---|---|---|---|---|---|---|---|---|---|
| | | | Time-point | Definition | Frequency # (%) | | iPET-neg | iPET-pos | At *n*-years | *p*-value |
| Li 2019 [222] | 129 | CHOP ×4 or R-CHOP ×4 | 4 cycles | ΔSUVmax<74% | 25 (32%) | Treatment unchanged | 84% | 31% | 2 years | 0.001 |
| Zhang 2015 [223] | 197 | R-CHOP×2 or R-CHOP×2 + RT | 2 cycles | IHP criteria | 87 (44.2%) | Therapy was performed as planned and was not altered due to IPET findings unless progression occurred | 75.8% | 38.2% | 3 years | <0.001 |
| Zhang 2015 [223] | 197 | R-CHOP×4 or R-CHOP×4 + RT | 4 cycles | IHP criteria | 68 (35%) | Therapy was performed as planned and was not altered due to IPET findings unless progression occurred | 75.3% | 24.7% | 3 years | <0.001 |

[a]The ΔSUVmax was however the only PET factor associated with overall survival

[b]After retrospective review according to D5PS, the 2-year PFS was highly different between D5PS score 4 and D5PS score 5 patients (88% versus 33%, $p = 0.0002$), given that treatment intensification was actually performed in the majority of them

[c]The 4-year PFS was 83% for the 12 patients (8%) with indeterminate result in iPET

[d]But only 57% for the 7% of patients with D5PS score 5, defined as uptake >3× liver and/or new lesions ($p = 0.01$). Interestingly, 13% of patients had D5PS score 5, defined as uptake >2× liver and/or new lesions and had a 2-year PFS ~67% (derived from survival curves)

[e]5-year PFS 70% versus 54% ($p = 0.01$) for patients with D5PS score 1–4 versus 5; the latter defined as uptake >2× liver and/or new lesions. Only 12% of the patients had D5PS score 5

iPET under R-CHOP-21 in PMLBCL are only derived from a small subgroup analysis of the PETAL trial [158]. A study from Memorial Sloan Kettering Cancer Center failed to show any impact of iPET on the outcome of PMLBCL, when treatment was modified in patients with positive findings: In detail, 51 patients received 4 cycles of accelerated R-$C_{1000}$HOP-14 and underwent iPET, which was negative in 53% of them [169]. A significant number of patients underwent biopsies of the iPET-positive mass, which were always negative [124]. Patients subsequently received non-cross resistant therapy with 3 cycles of ICE with or without rituximab and no additional RT. No difference in PFS emerged according to iPET result irrespective of the criterion used to define positivity. Similar results were reported by Lazarovici et al. in a study of 36 patients, in which 16/17 patients with positive iPET had negative biopsies [171]. However, none of the iPET-positive patients had D5PS score 5 and treatment (mostly R- or G-ACVBP) was modified according to iPET result.

In a retrospective study of 30 patients, R-VACOP-B ($n$ = 19) or 11 R-CHOP ($n$ = 11) was continued irrespective of iPET result without consolidative RT. [170] A positive iPET was observed in 47% of patients. Their 3-year PFS was 57% versus 94% for those with a negative iPET ($p$ = 0.015). However, there was a trend towards inferior prognostic performance of iPET after R-VACOP-B. In another Chinese retrospective study of 49 patients treated with R-da-EPOCH or R-CHOP, the rate of iPET positivity was 37% and 10/18 iPET-positive patients had D5PS score 5. Treatment was modified in 7/10 patients with score 5 and 1/8 with score 4. The 2-year PFS rate was 93% versus 69% versus 20% for patients with D5PS score 1–3, 4, and 5 respectively, with only score 5 conferring a clearly inferior outcome despite frequent treatment modification [172].

Finally, the previously described PETAL trial included a small subgroup of 42 patients with PMLBCL. Using the ΔSUVmax criterion, only 12% remained iPET-positive after R-CHOP×2. The 2-year FFTF was clearly superior for iPET-negative patients (89% versus 40%) despite treatment intensification in case of iPET positivity; however, the 2-year OS was virtually the same (97% versus 100%) [168]. Obviously, the effect of Burkitt-like treatment intensification could not be adequately evaluated with only 5 iPET-positive patients [168].

#### 14.4.3.3 T Cell Lymphomas

Interim PET positivity by the ΔSUVmax criterion is also a strong prognostic factor in patients with T cell lymphomas. The rarity of these subtypes has not permitted the development of separate trials. In a subgroup analysis of 76 patients with peripheral T cell lymphomas (ALCL, AITL, or PTCL-NOS) enrolled in the PETAL trial, 25% remained iPET-positive after CHOP×2 by the ΔSUVmax criterion. This percentage was 33% for PTCL, AILT, and ALK-ALCL combined, but only 1/21 patients with ALK+ ALCL had a positive iPET [173]. In the subgroup of 55 patients with PTCL, AILT, and ALK-ALCL, the SUVmax reduction criterion provided the best discrimination in terms of PFS at the cutoff of 50% (and not 66%) with 4-year PFS rates of 50% versus 0%. The same criterion at the cutoff of 66% and the D5PS (5 versus 1–4) provided very good, but slightly inferior discriminative capacity [173]. The extremely small number of events precluded an analysis in the 21 patients with ALK+ ALCL. However, treatment intensification with a Burkitt protocol failed to improve the outcome of iPET-positive patients, but this conclusion was based on the analysis of less than 20 patients and should be interpreted with caution [173, 174]. In extranodal NK/T cell lymphomas, iPET is also prognostically relevant [75], but data on potential treatment modification are lacking.

## 14.5 Impact of Interim and EOT-PET on Clinical Practice: Randomized Trials

Although the prognostic significance and the diagnostic accuracy of EOT-PET/CT have already been firmly established, studies evaluating PET-guided treatment decisions are only few

[83–86, 90, 91, 129–131, 140, 158, 175]. Evidence-based strategies for the implementation of iPET and/or EOT-PET are available only for HL and aggressive B cell lymphomas.

### 14.5.1 Hodgkin Lymphoma

#### 14.5.1.1 Radiotherapy Questions

Four recent randomized trials have focused on the possibility of omitting RT in localized stage HL after a negative PET/CT. The non-inferiority EORTC H10 has been the most informative of them [140, 175]. The published results of H10 suggest that RT cannot be safely spared after ABVD×2 in patients with stage I/II HL, who become strictly PET/CT-negative by the IHP criteria [77, 78] (roughly corresponding to D5PS scores 1–2), especially in those without adverse risk factors: In H10, patients who became PET/CT-negative after ABVD×2 were randomized to receive: (1) 1 or 2 further ABVD cycles (according to the absence or presence of risk factors) plus 30 Gy involved node RT (standard arm) or (2) 2 or 4 further ABVD cycles (according to the absence or presence of risk factors) without RT (experimental arm). The study was prematurely terminated due to excess relapses in the no-RT arms [175]. More mature results revealed a clear difference in terms of 5-year PFS for patients without adverse risk factors (99% versus 87%, hazard ratio 15.8 with 95% CI 3.8–66.1), but a non-significant one for those with ≥1 adverse factors, including bulky mediastinal masses (92% versus 90%, hazard ratio 1.45 with 95% CI 0.84–2.50). In any case however, non-inferiority of ABVD compared with combined modality could not be demonstrated for patients with a negative PET after ABVD×2 [140]. The design of the other 3 trials, namely RAPID, HD16, and HD17, rather resembled to an interim PET- than an EOT-PET-driven trial [83–86].

Overall, all published trials suggest that RT cannot be omitted after 2, 3, or 4 cycles of ABVD in patients with early favorable disease (stage I/II—no adverse prognostic factors) and a strictly negative PET after 2 or 3 ABVD cycles without relevant loss in disease control (generally 10–15% at 5 years; Table 14.2), although overall survival is not affected at all. Furthermore, it is not clear if omission of RT will be associated with an increased rate of very late relapses observed >5 years from initial diagnosis, which are typically not captured during the mid-term follow-up of randomized clinical trials [176]. On the contrary, in patients with early unfavorable disease (stage I/II and ≥ 1 adverse factors) the benefit from consolidative RT in case of a strictly negative iPET (D5PS scores 1–2) appears to be minimal. Thus, surprisingly, RT can be omitted in this unfavorable subgroup—even in patients with bulky disease—with minimal loss in disease control and no impact on overall survival, provided that a total of 6 ABVD cycles are given. After more intensive chemotherapy consisting of BEACOPP-escalated ×2 plus ABVD×2, RT can be omitted if EOT-PET is strictly negative without any loss even in disease control [85].

Whether RT can be omitted in patients with an iPET D5PS score 3 is unclear, since these patients were irradiated in the above randomized trials. However, both the RATHL [133] and the HD607 randomized trial [90, 91] included a considerable percentage of patients with early unfavorable stages and the outcomes without consolidative RT appeared to be comparable in the D5PS score 1–3 (iPET-negative) subgroup irrespective of the exact classification as 1, 2, or 3, again provided that 6 A(B)VD cycles were given. However, in the CALGB 50604 trial, after only 4 ABVD cycles and no consolidative RT, patients with non-bulky stage I/II HL with an iPET D5PS score 3 had numerically lower 3-year PFS compared to D5PS score 1–2 (77% versus 94%) [177].

In advanced stage HL, RT is not considered in EOT-PET-negative patients without bulky disease, while it can be omitted in case of iPET and EOT-PET negativity (D5PS score 1–3) after ABVD ×6 in patients with bulky disease defined as dmax ≥5 cm [90, 91]. It appears that this is independent from the size of bulky disease (even if ≥10 cm) although HD607 was not powered enough to address this specific subgroup question. As already mentioned, RT can be spared irrespective of the initial bulk in advanced HL patients with a negative PET and > 2.5 cm residual abnormalities (and obviously in those with smaller or no abnormalities), if this response has been achieved by intensive chemotherapy with BEACOPP-escalated or similar regimens, because >88% of them remain disease-free at 10 years [80, 87].

### 14.5.2 Chemotherapy Questions

Treatment intensification in the form of BEACOPP-escalated is recommended in patients with a positive iPET after ABVD ×2. There is clear evidence from the H10 trial that BEACOPP-escalated ×2 improves PFS and marginally overall survival in early unfavorable HL compared to ABVD ×2 plus the same consolidative RT. [140] Although not tested in any randomized trial of advanced HL, switching to 4–8 cycles of BEACOPP-escalated clearly improves PFS in iPET-positive patients with stages III/IV (or unfavorable II) [90, 91, 132–138]. The RATHL approach using BEACOPP-escalated ×4 or BEACOPP-14 ×6 appears reasonable in terms of preserved efficacy with the least possible toxicity.

Apart from starting with ABVD, another iPET-driven strategy involves starting with BEACOPP-escalated and de-escalating chemotherapy in case of a negative iPET. However, 2 different methods of de-escalation have been tested, as described above (sect. 14.4). Collectively, both the AHL 2011 and the HD18 trial suggest that, if BEACOPP-escalated is the initial choice, 6 cycles should be given to strictly iPET-positive patients, while de-escalation can be either a total of BEACOPP-escalated ×2 plus ABVD ×4 or a total of BEACOPP-escalated ×4. The optimal threshold to define iPET positivity (more strict or looser) needs to be defined further.

Overall, iPET-adapted therapy appears attractive and has been adopted in everyday practice in many institutions. Randomized trials are not yet mature enough to examine the presence of a potential overall survival benefit over ABVD. Whether an ABVD-first and escalation or BEACOPP-first and de-escalation is preferable is not clear [138].

### 14.5.3 Aggressive B Cell Lymphomas

#### 14.5.3.1 Radiotherapy Questions

Few prospective trials have evaluated the omission of RT after abbreviated chemoimmunotherapy regimens in DLBCL. Lamy et al. reported that RT can be omitted in patients with non-bulky (<7 cm), localized (stage I/II) DLBCL if a strictly negative PET was achieved after R-CHOP-14 ×4. Overall patients received 4 or 6 cycles of R-CHOP-14 according to baseline risk classification. The 5-year EFS was 92% vs. 89% for patients who were randomized to receive RT or not and relapse rates were similar [178]. Interestingly, PET positivity was defined visually as "18F-FDG uptake above the mediastinum or surrounding background in a location incompatible with normal anatomy or physiology," which is a very strict criterion for PET-negative status. In another prospective trial of 132 patients with non-bulky (<10 cm), localized (stage I/II) aggressive B cell lymphoma (mostly DLBCL), the rate of PET positivity, defined as D5PS score ≥ 4, was 11%. RT was omitted in patients with a negative iPET after R-CHOP-21 ×3 (D5PS score 1–3), who received R-CHOP ×4 in total without RT, while patients with positive iPET received involved field RT and subsequent radioimmunotherapy with ibritumomab tiuxetan. The 5-year PFS was 89% versus 86% for patients with iPET-negative or positive respectively after R-CHOP-21 ×3 [179]. Similarly, indirect comparison of the OPTIMAL>60 and the RICOVER60 trials suggests that RT can be spared in elderly patients with bulky DLBCL (>7.5 cm) who achieve a PET-negative status after R-CHOP-14-based immunochemotherapy with a 2-year PFS for all bulky patients of 79% (irrespective of PET status or RT) [114].

All the above data suggest that RT can be spared in localized, non-bulky DLBCL even after abbreviated immunochemotherapy in case of a negative PET after 3–4 cycles of immunochemotherapy. It can also be probably spared in bulky, PET-negative patients irrespective of stage, as has been suggested by the British Columbia retrospective experience as well [113].

In PMLBCL RT can be spared after R-da-EPOCH in patients with D5PS score 1–4 after

R-da-EPOCH based on the excellent results of a prospective trial [102, 103]. The results are also very encouraging after R-CHOP if RT is spared in patients with D5PS score 1–2 [97–99] or even score 3 [97]. However, there is still no evidence on this RT question from a randomized trial. The IELSG-37 trial is expected to shed light on this issue [180].

#### 14.5.3.2 Chemotherapy Questions

The only randomized trial in the field of aggressive lymphomas is PETAL, which failed to demonstrate any impact of intensified treatment in iPET-positive patients with aggressive lymphomas under initial treatment with R-CHOP [158]. In a recently published GAINED trial treatment was modified according to PET-2 and PET-4 results. The outcomes were similar for PET-2-negative/PET-4-negative patients who received intensive conventional immunochemotherapy and PET-2-positive/PET-4-negative patients, who received consolidation autologous stem cell transplantation, with 2-year PFS 90% versus 84%. The 2-year PFS was 62% for PET-4-positive patients. Although the above results suggest some improvement based on PET-driven therapy, this is not a randomized comparison of treatment strategies [181]. Thus, there is no established "more effective" treatment for iPET-positive patients with DLBCL, who have inferior outcomes.

## 14.6 PET in the Setting of Autologous Stem Cell Transplantation (ASCT)

The evaluation of PET in patients with lymphoma undergoing ASCT was introduced early in the course of utilization of PET in clinical practice. Generally, published studies have included mixed (HL and NHL) patient populations: Patients with positive pretransplant PET have inferior outcomes than those with negative studies. Pretransplant PET appears to be an independent predictor from established clinical risk scores at the time of relapse/progression [182]. In a meta-analysis of 12 studies, incorporating 630 patients with HL and aggressive NHL who underwent ASCT and had been evaluated with pre-high-dose chemotherapy PET examination, Terasawa et al. reported a summary sensitivity of 69%, summary specificity 81%, similar prognostic accuracy among studies, and shorter PFS for patients with positive PET scan [183]. Another meta-analysis reported hazard ratios of 3.2 (for disease progression) and 4.5 (for death) for patients with positive vs. negative pretransplant PET [184].

In relapsed/refractory HL, patients who become PET-negative with salvage chemotherapy and undergo ASCT have a long-term remission rate of 80–85% vs. 40–50% for those who remain PET-positive [185, 186], although the range for these figures among several published studies is much wider, as suggested in a another, more recent meta-analysis [187] (Fig. 14.8). These results demonstrate that failure to achieve a PET-negative status does not preclude ASCT in patients with HL, especially if they are chemosensitive by conventional imaging. However, more standardized protocols are required for evaluation of pretransplant PET/CT in patients undergoing ASCT: It is not clear whether pretransplant PET should be evaluated by the D5PS, SUVmax-based, or other criteria. As a general rule, the decision to proceed to ASCT in relapsed/refractory HL should be based rather on conventional chemosensitivity criteria than on PET evaluation.

The D5PS has been evaluated in several studies with patients with scores 4—and particularly those with score 5—carrying a worse prognosis [185, 188–191]. In addition the baseline MTV at initiation of salvage therapy is a strong prognostic factor [189], while the residual pretransplant MTV may also provide independent prognostic information within the unfavorable group of pretransplant PET-positive patients [188, 191]. The outcomes of PET-positive patients with low residual MTV are closer to those with a negative pretransplant PET than to patients with more bulky residuals [188, 191]. Although such sophisticated methods may provide very promising risk stratification, they are

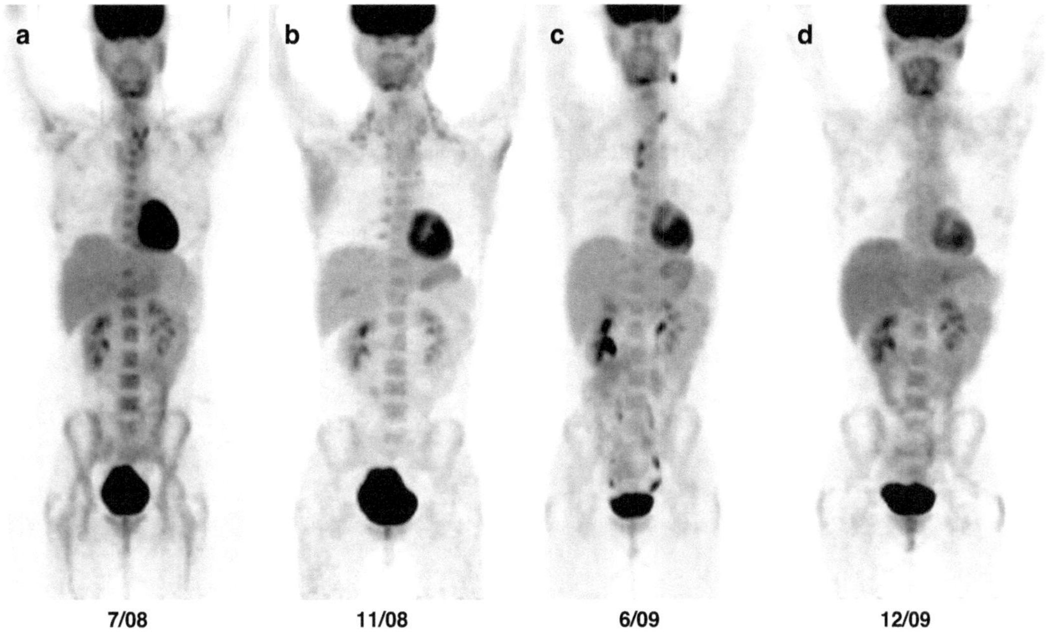


**Fig. 14.8** (**a**) 18 FDG-PET before autologous stem cell transplantation in a patient with relapsed Hodgkin lymphoma: hypermetabolic lymph nodes at the upper mediastinum. (**b**) 18 FDG-PET 4 weeks after autologous stem cell transplantation: negative. (**c**) Relapsing disease 6 months later. (**d**) The patient received additional radiation therapy and reached CR (PET negative)

not yet applicable in clinical practice and need further standardization and validation.

The probability of further progression after ASCT remains high in relapsed/refractory HL. As shown in the AETHERA trial, the probability of progression in high-risk patients can be significantly decreased by consolidative treatment with brentuximab vedotin, an anti-CD30 monoclonal antibody linked to a microtubule poisson. Brentuximab vedotin consolidation was highly beneficial in patients with a positive PET prior to ASCT but had minimal or no effect on those who had already achieved a PET-negative status [192]. These data should be interpreted with caution because pre-ASCT PET was not required by the protocol and, therefore, it was not performed in all patients and was not centrally and uniformly evaluated. Although this information was derived from an unplanned subgroup analysis, pre-ASCT PET might provide a clue to the optimal use of post-ASCT consolidation and should be further evaluated.

## 14.7 PET in the Era of Novel Agents

### 14.7.1 Programmed Death-1 (PD-1) Inhibitors

The introduction of Programmed Death-1 (PD-1) inhibitors nivolumab and pembrolizumab has provided very promising results in heavily pretreated patients with relapsed/refractory HL during the last few years [193–198]. Promising results have also been reported for PMLBCL [199, 200]. Apart from producing a high objective response rate with several durable remissions (>5 years) [197, 198] (Fig. 14.9a, b), PD-1 inhibitors may result in a transient tumor flare or pseudoprogression. For this reason, an attempt was made to modify the criteria for response assessment to PD-1 inhibitors by describing the LYRIC classification [201]. The description of these revised criteria is beyond the scope of this review.

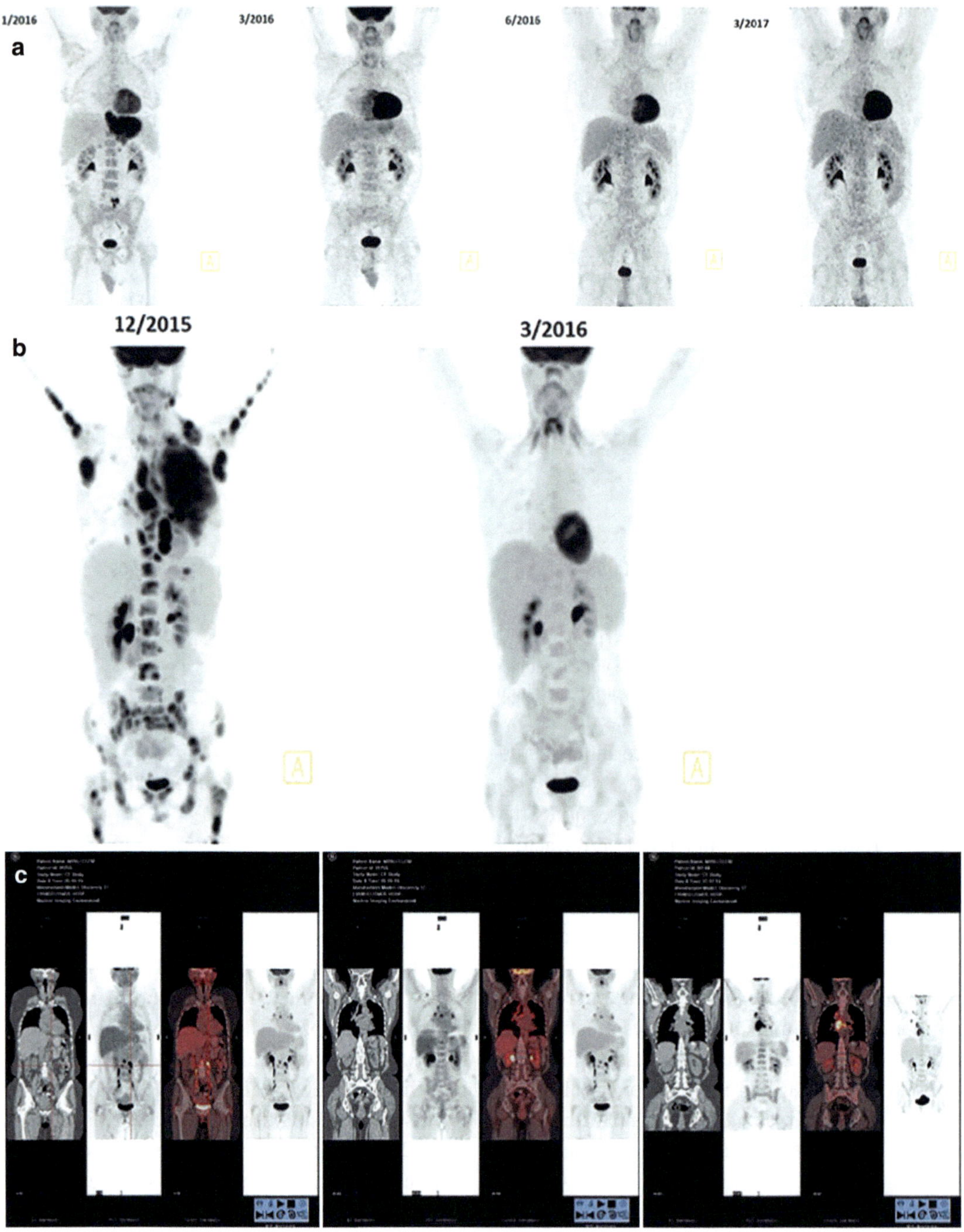
1/2016
a
3/2016
6/2016
3/2017
12/2015
b
3/2016
c

However, pseudoprogression appears to be a rather rare problem in relapsed/refractory HL, while new lesions may be also due to immune-related adverse events [202, 203].

As expected, PET/CT is superior to CT for response assessment during PD1 inhibitor treatment for relapsed/refractory HL uncovering more patients with complete metabolic responses [204, 205]. Responses are evident during the initial 2–3 months and correlate with PFS and overall survival [193, 195–198]. Based on the analysis of the KEYNOTE-087 trial for pembrolizumab the classification of responses appears to be similar irrespective of the use of the Cheson 2007 or the Lugano 2014 criteria [206]. Finally, it should be noted that some patients do not achieve an objective radiographic or PET-based response, but continue to receive clinical benefit for variable time periods despite episodes of disease progression [195]. This strategy of "treatment beyond progression" was formally assessed within the protocol of the CHECKMATE-205 trial of nivolumab.

**Fig. 14.9** (**a**) Fifty-two year old male with stage IIA classical Hodgkin lymphoma diagnosed on 2006, 10 years prior to this image, had a slow progression after ABVD × 6 + RT. He achieved a PR to IGEV salvage chemotherapy but declined ASCT approximately 5 years ago. Further ESHAP was too toxic and discontinued after 1 cycle. Brentuximab Vedotin was then instituted but the disease remained stable. The patient was initially unwilling and later ineligible for ASCT and remained on palliative therapy awaiting for a clinical trial with PD-1 inhibitor. Prior to PD-1 inhibitor initiation he had a very unusual disease localization with extensive esophagealgastric hypermetabolic mass (SUVmax 17.2), which caused dysphagia (left panel), regional small hypermetabolic lymph nodes (SUVmax 4.6) and hypermetabolic osseous/bone marrow involvement of the L4 vertebra. After the fourth PD-1 inhibitor infusion (pembrolizumab every 3 weeks) the patient had achieved a complete remission with a negative PET (second image from left, 3/2016). The patient remains in complete metabolic response (CMR) 27 months after the introduction of pembrolizumab (third and fourth images on the right, dated 6/2016 and 3/2017). (**b**) A 32 year old female with classical Hodgkin lymphoma, stage IIA, was diagnosed on 2012, 3 years prior to this image. After ABVD × 6 + RT she achieved a PR and subsequently relapsed. Although she did not respond to ESHAP salvage chemotherapy, she underwent ASCT, but progressed rapidly thereafter. She further received brentuximab vedotin, bendamustine and gemcitabine-vinorelbine with rapidly progressive disease after each modality. Prior to PD-1 inhibitor initiation she had very extensive disease with generalized hypermetabolic lymphadenopathy, bulky mediastinal (SUVmax 9.6) and left lung localization (SUVmax 6.6) and multiple bone marrow hypermetabolic foci (SUVmax 7.2) associated with a positive bone marrow biopsy and B-symptoms (left panel). After the fourth PD-1 inhibitor infusion (pembrolizumab every 3 weeks) the patient had achieved a complete metabolic response (CMR) with a negative PET (right panel). The patient remains in CMR 27 months after the introduction of anti-PD-1 therapy with pembrolizumab. (**c**) A 62 year old female with stage IIISXB nodular sclerosing classical Hodgkin lymphoma, was diagnosed approximately 2 years prior to this image. Despite a negative interim PET after ABVD × 2, she developed progressive disease after the seventh ABVD cycle. She failed to respond to IGEV and ESHAP salvage chemotherapy, always developing progressive disease with B-symptoms, pruritus and worsening anatomic findings, thus being unable to undergo ASCT. She also failed to respond to Brentuximab Vedotin and rapidly developed symptomatic progressive disease after 2 cycles of BEACOPP chemotherapy. On March 2016 she was started with the PD-1 inhibitor Nivolumab (3 mg/kg every 2 weeks). Serial CT and PET evaluations demonstrated lack of response, with some anatomic sites responding and others enlarging. However, the patient is asymptomatic and inflammatory markers (ESR, CRP and thrombocytosis) have been completely normalized. This type of sustained clinical response had never been achieved with conventional chemotherapy and Brentuximab Vedotin. It is now increasingly recognized that PD-1 inhibitors may induce relatively durable periods of meaningful clinical benefit in patients who have anatomically stable or slowly progressive disease [195]

### 14.7.2 Chimeric Antigen Receptor (CAR) T cells

CAR-T cells are autologous T cells, modified ex vivo to express receptors which combine antigen-binding and T cell activation properties. Currently CAR-T cell therapy is the most innovative and promising treatment approach for relapsed/refractory DLBCL and related aggressive lymphomas. Several studies have evaluated the prognostic role of PET/CT in the CAR-T cell treatment setting. Vercellino et al. highlighted the prognostic significance of TMTV, and aimed to create a prognostic model for early progression after CAR-T cell infusion by combining TMTV (>80 $cm^3$) and clinical characteristics related to tumor burden, at the time of treatment [207]. Another study aiming to explore the prognostic role of different baseline quantitative metrics also showed that high TMTV (≥25 $cm^3$) was associated with inferior PFS, whereas SUVmax was not of prognostic significance [208]. More studies are needed to define the optimal time point and prognostic role of PET/CT in patients treated with CAR-T cells.

## 14.8 Artificial Intelligence in F-FDG-PET/CT Scan

The recent applications of Artificial Intelligence (AI) in the field of medical imaging have created great expectations in cancer diagnostics and personalized treatment approaches. Machine Learning (ML) is a branch of AI that creates applications which learn “on their own” by recognizing patterns in input datasets. AI/ML in medical imaging encompasses a variety of applications (e.g., Convolutional Neural Networks—CNN) which aim to eliminate the various biases that may affect image interpretation by humans and produce results comparable to expert radiologists. As extensively discussed in this chapter, F-FDG-PET/CT imaging has been broadly used in staging and response assessment in malignant lymphomas. Until today, just a few studies related to the applications of AI in PET imaging of lymphoma have been published, but definitely, significant progress will be made during the forthcoming years.

Different methods and quantitative metrics (e.g., SUVmean, TMTV, TLG, etc.) in PET/CT have been used in order to quantify tumor burden, evaluate treatment response, and estimate prognosis. AI is expected to better manage these tasks, as its applications may permit automatic quantification and register multiple parts of the body at the same time [209]. The main tasks of AI applications in PET/CT image processing are detection, segmentation, and classification. Detection refers to localization of an area within a medical image which contains an object of interest [210]. Examples include automatically characterizing lymphoma lesions or defining areas of High Normal Activity (Hina) such as bladder and kidneys [211]. Furthermore, the use of radiomics in PET-CT scan has shown great results in separating sites with HiNA, inflammatory nonmalignant lesions, and malignant lesions as shown from Anunziata and Lartizien’s results [212, 213]. Segmentation is the process of demarcation and specific detection of the margins of an object of interest. Segmentation improves the ability of precise estimation of quantitative parameters and improves the methods of exact specification of tumor burden. It is very important to estimate the risk stratification of each patient and predict the therapy response. In order to accomplish this, radiomic features such as standardized uptake value (SUV) and total metabolic tumor volume (TMTV) are used [58, 214]. For example, TMTV and TLG could possibly be better estimated and in less time, through this procedure [215, 216]. Classification refers to the assignment of medical images into diagnostic or prognostic groups. Radiomics are usually used for this purpose in order to characterize lesions as normal or abnormal, or defining different histologic subtypes of lymphomas [216]. Classification could also lead to better prognostication, especially in procedures which highly depend on individual viewer’s experience, such as D5PS estimation [212].

The application of Delta radiomics, which compare the changes of a lesion before and after treatment may be a useful tool in order to estimate the therapy response and the prognosis of the patient [217]. It is crucial for the world's institutions to contribute to everyday clinical practice's amplification with AI algorithms in PET imaging [218].

Concluding, AI may provide promising and innovative tools for image processing, medical decision making, and prognostication. It is sure that several subjective and time-consuming procedures will be held automatically in the future. However, more time is needed to evaluate AI applications and produce reliable and robust results. Currently physician's critical thinking remains invaluable beyond any doubt.

## 14.9 The Role of PET/CT in the Follow-Up of Lymphomas

Once a negative PET/CT has been achieved, routine follow-up of patients with HL and aggressive B cell lymphomas with PET/CT is not recommended, because it does not affect survival and the risk of false positive findings outweighs any potential benefit of "earlier" identification of relapse and will lead to many unnecessary invasive procedures to exclude relapses. There is also no role for PET/CT in the follow-up of other lymphoma subtypes.

Information regarding PET/CT restaging for relapsing or refractory lymphoma is rather limited (Fig. 14.3b). PET/CT may have a particular role in patients, mainly those with HL, who could be candidates for local treatment with curative intent.

## 14.10 Conclusions

FDG-PET is a unique tool for the assessment of malignant lymphomas, demonstrating high accuracy and strong prognostic significance. The implementation of PET/CT has altered the definition of response to treatment and has already a major impact on staging and the design of treatment strategies. Although data are rapidly accumulating, the exact role of PET/CT in guiding treatment decisions, especially in the mid-treatment (interim) setting, needs to be defined by randomized trials, many of which are ongoing. Questions under investigation include the role of PET to decide about consolidation radiotherapy, the potential of improving outcomes by early treatment intensification in interim PET-positive patients, or conversely, the possibility of treatment reduction in patients with negative interim PET. Although some answers have already been obtained, evidence-based data on the appropriate use of PET in lymphomas are expected to be available shortly.

## References


1. Cheson BD, Fisher RI, Barrington SF, Cavalli F, Schwartz LH, Zucca E, et al. Recommendations for initial evaluation, staging, and response assessment of Hodgkin and non-Hodgkin lymphoma: the lugano classification. J Clin Oncol. 2014;32(27):3059–67.
2. Barrington SF, Mikhaeel NG, Kostakoglu L, Meignan M, Hutchings M, Müeller SP, et al. Role of Imaging in the staging and response assessment of lymphoma: consensus of the international conference on malignant lymphomas imaging working group. J Clin Oncol. 2014;32(27):3048.
3. d'Amore F, Gaulard P, Trümper L, Corradini P, Kim WS, Specht L, et al. Peripheral T-cell lymphomas: ESMO clinical practice guidelines for diagnosis, treatment and follow-up. Ann Oncol. 2015;26(Suppl 5):v108–15.
4. Dreyling M, Campo E, Hermine O, Jerkeman M, Le Gouill S, Rule S, et al. Newly diagnosed and relapsed mantle cell lymphoma: ESMO clinical practice guidelines for diagnosis, treatment and follow-up. Ann Oncol. 2017;28(suppl_4):iv62–71.
5. Dreyling M, Ghielmini M, Rule S, Salles G, Ladetto M, Tonino SH, et al. Newly diagnosed and relapsed follicular lymphoma: ESMO clinical practice guidelines for diagnosis, treatment and follow-up. Ann Oncol. 2021;32(3):298–308.
6. Zelenetz A, Gordon L, Chang J, Christian B, Abramson J, Advani R, et al. NCCN guidelines insights: B-cell lymphomas, version 3.2022. J Natl Compr Cancer Netw. 2022;17(6):650–61.
7. Horwitz SM, Ansell S, Ai WZ, Barnes J, Barta SK, Brammer J, et al. T-cell lymphomas, version 2.2022, NCCN clinical practice guidelines in oncology. J Natl Compr Cancer Netw. 2022;20(3):285–308.
8. Zucca E, Arcaini L, Buske C, Johnson PW, Ponzoni M, Radcrer M, et al. Marginal zone lymphomas: ESMO clinical practice guidelines for diagnosis, treatment and follow-up. Ann Oncol. 2020;31(1):17–29.

9. Ngeow JYY, Quek RHH, Ng DCE, Hee SW, Tao M, Lim LC, et al. High SUV uptake on FDG-PET/CT predicts for an aggressive B-cell lymphoma in a prospective study of primary FDG-PET/CT staging in lymphoma. Ann Oncol. 2009;20(9):1543–7.
10. Weiler-Sagie M, Bushelev O, Epelbaum R, Dann EJ, Haim N, Avivi I, et al. (18)F-FDG avidity in lymphoma readdressed: a study of 766 patients. J Nucl Med. 2010;51(1):25–30.
11. Barrington SF, Kirkwood AA, Franceschetto A, Fulham MJ, Roberts TH, Almquist H, et al. PET-CT for staging and early response: results from the response-adapted therapy in advanced Hodgkin lymphoma study. Blood. 2016;127(12):1531–8.
12. Angelopoulou M, Mosa E, Pangalis G, Rondogianni P, Chatziioannou S, Prassopoulos V, et al. The significance of PET/CT in the initial staging of Hodgkin lymphoma: experience outside clinical trials. Anticancer Res. 2017;37:5727–36.
13. Michallet AS, Sesques P, Rabe KG, Itti E, Tordot J, Tychyj-Pinel C, et al. An 18F-FDG-PET maximum standardized uptake value > 10 represents a novel valid marker for discerning Richter's syndrome. Leuk Lymphoma. 2016;57(6):1474–7.
14. Wang Y, Rabe KG, Bold MS, Shi M, Hanson CA, Schwager SM, et al. The role of 18F-FDG-PET in detecting Richter's transformation of chronic lymphocytic leukemia in patients receiving therapy with a B-cell receptor inhibitor. Haematologica. 2020;105(11):2675–8.
15. Eichenauer DA, Aleman BMP, André M, Federico M, Hutchings M, Illidge T, et al. Hodgkin lymphoma: esmo clinical practice guidelines for diagnosis, treatment and follow-up. Ann Oncol. 2018;29(Suppl 4):iv19–29.
16. El-Galaly TC, D'Amore F, Mylam KJ, Brown PDN, Bøgsted M, Bukh A, et al. Routine bone marrow biopsy has little or no therapeutic consequence for positron emission tomography/computed tomography-staged treatment-naive patients with Hodgkin lymphoma. J Clin Oncol. 2012;30(36):4508–14.
17. Vassilakopoulos TP, Rondogianni P, Prassopoulos V, Chatziioannou S, Moschogiannis M, Poziopoulos C et al. Comparative assessment of bone marrow involvement (BMI) by bone marrow biopsy (BMB) or positron emission tomography/computed tomography (PET/CT) in Hodgkin lymphoma (HL). Haematol Hematol J. 2014.
18. Zwarthoed C, El-Galaly TC, Canepari M, Ouvrier MJ, Viotti J, Ettaiche M, et al. Prognostic value of bone marrow tracer uptake pattern in baseline PET scans in Hodgkin lymphoma: results from an international collaborative study. J Nucl Med. 2017;58(8):1249–54.
19. Voltin CA, Goergen H, Baues C, Fuchs M, Mettler J, Kreissl S, et al. Value of bone marrow biopsy in Hodgkin lymphoma patients staged by FDG PET: results from the German Hodgkin study group trials HD16, HD17, and HD18. Ann Oncol. 2018;29(9):1926–31.
20. Pedersen MA, Gormsen LC, Kamper P, Wassberg C, Andersen MD, D'Amore AL, et al. Focal skeletal FDG uptake indicates poor prognosis in cHL regardless of extent and first-line chemotherapy. Br J Haematol. 2019;186(3):431–9. https://onlinelibrary.wiley.com/doi/10.1111/bjh.15933.
21. Adams HJA, Kwee TC, de Keizer B, Fijnheer R, de Klerk JMH, Littooij AS, et al. Systematic review and meta-analysis on the diagnostic performance of FDG-PET/CT in detecting bone marrow involvement in newly diagnosed Hodgkin lymphoma: is bone marrow biopsy still necessary? Ann Oncol. 2014;25(5):921–7.
22. Puccini B, Nassi L, Minoia C, Volpetti S, Ciancia R, Riccomagno PC, et al. Role of bone marrow biopsy in staging of patients with classical Hodgkin's lymphoma undergoing positron emission tomography/computed tomography. Ann Hematol. 2017;96(7):1147–53.
23. Vassilakopoulos TP, Angelopoulou MK, Constantinou N, Karmiris T, Repoussis P, Roussou P, et al. Development and validation of a clinical prediction rule for bone marrow involvement in patients with Hodgkin lymphoma. Blood. 2005;105(5):1875–80.
24. Sehn LH, Scott DW, Chhanabhai M, Berry B, Ruskova A, Berkahn L, et al. Impact of concordant and discordant bone marrow involvement on outcome in diffuse large B-cell lymphoma treated with R-CHOP. J Clin Oncol. 2011;29(11):1452–7.
25. Paone G, Itti E, Haioun C, Gaulard P, Dupuis J, Lin C, et al. Bone marrow involvement in diffuse large B-cell lymphoma: correlation between FDG-PET uptake and type of cellular infiltrate. Eur J Nucl Med Mol Imaging. 2009;36(5):745–50.
26. Hong J, Lee Y, Park Y, Kim SG, Hwang KH, Park SHS, et al. Role of FDG-PET/CT in detecting lymphomatous bone marrow involvement in patients with newly diagnosed diffuse large B-cell lymphoma. Ann Hematol. 2012;91(5):687–95.
27. Cerci JJ, Györke T, Fanti S, Paez D, Meneghetti JC, Redondo F, et al. Combined PET and biopsy evidence of marrow involvement improves prognostic prediction in diffuse large B-cell lymphoma. J Nucl Med. 2014;55(10):1591–7.
28. Berthet L, Cochet A, Kanoun S, Berriolo-Riedinger A, Humbert O, Toubeau M, et al. In newly diagnosed diffuse large B-cell lymphoma, determination of bone marrow involvement with 18F-FDG PET/CT provides better diagnostic performance and prognostic stratification than does biopsy. J Nucl Med. 2013;54(8):1244–50.
29. Adams HJA, Kwee TC, Fijnheer R, Dubois SV, Nievelstein RAJ, de Klerk JMH. Bone marrow 18F-fluoro-2-deoxy-D-glucose positron emission tomography/computed tomography cannot replace bone marrow biopsy in diffuse large B-cell lymphoma. Am J Hematol. 2014;89(7):726–31.
30. Khan AB, Barrington SF, Mikhaeel NG, Hunt AA, Cameron L, Morris T, et al. PET-CT staging

of DLBCL accurately identifies and provides new insight into the clinical significance of bone marrow involvement. Blood. 2013;122(1):61–7.

31. Adams HJA, Kwee TC. Do not abandon the bone marrow biopsy yet in diffuse large B-cell lymphoma. J Clin Oncol. 2015;33(10):1217.
32. Andreou JA, Kosmidis PA, Gouliamos AD, Prassopoulos V, Vassilakopoulos TPVE. PET/CT in lymphomas: a case-based Atlas. Cham: Springer International; 2016.
33. Kaddu-Mulindwa D, Altmann B, Held G, Angel S, Stilgenbauer S, Thurner L, et al. FDG PET/CT to detect bone marrow involvement in the initial staging of patients with aggressive non-Hodgkin lymphoma: results from the prospective, multicenter PETAL and OPTIMAL>60 trials. Eur J Nucl Med Mol Imaging. 2021;48(11):3550–9.
34. Zelenetz AD, Gordon LI, Abramson JS, Advani RH, Bartlett NL, Caimi PF, et al. NCCN guidelines insights: B-cell lymphomas, version 3.2019. J Natl Compr Cancer Netw. 2019;17(6):650–61.
35. Tilly H, Gomes da Silva M, Vitolo U, Jack A, Meignan M, Lopez-Guillermo A, et al. Diffuse large B-cell lymphoma (DLBCL): ESMO clinical practice guidelines for diagnosis, treatment and follow-up. Ann Oncol. 2015;26:vii78–82.
36. Alzahrani M, El-Galaly TC, Hutchings M, Hansen JW, Loft A, Johnsen HE, et al. The value of routine bone marrow biopsy in patients with diffuse large B-cell lymphoma staged with PET/CT: a Danish-Canadian study. Ann Oncol. 2016;27(6):1095–9.
37. Vassilakopoulos TP, Prassopoulos V, Rondogianni P, Chatziioannou S, Konstantopoulos K, Angelopoulou MK. Role of FDG-PET/CT in staging and first-line treatment of Hodgkin and aggressive B-cell lymphomas. Mag Eur Med Oncol. 2015;2(8):105–14.
38. Vassilakopoulos TP, Pangalis GA, Katsigiannis A, Papageorgiou SG, Constantinou N, Terpos E, et al. Rituximab, cyclophosphamide, doxorubicin, vincristine, and prednisone with or without radiotherapy in primary mediastinal large B-cell lymphoma: the emerging standard of care. Oncologist. 2012;17(2):239–49.
39. Martelli M, Ceriani L, Zucca E, Zinzani PL, Ferreri AJM, Vitolo U, et al. [18F]fluorodeoxyglucose positron emission tomography predicts survival after chemoimmunotherapy for primary mediastinal large B-cell lymphoma: results of the International Extranodal Lymphoma Study Group IELSG-26 Study. J Clin Oncol. 2014;32(17):1769–75.
40. Meignan M, Itti E, Gallamini A, Younes A. FDG PET/CT imaging as a biomarker in lymphoma. Eur J Nucl Med Mol Imaging. 2015;42(4):623–33.
41. Kanoun S, Rossi C, Berriolo-Riedinger A, Dygai-Cochet I, Cochet A, Humbert O, et al. Baseline metabolic tumour volume is an independent prognostic factor in Hodgkin lymphoma. Eur J Nucl Med Mol Imaging. 2014;41(9):1735–43.
42. Song MK, Chung JS, Lee JJ, Jeong SY, Lee SM, Hong JS, et al. Metabolic tumor volume by positron emission tomography/computed tomography as a clinical parameter to determine therapeutic modality for early stage Hodgkin's lymphoma. Cancer Sci. 2013;104(12):1656–61.
43. Cottereau AS, Versari A, Loft A, Casasnovas O, Bellei M, Ricci R, et al. Prognostic value of baseline metabolic tumor volume in early-stage Hodgkin lymphoma in the standard arm of the H10 trial. Blood. 2018;131(13):1456–63.
44. Akhtari M, Milgrom SA, Pinnix CC, Reddy JP, Dong W, Smith GL, et al. Reclassifying patients with early-stage Hodgkin lymphoma based on functional radiographic markers at presentation. Blood. 2018;131(1):84–94.
45. Barrington SF, Kirkwood AA, Pike LC, Guezennec C, Li H, Blanc M, et al. New prognostic score incorporating MTV predicts treatment failure in advanced Hodgkin lymphoma. Hematol Oncol. 2021;39(S2)
46. Gallamini A, Rambaldi A, Patti C, Romano A, Viviani S, Bolis S, et al. Baseline metabolic tumor volume and IPS predict ABVD in advanced- stage Hodgkin lymphoma with a negative interim PET scan after 2 chemotherapy cycles. A retrospective analysis from the GITIL/FIL HD0607 TRIAL. Hematol Oncol. 2021;39(S2):47–8.
47. Pinochet P, Texte E, Stamatoullas-Bastard A, Vera P, Mihailescu SD, Becker S. Prognostic value of baseline metabolic tumour volume in advanced-stage Hodgkin's lymphoma. Sci Rep. 2021;11(1):23195.
48. Pike LC, Kirkwood AA, Patrick P, Radford J, Burton C, Stevens L, et al. Can baseline PET-CT features predict outcomes in advanced Hodgkin lymphoma? A prospective evaluation of UK patients in the RATHL trial (CRUK/07/033). Hematol Oncol. 2017;9:37–8.
49. Song MK, Chung JS, Shin HJ, Lee SM, Lee SE, Lee HS, et al. Clinical significance of metabolic tumor volume by PET/CT in stages II and III of diffuse large B cell lymphoma without extranodal site involvement. Ann Hematol. 2012;91(5):697–703.
50. Sasanelli M, Meignan M, Haioun C, Berriolo-Riedinger A, Casasnovas RO, Biggi A, et al. Pretherapy metabolic tumour volume is an independent predictor of outcome in patients with diffuse large B-cell lymphoma. Eur J Nucl Med Mol Imaging. 2014;41(11):2017–22.
51. Mikhaeel NG, Smith D, Dunn JT, Phillips M, Møller H, Fields PA, et al. Combination of baseline metabolic tumour volume and early response on PET/CT improves progression-free survival prediction in DLBCL. Eur J Nucl Med Mol Imaging. 2016;43(7):1209.
52. Song MK, Yang DH, Lee GW, Lim SN, Shin S, Pak KJ, et al. High total metabolic tumor volume in PET/CT predicts worse prognosis in diffuse large B cell lymphoma patients with bone marrow involvement in rituximab era. Leuk Res. 2016;42:1–6.
53. Cottereau AS, Lanic H, Mareschal S, Meignan M, Vera P, Tilly H, et al. Molecular profile and FDG-PET/CT total metabolic tumor volume improve risk classification at diagnosis for patients with

diffuse large B-cell lymphoma. Clin Cancer Res. 2016;22(15):3801–9.
54. Kim TM, Paeng JC, Chun IK, Keam B, Jeon YK, Lee SH, et al. Total lesion glycolysis in positron emission tomography is a better predictor of outcome than the international prognostic index for patients with diffuse large B cell lymphoma. Cancer. 2013;119(6):1195–202.
55. Zhou M, Chen Y, Huang H, Zhou X, Liu J, Huang G. Prognostic value of total lesion glycolysis of baseline 18F-fluorodeoxyglucose positron emission tomography/computed tomography in diffuse large B-cell lymphoma. Oncotarget. 2016;7(50):83544.
56. Mikhaeel NG, Heymans MW, Eertink JJ, de Vet HCW, Boellaard R, Dührsen U, et al. Proposed New dynamic prognostic index for diffuse large B-cell lymphoma: international metabolic prognostic index. J Clin Oncol. 2022;40:JCO2102063.
57. Kostakoglu L, Mattiello F, Martelli M, Sehn LH, Belada D, Ghiggi C, et al. Total metabolic tumor volume as a survival predictor for patients with diffuse large B-cell lymphoma in the GOYA study. Haematologica. 2020;107(7):1633–42.
58. Vercellino L, Cottereau AS, Casasnovas O, Tilly H, Feugier P, Chartier L, et al. High total metabolic tumor volume at baseline predicts survival independent of response to therapy. Blood. 2020;135(16):1396–405.
59. Ceriani L, Martelli M, Zinzani PL, Ferreri AJM, Botto B, Stelitano C, et al. Utility of baseline 18FDG-PET/CT functional parameters in defining prognosis of primary mediastinal (thymic) large B-cell lymphoma. Blood. 2015;126(8):950–6.
60. Camus V, Rossi C, Sesques P, Lequesne J, Tonnelet D, Haioun C, et al. Outcomes after first-line immunochemotherapy for primary mediastinal B-cell lymphoma: a LYSA study. Blood Adv. 2021;5(19):3862–72.
61. Pinnix CC, Ng AK, Dabaja BS, Milgrom SA, Gunther JR, David Fuller C, et al. Positron emission tomography-computed tomography predictors of progression after DA-R-EPOCH for PMBCL. Blood Adv. 2018;2(11):1334–43.
62. Cottereau AS, Nioche C, Dirand AS, Clerc J, Morschhauser F, Casasnovas O, et al. 18 F-FDG PET dissemination features in diffuse large B-cell lymphoma are predictive of outcome. J Nucl Med. 2020;61(1):40–5.
63. Gallamini A, Rambaldi A, Patti C, Romano A, Viviani S, Silvia B, et al. Lesion dissemination in baseline PET/CT (D-MAX) and IPS score predict ABVD treatment outcome in PET-2 negative advanced-stage Hodgkin lymphoma patients enrolled in the prospective GITIL/FIL HD0607 trial. Blood. 2021;138:2443.
64. Cottereau AS, Meignan M, Nioche C, Capobianco N, Clerc J, Chartier L, et al. Risk stratification in diffuse large B-cell lymphoma using lesion dissemination and metabolic tumor burden calculated from baseline PET/CT. Ann Oncol. 2021;32(3): 404–11.
65. Ceriani L, Milan L, Martelli M, Ferreri AJM, Cascione L, Zinzani PL, et al. Metabolic heterogeneity on baseline 18FDG-PET/CT scan is a predictor of outcome in primary mediastinal B-cell lymphoma. Blood. 2018;132(2):179–86.
66. Senjo H, Hirata K, Izumiyama K, Minauchi K, Tsukamoto E, Itoh K, et al. High metabolic heterogeneity on baseline 18FDG-PET/CT scan as a poor prognostic factor for newly diagnosed diffuse large B-cell lymphoma. Blood Adv. 2020;4(10):2286–96.
67. Genta S, Ghilardi G, Cascione L, Juskevicius D, Tzankov A, Schär S, et al. Integration of baseline metabolic parameters and mutational profiles predicts long-term response to first-line therapy in DLBCL patients: a post Hoc analysis of the SAKK38/07 study. Cancers (Basel). 2022;14(4):1018.
68. Meignan M, Cottereau AS, Versari A, Chartier L, Dupuis J, Boussetta S, et al. Baseline metabolic tumor volume predicts outcome in high-tumor-burden follicular lymphoma: a pooled analysis of three multicenter studies. J Clin Oncol. 2016;34(30):3618–26.
69. Delfau-Larue MH, Van Der Gucht A, Dupuis J, Jais JP, Nel I, Beldi-Ferchiou A, et al. Total metabolic tumor volume, circulating tumor cells, cell-free DNA: distinct prognostic value in follicular lymphoma. Blood Adv. 2018;2(7):807–16.
70. Barrington SF, Trotman J, Sahin D, Belada D, Davies A, MacEwan R, et al. Baseline PET-derived metabolic tumor volume metrics did not predict outcomes in follicular lymphoma patients treated with first-line immunochemotherapy and antibody maintenance in the phase III GALLIUM study. Blood. 2018;132(Supplement 1):2882.
71. Albano D, Bosio G, Bianchetti N, Pagani C, Re A, Tucci A, et al. Prognostic role of baseline 18F-FDG PET/CT metabolic parameters in mantle cell lymphoma. Ann Nucl Med. 2019;33(7):449–58.
72. Cottereau BS, Broussais F, Casasnovas O, Kanoun S, Roques M, et al. Prognostic value of baseline total metabolic tumor volume (TMTV0) measured on FDG-PET/CT in patients with peripheral T-cell lymphoma (PTCL). Ann Oncol. 2016;27(4):719–24.
73. Cottereau AS, El-Galaly TC, Becker S, Broussais F, Petersen LJ, Bonnet C, et al. Predictive value of PET response combined with baseline metabolic tumor volume in peripheral T-cell lymphoma patients. J Nucl Med. 2018;59(4):589–95.
74. Kitadate A, Narita K, Fukumoto K, Terao T, Tsushima T, Kobayashi H, et al. Baseline total lesion glycolysis combined with interim positron emission tomography-computed tomography is a robust predictor of outcome in patients with peripheral T-cell lymphoma. Cancer Med. 2020;9(15):5509–18.
75. Chang Y, Fu X, Sun Z, Xie X, Wang R, Li Z, et al. Utility of baseline, interim and end-of-treatment 18F-FDG PET/CT in extranodal natural killer/T--cell lymphoma patients treated with L-asparaginase/ pegaspargase. Sci Rep. 2017;7(1):1–12.
76. Juweid ME, Wiseman GA, Vose JM, Ritchie JM, Menda Y, Wooldridge JE, et al. Response assessment of aggressive non-Hodgkin's lymphoma

by integrated international workshop criteria and fluorine-18-fluorodeoxyglucose positron emission tomography. J Clin Oncol. 2005;23(21):4652–61.

77. Cheson BD, Pfistner B, Juweid ME, Gascoyne RD, Specht L, Horning SJ, et al. Revised response criteria for malignant lymphoma. J Clin Oncol. 2007;25(5):579–86.
78. Juweid ME, Stroobants S, Hoekstra OS, Mottaghy FM, Dietlein M, Guermazi A, et al. Use of positron emission tomography for response assessment of lymphoma: consensus of the imaging subcommittee of international harmonization project in lymphoma. J Clin Oncol. 2007;25(5):571–8.
79. Vassilakopoulos T, Pangalis GA, Boutsikas G, Rontogianni P, Masouridis S, Prassopoulos V, et al. Prognostic factors in patients with Hodgkin lymphoma (HL) and a negative PET/CT after ABVD chemotherapy: potential applications for the design of follow-up strategies. Haematol Hematol J. 2012;97(Suppl 1):218.
80. Engert A, Haverkamp H, Kobe C, Markova J, Renner C, Ho A, et al. Reduced-intensity chemotherapy and PET-guided radiotherapy in patients with advanced stage Hodgkin's lymphoma (HD15 trial): a randomised, open-label, phase 3 non-inferiority trial. Lancet. 2012;379(9828):1791–9.
81. Barnes JA, LaCasce AS, Zukotynski K, Israel D, Feng Y, Neuberg D, et al. End-of-treatment but not interim PET scan predicts outcome in nonbulky limited-stage Hodgkin's lymphoma. Ann Oncol. 2011;22(4):910–5.
82. Sher DJ, Mauch PM, Van Den Abbeele A, LaCasce AS, Czerminski J, Ng AK. Prognostic significance of mid- and post-ABVD PET imaging in Hodgkin's lymphoma: the importance of involved-field radiotherapy. Ann Oncol. 2009;20(11):1848–53.
83. Radford J, Illidge T, Counsell N, Hancock B, Pettengell R, Johnson P, et al. Results of a trial of PET-directed therapy for early-stage Hodgkin's lymphoma. N Engl J Med. 2015;372(17):1598–607.
84. Fuchs M, Goergen H, Kobe C, Kuhnert G, Lohri A, Greil R, et al. Positron emission tomography-guided treatment in early-stage favorable Hodgkin lymphoma: final results of the international, randomized phase III HD16 trial by the German Hodgkin study group. J Clin Oncol. 2019;37(31):2835–45.
85. Borchmann P, Plütschow A, Görgen H, Kobe C, Greil R, Meissner J, et al. PET-guided omission of radiotherapy in early-stage unfavourable Hodgkin lymphoma (GHSG HD17): a multicentre, open-label, randomised, phase 3 trial. Lancet Oncol. 2021;22:223–34.
86. Borchmann P, Plütschow A, Görgen H. PET-guided omission of radiotherapy in Hodgkin lymphoma: authors' reply. Lancet Oncol. 2021;22(5):e182.
87. Engert A, Goergen H, Markova J, Pabst T, Meissner J, Zijlstra JM, et al. Reduced-intensity chemotherapy in patients with advanced-stage Hodgkin lymphoma: updated results of the open-label, international, randomised phase 3 HD15 trial by the German Hodgkin study group. HemaSphere. 2017;1(1):e5.
88. Barrington SF, Phillips EH, Counsell N, Hancock B, Pettengell R, Johnson P, et al. Positron emission tomography score has greater prognostic significance than pretreatment risk stratification in early-stage Hodgkin lymphoma in the UK RAPID Study. J Clin Oncol. 2019;37(20):1732–41.
89. Hartridge-Lambert SK, Schöder H, Lim RC, Maragulia JC, Portlock CS. ABVD alone and a PET scan complete remission negates the need for radiologic surveillance in early-stage, nonbulky Hodgkin lymphoma. Cancer. 2013;119(6):1203–9.
90. Gallamini A, Tarella C, Viviani S, Rossi A, Patti C, Mule A, et al. Early chemotherapy intensification with escalated BEACOPP in patients with advanced-stage Hodgkin lymphoma with a positive interim positron emission tomography/computed tomography scan after two ABVD cycles: long-term results of the GITIL/FIL HD 0607 tria. J Clin Oncol. 2018;36(5):454–62.
91. Gallamini A, Rossi A, Patti C, Picardi M, Romano A, Cantonetti M, et al. Consolidation radiotherapy could be safely omitted in advanced Hodgkin lymphoma with large nodal mass in complete metabolic response after ABVD: final analysis of the randomized GITIL/FIL HD0607 trial. J Clin Oncol. 2020;38(33):3905–13.
92. Vassilakopoulos TP, Rontogianni P, Pangalis G, Boutsikas G, Prassopoulos V, Masouridis S, et al. Outcome and prognostic factors in patients with Hodgkin lymphoma (HL) who remain PET/CT-positive after ABVD combination chemotherapy: potential applications for the design of subsequent treatment. Haematologica. 2012;97(s1):562.
93. Kobe C, Kuhnert G, Kahraman D, Haverkamp H, Eich HT, Franke M, et al. Assessment of tumor size reduction improves outcome prediction of positron emission tomography/computed tomography after chemotherapy in advanced-stage Hodgkin lymphoma. J Clin Oncol. 2014;32(17):1776–81.
94. Vassilakopoulos TP, Pangalis GA, Polliack A. A "PET" topic in primary mediastinal large B-cell lymphoma: positive or negative, and how to handle it in the end. Leuk Lymphoma. 2015;56(1):3–5.
95. Pinnix CC, Dabaja B, Ahmed MA, Chuang HH, Costelloe C, Wogan CF, et al. Single-institution experience in the treatment of primary mediastinal B cell lymphoma treated with immunochemotherapy in the setting of response assessment by 18fluorodeoxyglucose positron emission tomography. Int J Radiat Oncol Biol Phys. 2015;92(1):113–21.
96. Filippi AR, Piva C, Giunta F, Bellò M, Chiappella A, Caracciolo D, et al. Radiation therapy in primary mediastinal B-cell lymphoma with positron emission tomography positivity after rituximab chemotherapy. Int J Radiat Oncol Biol Phys. 2013;87(2):311–6.
97. Hayden AR, Tonseth P, Lee DG, Villa D, Gerrie AS, Scott DW, et al. Outcome of primary mediastinal large

B-cell lymphoma using R-CHOP: impact of a PET-adapted approach. Blood. 2020;136(24):2803–11.
98. Vassilakopoulos TP, Papageorgiou SG, Angelopoulou MK, Chatziioannou S, Prassopoulos V, Karakatsanis S, et al. Positron emission tomography after response to rituximab-CHOP in primary mediastinal large B-cell lymphoma: impact on outcomes and radiotherapy strategies. Ann Hematol. 2021;100(9):2279–92.
99. Vassilakopoulos TP, Pangalis GA, Chatziioannou S, Papageorgiou S, Angelopoulou MK, Galani Z, et al. PET/CT in primary mediastinal large B-cell lymphoma responding to rituximab-CHOP: An analysis of 106 patients regarding prognostic significance and implications for subsequent radiotherapy. Leukemia. 2016;30(1):238–42.
100. Filippi AR, Piva C, Levis M, Chiappella A, Caracciolo D, Bellò M, et al. Prognostic role of pre-radiation therapy (18)F-fluorodeoxyglucose positron emission tomography for primary mediastinal B-cell lymphomas treated with R-CHOP or R-CHOP-like chemotherapy plus radiation. Int J Radiat Oncol Biol Phys. 2016;95(4):1239–43.
101. Ceriani L, Martelli M, Gospodarowicz MK, Ricardi U, Ferreri AJM, Chiappella A, et al. Positron emission tomography/computed tomography assessment after immunochemotherapy and irradiation using the lugano classification criteria in the IELSG-26 study of primary mediastinal B-cell lymphoma. Int J Radiat Oncol Biol Phys. 2017;97(1):42–9.
102. Dunleavy K, Pittaluga S, Maeda LS, Advani R, Chen CC, Hessler J, et al. Dose-adjusted EPOCH-rituximab therapy in primary mediastinal B-cell lymphoma. N Engl J Med. 2013;368(15):1408–16.
103. Melani C, Advani R, Roschewski M, Walters KM, Chen CC, Baratto L, et al. End-of-treatment and serial PET imaging in primary mediastinal B-cell lymphoma following dose-adjusted EPOCH-R: a paradigm shift in clinical decision making. Haematologica. 2018;103(8):1337–44.
104. Vassilakopoulos T, Chatzidimitriou C, Mellios Z, Verigou E, Papageorgiou S, Giatra H, et al. PET-scan for response assessment after Rituximab-dose-Adjusted-EPOCH (R-DA-EPOCH) in Primary Mediastinal Large B-Cell Lymphoma (PMLBCL): clinical and prognostic significance. HemaSphere. 2019;3(S1):494.
105. Vassilakopoulos T, Piperidou A, Mellios Z, Verigou E, Kalpadakis C, Katodritou E, et al. PET/CT imaging scan for response assessment and treatment guidance after Rituximab-Dose-Adjusted-EPOCH (R-DA-EPOCH) in Primary Mediastinal Large B-Cell Lymphoma (PMLBCL): the hellenic experience on 107 patients. HemaSphere. 2022;6:1115–6.
106. Kanemasa Y, Shimoyama T, Sasaki Y, Tamura M, Sawada T, Omuro Y, et al. Analysis of prognostic value of complete response by PET-CT and further stratification by clinical and biological markers in DLBCL patients. Med Oncol. 2017;34(2):29.
107. Thomas A, Gingrich RD, Smith BJ, Jacobus L, Ristow K, Allmer C, et al. 18-Fluoro-deoxyglucose positron emission tomography report interpretation as predictor of outcome in diffuse large B-cell lymphoma including analysis of "indeterminate" reports. Leuk Lymphoma. 2010;51(3):439–46.
108. Dabaja BS, Phan J, Mawlawi O, Medeiros LJ, Etzel C, Liang FW, et al. Clinical implications of positron emission tomography-negative residual computed tomography masses after chemotherapy for diffuse large B-cell lymphoma. Leuk Lymphoma. 2013;54(12):2631–8.
109. Vassilakopoulos T, Kanellopoulos A, Papageorgiou S, Pangalis G, Anastasopoulou A, Moschogiannis M, et al. Clinical implications and prognostic significance of positron emission tomography (PET/CT) in patients with diffuse large B-cell lymphoma (DLBCL) after R-CHOP chemoimmunotherapy. Haematol Hematol J. 2014;99(Suppl 1):Abstract PB1831.
110. Witzig TE, Tobinai K, Rigacci L, Ikeda T, Vanazzi A, Hino M, et al. Adjuvant everolimus in high-risk diffuse large B-cell lymphoma: final results from the PILLAR-2 randomized phase III trial. Ann Oncol. 2018;29(3):707–14.
111. Mamot C, Klingbiel D, Hitz F, Renner C, Pabst T, Driessen C, et al. Final results of a prospective evaluation of the predictive value of interim positron emission tomography in patients with diffuse large b-cell lymphoma treated with R-CHOP-14 (SAKK 38/07). J Clin Oncol. 2015;33(23):2523–9.
112. Kostakoglu L, Martelli M, Sehn LH, Belada D, Carella AM, Chua N, et al. End-of-treatment PET/CT predicts PFS and OS in DLBCL after first-line treatment: results from GOYA. Blood Adv. 2021;5(5):1283–90.
113. Freeman CL, Savage KJ, Villa DR, Scott DW, Srour L, Gerrie AS, et al. Long-term results of PET-guided radiation in patients with advanced-stage diffuse large B-cell lymphoma treated with R-CHOP. Blood. 2021;137(7):929–38.
114. Pfreundschuh M, Christofyllakis K, Altmann B, Ziepert M, Haenel M, Viardot A, et al. Radiotherapy to bulky disease PET-negative after immunochemotherapy in elderly DLBCL patients: results of a planned interim analysis of the first 187 patients with bulky disease treated in the OPTIMAL>60 study of the DSHNHL. J Clin Oncol. 2017;35:7506.
115. Dupuis J, Berriolo-Riedinger A, Julian A, Brice P, Tychyj-Pinel C, Tilly H, et al. Impact of [(18)F]fluorodeoxyglucose positron emission tomography response evaluation in patients with high-tumor burden follicular lymphoma treated with immunochemotherapy: a prospective study from the Groupe d'Etudes des Lymphomes de l'Adulte and GOELAMS. J Clin Oncol. 2012;30(35):4317–22.
116. Trotman J, Luminari S, Boussetta S, Versari A, Dupuis J, Tychyj C, et al. Prognostic value of PET-CT after first-line therapy in patients with follicular lymphoma: a pooled analysis of central scan review in three multicentre studies. Lancet Haematol. 2014;1(1):e17–27.

117. Trotman J, Barrington SF, Belada D, Meignan M, MacEwan R, Owen C, et al. Prognostic value of end-of-induction PET response after first-line immunochemotherapy for follicular lymphoma (GALLIUM): secondary analysis of a randomised, phase 3 trial. Lancet Oncol. 2018;19(11):1530–42.
118. Lamonica D, Graf DA, Munteanu MC, Czuczman MS. 18F-FDG PET for measurement of response and prediction of outcome to relapsed or refractory mantle cell lymphoma therapy with bendamustine-rituximab. J Nucl Med. 2017;58(1):62–8.
119. Klener P, Fronkova E, Belada D, Forsterova K, Pytlik R, Kalinova M, et al. Alternating R-CHOP and R-cytarabine is a safe and effective regimen for transplant-ineligible patients with a newly diagnosed mantle cell lymphoma. Hematol Oncol. 2018;36(1):110–5.
120. Bailly C, Carlier T, Berriolo-Riedinger A, Casasnovas O, Gyan E, Meignan M, et al. Prognostic value of FDG-PET in patients with mantle cell lymphoma: results from the LyMa-PET project. Haematologica. 2020;105(1):e33–6.
121. El-Galaly TC, Pedersen MB, Hutchings M, Mylam KJ, Madsen J, Gang AO, et al. Utility of interim and end-of-treatment PET/CT in peripheral T-cell lymphomas: A review of 124 patients. Am J Hematol. 2015;90(11):975–80.
122. Hutchings M, Loft A, Hansen M, Pedersen LM, Buhl T, Jurlander J, et al. FDG-PET after two cycles of chemotherapy predicts treatment failure and progression-free survival in Hodgkin lymphoma. Blood. 2006;107(1):52–9.
123. Gallamini A, Hutchings M, Rigacci L, Specht L, Merli F, Hansen M, et al. Early interim 2-[18F] fluoro-2-deoxy-D-glucose positron emission tomography is prognostically superior to international prognostic score in advanced-stage Hodgkin's lymphoma: a report from a joint Italian-Danish study. J Clin Oncol. 2007;25(24):3746–52.
124. Moskowitz CH, Schöder H, Teruya-Feldstein J, Sima C, Iasonos A, Portlock CS, et al. Risk-adapted dose-dense immunochemotherapy determined by interim FDG-PET in advanced-stage diffuse large B-cell lymphoma. J Clin Oncol. 2010;28(11):1896–903.
125. Gallamini A, Barrington SF, Biggi A, Chauvie S, Kostakoglu L, Gregianin M, et al. The predictive role of interim positron emission tomography for Hodgkin lymphoma treatment outcome is confirmed using the interpretation criteria of the Deauville five-point scale. Haematologica. 2014;99(6):1107–13.
126. Kostakoglu L, Schöder H, Johnson JL, Hall NC, Schwartz LH, Straus DJ, et al. Interim FDG PET imaging in stage I/II non-bulky Hodgkin lymphoma: would using combined PET and CT criteria better predict response than each test alone? Leuk Lymphoma. 2012;53(11):2143–50.
127. Casasnovas RO, Bouabdallah R, Brice P, Lazarovici J, Ghesquieres H, Stamatoullas A, et al. PET-adapted treatment for newly diagnosed advanced Hodgkin lymphoma (AHL2011): a randomised, multicentre, non-inferiority, phase 3 study. Lancet Oncol. 2019;20(2):202–15.
128. Casasnovas R-O, Bouabdallah R, Brice P, Lazarovici J, Ghesquieres H, Stamatoullas A, et al. Positron emission tomography–driven strategy in advanced Hodgkin lymphoma: prolonged follow-up of the AHL2011 phase III lymphoma study association study. J Clin Oncol. 2022;40(10):1091–101.
129. Kreissl S, Goergen H, Buehnen I, Kobe C, Moccia A, Greil R, et al. PET-guided eBEACOPP treatment of advanced-stage Hodgkin lymphoma (HD18): follow-up analysis of an international, open-label, randomised, phase 3 trial. Lancet Haematol. 2021;8(6):e398–409.
130. Borchmann P, Goergen H, Kobe C, Lohri A, Greil R, Eichenauer DA, et al. PET-guided treatment in patients with advanced-stage Hodgkin's lymphoma (HD18): final results of an open-label, international, randomised phase 3 trial by the German Hodgkin study group. Lancet. 2017;390(10114):2790–802.
131. Borchmann P, Haverkamp H, Lohri A, Mey U, Kreissl S, Greil R, et al. Progression-free survival of early interim PET-positive patients with advanced stage Hodgkin's lymphoma treated with BEACOPP escalated alone or in combination with rituximab (HD18): an open-label, international, randomised phase 3 study by the German Hodg. Lancet Oncol. 2017;18(4):454–63.
132. Gallamini A, Patti C, Viviani S, Rossi A, Fiore F, Di Raimondo F, et al. Early chemotherapy intensification with BEACOPP in advanced-stage Hodgkin lymphoma patients with a interim-PET positive after two ABVD courses. Br J Haematol. 2011;152(5):551–60.
133. Johnson P, Federico M, Kirkwood A, Fosså A, Berkahn L, Carella A, et al. Adapted treatment guided by interim PET-CT Scan in advanced Hodgkin's lymphoma. N Engl J Med. 2016;374(25):2419–29.
134. Press OW, Li H, Schöder H, Straus DJ, Moskowitz CH, LeBlanc M, et al. US intergroup trial of response-adapted therapy for stage III to IV Hodgkin lymphoma using early interim fluorodeoxyglucose-positron emission tomography imaging: Southwest oncology group S0816. J Clin Oncol. 2016;34(17):2020–7.
135. Ganesan P, Rajendranath R, Kannan K, Radhakrishnan V, Ganesan TS, Udupa K, et al. Phase II study of interim PET-CT-guided response-adapted therapy in advanced Hodgkin's lymphoma. Ann Oncol. 2015;26(6):1170–4.
136. Vassilakopoulos T, Rontogianni F, Boutsikas G, Assimakopoulos I, Chatziioannou S, Moschogiannis M, et al. PET/CT for the early interim evaluation of response in advanced Hodgkin lymphoma after ABVDx2: effective salvage with BEACOPP but low negative predictive value for stage IV. Hematol Oncol. 2015;33(s1):abstr 463.
137. Stephens DM, Li H, Schoder H, Straus DJ, Moskowitz CH, LeBlanc M, et al. Five-year follow-up of SWOG S0816: limitations and values of a

PET-adapted approach with stage III/IV Hodgkin lymphoma. Blood. 2019;134(15):1238–46.
138. Vassilakopoulos TP, Johnson PWM. Treatment of advanced-stage Hodgkin lymphoma. Semin Hematol. 2016;53(3):171–9.
139. Zinzani PL, Broccoli A, Gioia DM, Castagnoli A, Ciccone G, Evangelista A, et al. Interim positron emission tomography response-adapted therapy in advanced-stage Hodgkin Lymphoma: final results of the phase II part of the HD0801 study. J Clin Oncol. 2016;34(12):1376–85.
140. André MPE, Girinsky T, Federico M, Reman O, Fortpied C, Gotti M, et al. Early positron emission tomography response-adapted treatment in stage I and II Hodgkin lymphoma: final results of the randomized EORTC/LYSA/FIL H10 trial. J Clin Oncol. 2017;35(16):1786–96.
141. Cottereau AS, Versari A, Loft A, Casasnovas O, et al. Deuville score evaluation of PET2 positive patients included in the H10 trial. In: 7th International Workshop on PET in Lymphoma and Myeloma; 2018.
142. Oki Y, Chuang H, Chasen B, Jessop A, Pan T, Fanale M, et al. The prognostic value of interim positron emission tomography scan in patients with classical Hodgkin lymphoma. Br J Haematol. 2014;165(1):112–6.
143. Cimino G, Zaucha JM, Cirillo S, Saviolo C, Hutchings M, El-Galaly TC, et al. The complementary prognostic role of baseline and interim PET in predicting treatment outcome in advanced-stage Hodgkin lymphoma. Blood. 2014;124(21):4405.
144. Lopez-Alonso R, Qi S, Mashiach T, Weiler-Sagie M, Yahalom J, Dann EJ. The presence of a bulky mediastinal mass of 7 cm or greater in diameter confers an adverse prognosis to patients with advanced Hodgkin lymphoma in case of negative interim PET/CT. Leuk Lymphoma. 2021;62(6):1313–24.
145. Illidge TM, Phillips EH, Counsell N, Pettengell R, Johnson PWM, Culligan DJ, et al. Maximum tumor diameter is associated with event-free survival in PET-negative patients with stage I/IIA Hodgkin lymphoma. Blood Adv. 2020;4(1):203–6.
146. Rigacci L, Puccini B, Broccoli A, Dona M, Gotti M, Evangelista A, et al. Clinical characteristics of interim-PET negative patients with a positive end PET from the prospective HD08-01 FIL study. Ann Hematol. 2020;99(2):283–91.
147. Bari A, Marcheselli R, Sacchi S, Re A, Pagani C, Tucci A, et al. The classic prognostic factors in advanced Hodgkin's lymphoma patients are losing their meaning at the time of Pet-guided treatments. Ann Hematol. 2020;99(2):277–82.
148. Romano A, Pavoni C, Di Raimondo F, Tarella C, Viviani S, Rossi A, et al. The neutrophil to lymphocyte ratio (NLR) and the presence of large nodal mass are independent predictors of early response: a subanalysis of the prospective phase II PET-2-adapted HD0607 trial. Cancer Med. 2020;9(23):8735–46.
149. Agostinelli C, Gallamini A, Stracqualursi L, Agati P, Tripodo C, Fuligni F, et al. The combined role of biomarkers and interim PET scan in prediction of treatment outcome in classical Hodgkin's lymphoma: a retrospective, European, multicentre cohort study. Lancet Haematol. 2016;3(10):e467–79.
150. Viviani S, Mazzocchi A, Pavoni C, Taverna F, Rossi A, Patti C, et al. Early serum TARC reduction predicts prognosis in advanced-stage Hodgkin lymphoma patients treated with a PET-adapted strategy. Hematol Oncol. 2020;38(4):501–8.
151. Itti E, Meignan M, Berriolo-Riedinger A, Biggi A, Cashen AF, Véra P, et al. An international confirmatory study of the prognostic value of early PET/CT in diffuse large B-cell lymphoma: comparison between Deauville criteria and ΔSUVmax. Eur J Nucl Med Mol Imaging. 2013;40(9):1312–20.
152. Schöder H, Polley MYC, Knopp MV, Hall N, Kostakoglu L, Zhang J, et al. Prognostic value of interim FDG-PET in diffuse large cell lymphoma: results from the CALGB 50303 clinical trial. Blood. 2020;135(25):2224–34.
153. Mikhaeel NG, Cunningham D, Counsell N, McMillan A, Radford JA, Ardeshna KM, et al. FDG-PET/CT after two cycles of R-CHOP in DLBCL predicts complete remission but has limited value in identifying patients with poor outcome–final result of a UK National Cancer Research Institute prospective study. Br J Haematol. 2021;192(3):504–13.
154. Zucca E, Cascione L, Ruberto T, Facchinelli D, Schär S, Hayoz S, et al. Prognostic models integrating quantitative parameters from baseline and interim positron emission computed tomography in patients with diffuse large B-cell lymphoma: post-hoc analysis from the SAKK38/07 clinical trial. Hematol Oncol. 2020;38(5):715–25.
155. Casasnovas RO, Meignan M, Berriolo-Riedinger A, Bardet S, Julian A, Thieblemont C, et al. SUVmax reduction improves early prognosis value of interim positron emission tomography scans in diffuse large B-cell lymphoma. Blood. 2011;118(1):37–43.
156. Casasnovas RO, Ysebaert L, Thieblemont C, Bachy E, Feugier P, Delmer A, et al. FDG-PET-driven consolidation strategy in diffuse large B-cell lymphoma: final results of a randomized phase 2 study. Blood. 2017;130(11):1315–26.
157. Pardal E, Coronado M, Martín A, Grande C, Marín-Niebla A, Panizo C, et al. Intensification treatment based on early FDG-PET in patients with high-risk diffuse large B-cell lymphoma: a phase II GELTAMO trial. Br J Haematol. 2014;167(3):327–36.
158. Dührsen U, Müller S, Hertenstein B, Thomssen H, Kotzerke J, Mesters R, et al. Positron emission tomography-guided therapy of aggressive Non-Hodgkin lymphomas (PETAL): a multicenter, randomized phase III trial. J Clin Oncol. 2018;36(20):2024–34.
159. Kurch L, Hüttmann A, Georgi TW, Rekowski J, Sabri O, Schmitz C, et al. Interim PET in diffuse large B-cell lymphoma. J Nucl Med. 2021;62(8):1068–74.

160. Schmitz C, Hüttmann A, Müller SP, Hanoun M, Boellaard R, Brinkmann M, et al. Dynamic risk assessment based on positron emission tomography scanning in diffuse large B-cell lymphoma: post-hoc analysis from the PETAL trial. Eur J Cancer. 2020;124:25–36.
161. Meignan M, Gallamini A. ΔSUVmax for interim PET in DLBCL: old is new. Blood. 2020;135(25):2202–3.
162. Yim SK, Yhim HY, Han YH, Jeon SY, Lee NR, Song EK, et al. Early risk stratification for diffuse large B-cell lymphoma integrating interim Deauville score and international prognostic index. Ann Hematol. 2019;98(12):2739–48.
163. Wight J, Wai SH, Shen E, Lee ST, Berlangieri S, Fancourt T, et al. Predicting primary treatment failure using interim FDG-PET scanning in diffuse large B-cell lymphoma. Eur J Haematol. 2021;107(4):475–83.
164. Safar V, Dupuis J, Itti E, Jardin F, Fruchart C, Bardet S, et al. Interim [18F]fluorodeoxyglucose positron emission tomography scan in diffuse large B-cell lymphoma treated with anthracycline-based chemotherapy plus rituximab. J Clin Oncol. 2012;30(2):184–90.
165. Hertzberg M, Gandhi MK, Trotman J, Butcher B, Taper J, Johnston A, et al. Early treatment intensification with R-ICE and 90Y-ibritumomab tiuxetan (Zevalin)-BEAM stem cell transplantation in patients with high-risk diffuse large B-cell lymphoma patients and positive interim PET after 4 cycles of R-CHOP-14. Haematologica. 2017;102(2):356–63.
166. Swinnen LJ, Li H, Quon A, Gascoyne R, Hong F, Ranheim EA, et al. Response-adapted therapy for aggressive non-Hodgkin's lymphomas based on early [18F] FDG-PET scanning: ECOG-ACRIN cancer research group study (E3404). Br J Haematol. 2015;170(1):56–65.
167. Sehn LH, Hardy ELG, Gill KK, Al-Tourah AJ, Shustik J, Macpherson NA, et al. Phase 2 trial of interim PET scan-tailored therapy in patients with advanced stage Diffuse Large B-Cell Lymphoma (DLBCL) in British Columbia (BC). Blood. 2014;124(21):392.
168. Duehrsen U, Müller SP, Rekowski J, Hertenstein B, Franzius C, Mesters R, et al. Positron Emission Tomography (PET) guided therapy of Aggressive lymphomas-interim PET-based outcome prediction and treatment changes in patients with B cell lymphomas participating in the PETAL trial. Blood. 2016;128(22):1857.
169. Moskowitz C, Hamlin PA, Maragulia J, Meikle J, Zelenetz AD. Sequential dose-dense RCHOP followed by ICE consolidation (MSKCC protocol 01–142) without radiotherapy for patients with primary mediastinal large B cell lymphoma. Blood. 2010;116(21):420.
170. Avigdor A, Sirotkin T, Kedmi M, Ribakovsy E, Berkowicz M, Davidovitz Y, et al. The impact of R-VACOP-B and interim FDG-PET/CT on outcome in primary mediastinal large B cell lymphoma. Ann Hematol. 2014;93(8):1297–304.
171. Lazarovici J, Terroir M, Arfi-Rouche J, Michot JM, Mussot S, Florea V, et al. Poor predictive value of positive interim FDG-PET/CT in primary mediastinal large B-cell lymphoma. Eur J Nucl Med Mol Imaging. 2017;44(12):2018–24.
172. Qin W, Jiang X, You J, Guo R, Shi Q, Dong L, et al. Deauville score evaluation of interim PET/CT in primary mediastinal large B-cell lymphoma. Eur J Nucl Med Mol Imaging. 2021;48(11):3347–50.
173. Schmitz C, Rekowski J, Müller SP, Hertenstein B, Franzius C, Ganser A, et al. Baseline and interim PET-based outcome prediction in peripheral T-cell lymphoma: a subgroup analysis of the PETAL trial. Hematol Oncol. 2020;38(3):244–56.
174. Huttmann A, Müller SP, Rekowski J, Hertenstein B, Franzius C, Franzke A, et al. Positron emission tomography (PET) guided therapy of aggressive lymphomas–interim PET-based outcome prediction and treatment changes in patients with T cell lymphomas participating in the PETAL trial. Blood. 2016;128:185.
175. Raemaekers JMM, André MPE, Federico M, Girinsky T, Oumedaly R, Brusamolino E, et al. Omitting radiotherapy in early positron emission tomography-negative stage I/II Hodgkin lymphoma is associated with an increased risk of early relapse: clinical results of the preplanned interim analysis of the randomized EORTC/LYSA/FIL H10 trial. J Clin Oncol. 2014;32(12):1188–94.
176. Vassilakopoulos TP, Kravvariti E, Panitsas F, Angelopoulou MK, Liaskas A, Kontopidou FN, et al. Very late relapses in Hodgkin lymphoma treated with chemotherapy with or without radiotherapy: linear pattern and distinct prognostic factors. Blood Cancer J. 2022;12(7):102.
177. Straus DJ, Jung SH, Pitcher B, Kostakoglu L, Grecula JC, Hsi ED, et al. CALGB 50604: risk-adapted treatment of nonbulky early-stage Hodgkin lymphoma based on interim PET. Blood. 2018;132(10):1013–21.
178. Lamy T, Damaj G, Soubeyran P, Gyan E, Cartron G, Bouabdallah K, et al. R-CHOP 14 with or without radiotherapy in nonbulky limited-stage diffuse large B-cell lymphoma. Blood. 2018;131(2):174–81.
179. Persky DO, Li H, Stephens DM, Park SI, Bartlett NL, Swinnen LJ, et al. Positron emission tomography-directed therapy for patients with limited-stage diffuse large B-cell lymphoma: results of intergroup national clinical trials network study S1001. J Clin Oncol. 2020;38(26):3003–11.
180. Martelli M, Zucca E, Gospodarowicz M, Johnson PWM, Ricardi U, et al. A randomized, multicentre, two-arm phase III comparative study assessing the role of mediastinal radiotherapy after rituximab-containing chemotherapy regimens to patients with newly diagnosed primary mediastinal large B-cell lymphoma (PMLBCL): The IELSG-3. Hematol Oncol. 2013;31(S1):140.
181. Le Gouill S, Ghesquières H, Oberic L, Morschhauser F, Tilly H, Ribrag V, et al. Obinutuzumab vs

rituximab for advanced DLBCL: a PET-guided and randomized phase 3 study by LYSA. Blood. 2021;137(17):2307–20.
182. Schot BW, Zijlstra JM, Sluiter WJ, Van Imhoff GW, Pruim J, Vaalburg W, et al. Early FDG-PET assessment in combination with clinical risk scores determines prognosis in recurring lymphoma. Blood. 2007;109(2):486–91.
183. Terasawa T, Lau J, Bardet S, Couturier O, Hotta T, Hutchings M, et al. Fluorine-18-fluorodeoxyglucose positron emission tomography for interim response assessment of advanced-stage Hodgkin's lymphoma and diffuse large B-cell lymphoma: a systematic review. J Clin Oncol. 2009;27(11):1906–14.
184. Poulou LS, Thanos L, Ziakas PD. Unifying the predictive value of pretransplant FDG PET in patients with lymphoma: a review and meta-analysis of published trials. Eur J Nucl Med Mol Imaging. 2010;37(1):156–62.
185. Angelopoulou M, Moschogiannis M, Rondogianni P, Tsirkinidis P, Nikaki A, Chatziioannou S, et al. PET/CT in the setting of Autologous Stem Cell Transplantation (ASCT) for relapsed/refractory Hodgkin Lymphoma (HL): performance of various interpretation systems. Haematol Hematol J. 2013;98(s2):Abstract P119.
186. Moskowitz AJ, Yahalom J, Kewalramani T, Maragulia JC, Vanak JM, Zelenetz AD, et al. Pretransplantation functional imaging predicts outcome following autologous stem cell transplantation for relapsed and refractory Hodgkin lymphoma. Blood. 2010;116(23):4934–7.
187. Adams HJA, Kwee TC. Prognostic value of pretransplant FDG-PET in refractory/relapsed Hodgkin lymphoma treated with autologous stem cell transplantation: systematic review and meta-analysis. Ann Hematol. 2016;95(5):695–706.
188. Yhim HY, Eshet Y, Metser U, Lajkosz K, Cooper M, Prica A, et al. Risk stratification for relapsed/refractory classical Hodgkin lymphoma integrating pretransplant Deauville score and residual metabolic tumor volume. Am J Hematol. 2022;97(5):583–91.
189. Moskowitz AJ, Schöder H, Gavane S, Thoren KL, Fleisher M, Yahalom J, et al. Prognostic significance of baseline metabolic tumor volume in relapsed and refractory Hodgkin lymphoma. Blood. 2017;130(20):2196–203.
190. Damlaj M, Ghazi S, Syed G, Pasha T, Gmati G, Salama H, et al. Pre-autologous transplantation PET/CT using Deauville criteria is an independent predictor of progression in relapsed refractory classical Hodgkin lymphoma. Bone Marrow Transplant. 2017;52(9):1342–4.
191. Procházka V, Gawande RS, Cayci Z, Froelich JW, Cao Q, Wilke C, et al. Positron emission tomography-based assessment of metabolic tumor volume predicts survival after autologous hematopoietic cell transplantation for Hodgkin lymphoma. Biol Blood Marrow Transplant. 2018;24(1):64–70.
192. Moskowitz CH, Nademanee A, Masszi T, Agura E, Holowiecki J, Abidi MH, et al. Brentuximab vedotin as consolidation therapy after autologous stem-cell transplantation in patients with Hodgkin's lymphoma at risk of relapse or progression (AETHERA): a randomised, double-blind, placebo-controlled, phase 3 trial. Lancet. 2015;385(9980):1853–62.
193. Younes A, Santoro A, Shipp M, Zinzani PL, Timmerman JM, Ansell S, et al. Nivolumab for classical Hodgkin's lymphoma after failure of both autologous stem-cell transplantation and brentuximab vedotin: a multicentre, multicohort, single-arm phase 2 trial. Lancet Oncol. 2016;17(9):1283–94.
194. Chen R, Zinzani PL, Fanale MA, Armand P, Johnson NA, Brice P, et al. Phase II Study of the efficacy and safety of pembrolizumab for relapsed/refractory classic Hodgkin lymphoma. J Clin Oncol. 2017;35(19):2125–32.
195. Armand P, Engert A, Younes A, Fanale M, Santoro A, Zinzani PL, et al. Nivolumab for relapsed/refractory classic Hodgkin lymphoma after failure of autologous hematopoietic cell transplantation: extended follow-up of the multicohort single-arm phase II CheckMate 205 Trial. J Clin Oncol. 2018;36(14):1428–39.
196. Chen R, Zinzani PL, Lee HJ, Armand P, Johnson NA, Brice P, et al. Pembrolizumab in relapsed or refractory Hodgkin lymphoma: 2-year follow-up of KEYNOTE-087. Blood. 2019;134(14):1144–53.
197. Ansell SM, Bröckelmann PJ, Von KG, Lee HJ, et al. Nivolumab for Relapsed or Refractory(R/R) Classical Hodgkin Lymphoma(CHL) after autologous transplantation: 5-year overall survival from phase 2 CHECKMATE 205 study. In: International Conference on Malignant Lymphoma; 2021. p. 122–5.
198. Armand P, Pier Luigi Zinzani M, Lee HJ, Johnson N, Al E. Five-year follow-up of keynote-087: pembrolizumab monotherapy in Relapsed/Refractory classical Hodgkin lymphoma (R/R cHL). Blood. 2021;138(Supplement 1):1366.
199. Zinzani PL, Santoro A, Gritti G, Brice P, Barr PM, Kuruvilla J, et al. Nivolumab combined With brentuximab vedotin for relapsed/refractory primary mediastinal large B-cell lymphoma: efficacy and safety from the phase II CheckMate 436 study. J Clin Oncol. 2019;37(33):3081–9.
200. Armand P, Rodig S, Melnichenko V, Thieblemont C, Bouabdallah K, Tumyan G, et al. Pembrolizumab in relapsed or refractory primary Mediastinal large B-cell lymphoma. J Clin Oncol. 2019;37(34):3291–9.
201. Cheson BD, Ansell S, Schwartz L, Gordon LI, Advani R, Jacene HA, et al. Refinement of the lugano classification lymphoma response criteria in the era of immunomodulatory therapy. Blood. 2016;128(21):2489–96.
202. Dercle L, Seban RD, Lazarovici J, Schwartz LH, Houot R, Ammari S, et al. 18F-FDG PET and CT scans detect new imaging patterns of response and progression in patients with Hodgkin lymphoma treated by anti–programmed death 1 immune checkpoint inhibitor. J Nucl Med. 2018;59(1):15–24.

203. Dercle L, Mokrane FZ, Schiano de Colella JM, Stamatoullas A, Morschhauser F, Brice P, et al. Unconventional immune-related phenomena observed using 18F-FDG PET/CT in Hodgkin lymphoma treated with anti PD-1 monoclonal antibodies. Eur J Nucl Med Mol Imaging. 2019;46(6):1391–2.
204. Mokrane FZ, Chen A, Schwartz LH, Morschhauser F, Stamatoullas A, De Colella JMS, et al. Performance of CT compared with 18F-FDG PET in predicting the efficacy of nivolumab in relapsed or Refractory Hodgkin lymphoma. Radiology. 2020;295(3):651–61.
205. Chen A, Mokrane FZ, Schwartz LH, Morschhauser F, Stamatoullas A, Schiano de Colella JM, et al. early 18 f-fdg pet/ct response predicts survival in relapsed or refractory Hodgkin lymphoma treated with Nivolumab. J Nucl Med. 2020;61(5):649–54.
206. Moskowitz CH, Chen RW, Armand P, Zinzani PL, Vassilakopoulos TP, Goldmacher GV, et al. Pembrolizumab antitumor activity in relapsed/refractory Classical Hodgkin lymphoma in keynote-087: revised response criteria for malignant lymphoma 2007 criteria versus Lugano 2014 classification. Blood. 2017;130(Supplement 1):4085.
207. Vercellino L, Di Blasi R, Kanoun S, Tessoulin B, Rossi C, D'Aveni-Piney M, et al. Predictive factors of early progression after CAR T-cell therapy in relapsed/refractory diffuse large B-cell lymphoma. Blood Adv. 2020;4(22):5607–15.
208. Iacoboni G, Simó M, Villacampa G, Catalá E, Carpio C, Díaz-Lagares C, et al. Prognostic impact of total metabolic tumor volume in large B-cell lymphoma patients receiving CAR T-cell therapy. Ann Hematol. 2021;100(9):2303–10.
209. Bi L, Kim J, Kumar A, Wen L, Feng D, Fulham M. Automatic detection and classification of regions of FDG uptake in whole-body PET-CT lymphoma studies. Comput Med Imaging Graph. 2017;60:3–10.
210. Barrington SF, Meignan M. Time to prepare for risk adaptation in lymphoma by standardizing measurement of metabolic tumor burden. J Nucl Med. 2019;60(8):1096–102.
211. Sibille L, Seifert R, Avramovic N, Vehren T, Spottiswoode B, Zuehlsdorff S, et al. 18 F-FDG PET/CT Uptake classification in lymphoma and lung cancer by Using deep convolutional neural networks. Radiology. 2020;294(2):445–52.
212. Annunziata S, Pelliccioni A, Hohaus S, Maiolo E, Cuccaro A, Giordano A. The prognostic role of end-of-treatment FDG-PET/CT in diffuse large B cell lymphoma: a pilot study application of neural networks to predict time-to-event. Ann Nucl Med. 2021;35(1):102–10.
213. Lartizien C, Rogez M, Niaf E, Ricard F. Computer-aided staging of lymphoma patients with FDG PET/CT imaging based on textural information. IEEE J Biomed Heal inform. 2014;18(3):946–55.
214. Guo B, Tan X, Ke Q, Cen H. Prognostic value of baseline metabolic tumor volume and total lesion glycolysis in patients with lymphoma: a meta-analysis. PLoS One. 2019;14(1):e0210224.
215. Yu Y, Decazes P, Lapuyade-Lahorgue J, Gardin I, Vera P, Ruan S. Semi-automatic lymphoma detection and segmentation using fully conditional random fields. Comput Med Imaging Graph. 2018; 70:1–7.
216. Kostakoglu L, Chauvie S. PET-derived quantitative metrics for response and prognosis in lymphoma. PET Clin. 2019;14(3):317–29.
217. Alahmari SS, Cherezov D, Goldgof DB, Hall LO, Gillies RJ, Schabath MB. Delta radiomics improves pulmonary nodule malignancy prediction in lung cancer screening. IEEE Access. 2018;6:77796–806.
218. Hasani N, Paravastu SS, Farhadi F, Yousefirizi F, Morris MA, Rahmim A, et al. Artificial Intelligence in lymphoma PET imaging: a scoping review (current trends and future directions). PET Clin. 2022;17(1):145–74.
219. De Oliveira CR, Neto AH, Siqueira S, De Padua Covas Lage LA, De Paula HM, Coutinho AM, et al. Interim fluorine-18 fluorodeoxyglucose PET-computed tomography and cell of origin by immunohistochemistry predicts progression-free and overall survival in diffuse large B-cell lymphoma patients in the rituximab era. Nucl Med Commun. 2016;37(10):1095–101.
220. Jiang M, Chen P, Ruan X, Xu W, Li T, Wu L, et al. Interim 18F-FDG PET/CT and BCL2 for predicting the prognosis of patients with diffuse large B-cell lymphoma in the rituximab era. Nucl Med Commun. 2018;39(2):147–53.
221. Kim J, Lee JO, Paik JH, Lee WW, Kim SE, Song YS. Different predictive values of interim 18 F-FDG PET/CT in germinal center like and non-germinal center like diffuse large B-cell lymphoma. Ann Nucl Med. 2017;31(1):1–11.
222. Li X, Sun X, Li J, Liu Z, Mi M, Zhu F, et al. Interim PET/CT based on visual and semiquantitative analysis predicts survival in patients with diffuse large B-cell lymphoma. Cancer Med. 2019;8(11):5012–22.
223. Zhang X, Fan W, Xia ZJ, Hu YY, Lin XP, Zhang YR, et al. Use of subsequent PET/CT in diffuse large B-cell lymphoma patients in complete remission following primary therapy. Chin J Cancer. 2015;34(2):70–8.

GPSR Compliance

*The European Union's (EU) General Product Safety Regulation (GPSR) is a set of rules that requires consumer products to be safe and our obligations to ensure this.*

*If you have any concerns about our products, you can contact us on ProductSafety@springernature.com*

In case Publisher is established outside the EU, the EU authorized representative is:

Springer Nature Customer Service Center GmbH
Europaplatz 3
69115 Heidelberg, Germany

**Batch number: 10731385**

Printed by Printforce, the Netherlands